Neurons and Interneuronal Connections of the Central Visual System

Neurons and Interneuronal Connections of the Central Visual System

Ekaterina G. Shkol'nik-Yarros
Brain Institute
Academy of Medical Sciences of the USSR
Moscow, USSR

Translated from Russian by
Basil Haigh

Translation Editor
Robert W. Doty
Center for Brain Research
University of Rochester
Rochester, New York

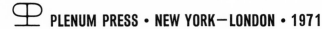 **PLENUM PRESS** • **NEW YORK–LONDON** • **1971**

The original Russian text, published by Meditsina Press in 1965
for the Academy of Medical Sciences of the USSR, has been corrected
by the author for the present edition. The English translation
is published under an agreement with Mezhdunarodnaya Kniga, the
Soviet book export agency.

Е. Г. ШКОЛЬНИК-ЯРРОС

НЕЙРОНЫ И МЕЖНЕЙРОННЫЕ СВЯЗИ—ЗРИТЕЛЬНЫЙ АНАЛИЗАТОР
NEIRONY I MEZHNEIRONNYE SVYAZI — ZRITEL'NYI ANALIZATOR

Library of Congress Catalog Card Number 69-18115
SBN 306-30429-5

© 1971 Plenum Press, New York
A Division of Plenum Publishing Corporation
227 West 17th Street, New York, N.Y. 10011

United Kingdom edition published by Plenum Press, London
A Division of Plenum Publishing Company, Ltd.
Davis House (4th Floor), 8 Scrubs Lane, Harlesden, NW10 6SE, England

Printed in the United States of America

PREFACE

This century has witnessed the creation of new sciences extending the frontiers of knowledge to an unprecedented degree. We have seen the birth of cybernetics and bionics, bringing together such apparently distantly related branches of science as neurohistology and automation, synaptology and electronics. The electron microscope has resolved tissues almost down to the molecular level, and histochemistry has led to the fine analysis of brain structure.

However, before these and other new sciences can develop properly and scientifically, a precise knowledge of the structure of the material with which they are concerned is absolutely essential. That is why the need exists at the present time for a detailed study of the larger units, i.e., the neurons, their interrelationships and the pathways by which excitation is conducted. Biologists, neurologists, physicists, and specialists in other technical disciplines will find this study highly useful.

During recent years many advances have been made in knowledge of the central visual system and its pathways. Above all, it has been found that the visual system is very extensive. The optic tract is connected, not only with the lateral geniculate body, but with the superior colliculus and the pulvinar. Besides the discovery of these principal pathways, connections have also been studied with the hypothalamus, the pretectal region, the medial geniculate body, subthalamus, and other parts of the brain stem. The visual system is thus connected with the reflex apparatus, the autonomic nervous system, and the auditory and reticular systems. At the cortical level, visual representation likewise has been shown not to be confined to the typical visual center in Area 17. The discovery of these complex and extensive connections at cortical and subcortical levels has considerably broadened present concepts of analyzers in general and of the visual analyzer in particular.

Refined electrophysiological investigations in recent years have revealed remarkable facts concerning the convergence of excitation on visual cortical neurons. The same neuron can apparently receive not only specific visual impulses, but also impulses of a different character, such as vestibular, auditory, etc. It has also been found that neurons reacting to onset and cessation of light and to changes in the direction of movement exist not only in the retina but also in the cortex (Jung *et al.*; Hubel and Wiesel), and that many other types of neurons can be distinguished by their response to excitation of the visual receptor. Recent microelectrode studies of De Valois and co-workers are developing in the same direction. They have shown that neurons of the lateral geniculate body in primates do not respond equally to colored stimuli.

What is revealed by these new data concerning the organization of analyzers? Is it possible to correlate the anatomical and physiological facts? With the gradual accumulation of facts concerning neurons of the central visual system, problems have arisen which have been partially solved or have given rise to other new problems: by comparison with other analyzers, does the structure of the visual analyzer exhibit specificity? Are the attempts to regard the retina as connected with the brain only by centripetal fibers valid? Can a morphological basis for color vision be found in the structure of the brain?

These and many other questions can be answered most satisfactorily and completely by a systematic investigation of the neurons and interneuronal connections of the central visual system, and this was the main purpose of the work described in this volume, most of which was done between 1947 and 1960.

As a foundation for my research, carried on at the Brain Institute, Academy of Medical Sciences of the U.S.S.R., I have been fortunate in having the experience of members of the Institute's staff, gained during many years of investigating the phylogeny and ontogeny of the brain and its neuronal structure. I particularly wish to express my sincere thanks to Professor G.I. Polyakov, to T.A. Leontovich, and to G.P. Zhukova for their unswerving and friendly support and for their helpful criticisms.

I am also grateful to A. A. Kudryashev and M. A. Vinogradova, of the Photographic Laboratory of the Brain Institute and to laboratory artists A. V. Chekurova, V. A. Nilova, and R. I. Minakova for preparing the photographs and drawings for publication. The illustrations were made by means of a drawing apparatus; the cortex and lateral geniculate body are represented as composite drawings from series of sections impregnated by Golgi's method.

I also wish to thank A. S. Novokhatskii, V. G. Skrebitskii, and I. M. Feigenberg for their valuable comments during preparation of the manuscript for publication.

E.G. SHKOL'NIK-YARROS

CONTENTS

Chapter 1

NEURONS OF THE
CENTRAL VISUAL SYSTEM

THE CORTEX AND LATERAL GENICULATE BODY

Progressive development of the cerebral cortex in mammals in the course of evolution takes place through many interdependent processes. The surface area of the cortex is increased by the formation of fissures and gyri. The fissures and gyri are formed as a result of an increase in the number of neurons and of their long processes forming the white matter. The mass of white matter is increased, particularly on account of association pathways, and this in turn is connected with an increase in the number of pyramidal cells in the cortex. Considerable differentiation takes place in the cortex, with the appearance of new areas and subareas and their corresponding new connections, for thousands of association, commissural, and projection fibers arise from every point of the cortex. As the brain develops, and increases in complexity in response to adaptation to the external environment, the number of layers in the cortex changes. Changes in the architectonics of the brain and in the structure of its layers are a manifestation of neuronal specialization corresponding to the areas and lobes of the brain.

Within the limits of the visual system, differences are found in cortical structure depending on the level of development of the nervous system and the state of visual function.

It must also be emphasized that this process of progressive development does not take place equally at all levels of the visual system. The extremely fine specialization of the eyes of many fish (Detwiler, 1955) and the fine differentiation of the retina in many birds are well known. The accurate swoop of a predatory bird from a height while seeking food, and the precise coordination of vision with movements and vestibular responses are characteristic of vision in birds. It is not surprising that in many vertebrates the eye is larger than the brain (Fig. 1); at lower levels of evolution the peripheral

1

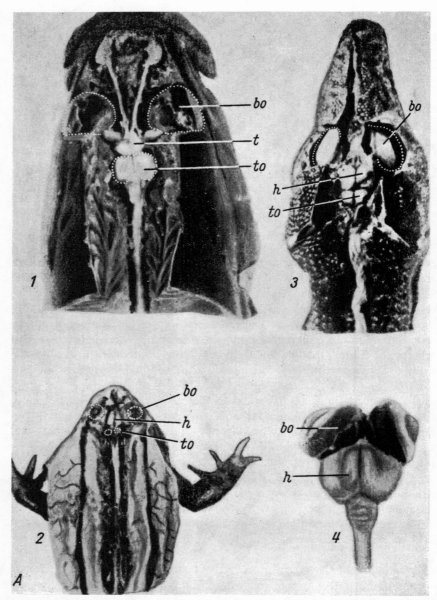

Fig. 1. Relative size of the eye and brain in some vertebrates, mammals, and man. A: 1, fish; 2, frog; 3, lizard (monitor); 4, bird (fowl); to, tectum opticum; bo, bulbus oculi; t, telencephalon; h, hemisphere.

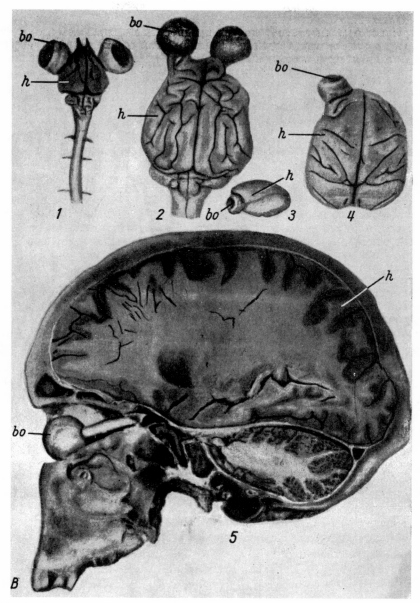

Fig. 1. (Continued) B: 1, rabbit; 2, dog; 3, marmoset (lateral surface of hemisphere); 4, macaque; 5, man (sagittal section through skull and hemisphere). Remainder of legend as in A. (Zvorykin and Shkol'nik-Yarros, 1953.)

visual system is more important than the central (Zvorykin and Shkol'nik-Yarros, 1953).

In the course of adaptation to the external environment, considerable change has taken place in the visual system of higher mammals, for while the peripheral part of the system has diminished relatively in size, the central portions have grown enormously. Man and other primates do not possess the two foveae centrales in the retina and the double accommodation apparatus characteristic of certain birds. Man does not possess the complex (15 layers) structure of the optic lobe of the mesencephalon (superior colliculus) typical of birds (Cajal, 1909–1911). However, as Friedrich Engels stated so pertinently: "the eagle can see much farther than man, but the human eye can detect far more in things than the eye of the eagle."* What is the essence of this progressive improvement in the human visual system?

Before describing my own results concerning neuronal structure of the cortex and lateral geniculate body, I shall give a short survey of the literature on the cytoarchitectonics and neurons of these formations.

Cytoarchitectonic studies have made a very valuable contribution to knowledge of the structure of the visual system. Basic facts essential for further study can be found in the writings of Meynert (1867, 1869), Betz (1873, 1874), Campbell (1905), Brodmann (1909), Aluf (1929), Filimonov (1932, 1933), Preobrazhenskaya (1939, 1948, 1955, 1962), Poemnyi (1940), Bonin (1942), and others.

For my own work, the main conclusion to be drawn from the investigations cited above is as follows: the lower the level of development of the mammal, the smaller the size of parts of the visual cortex surrounding Area 17. According to Brodmann, in the hedgehog Areas 18 and 19 are completely absent, in the rabbit Area 18 is very small, and in carnivores it is relatively larger than in rodents. In primates (Filimonov, 1933) and, in particular, in man, as may be seen from the map produced by the Brain Institute, Academy of Medical Sciences of the U.S.S.R., the area of the occipital cortex has increased in size many times over on account of Areas 18 and 19.

Yet it is these phylogenetically new areas, of the greatest interest at present, which have been least investigated from the standpoint of neuronal structure and connections.

At present, information on the neuronal structure of Area 17 and the lateral geniculate body in different mammals likewise is extremely deficient and at times erroneous. Neurons of Area 17 have been most fully studied in man (Cajal, 1900, 1911). In the visual cortex Cajal distinguished nine layers: (1) plexiform, (2) layer of small pyramidal cells, (3) layer of medium-sized

---

* Friedrich Engels. *Dialectics of Nature* [in Russian], Izd. Polit. Lit., Moscow (1964), p. 148.

pyramidal cells, (4) layer of large stellate cells, (5) layer of small stellate cells, (6) layer of small pyramidal cells with an ascending axon, (7) layer of giant pyramidal cells, (8) layer of medium-sized pyramidal cells with an arcuate axon, (9) layer of fusiform and triangular cells. In his description of the composition of the layers, Cajal went into very considerable detail.* He emphasized the special structure of the visual cortex, characterized by the presence of stellate cells with a descending axon, a plexus of visual fibers, layers 6 and 8 consisting of cells with an arcuate axon, and giant pyramidal cells of Meynert. It is also important to note his remarks that the pyramidal cells of layers 4 and 5 are connected both with visual stimulation and with the association pathways of layer 1, so that they can give two types of discharge. In his opinion the role of the small stellate cells with a short axon is to increase the intensity of visual excitation which they transfer to stellate cells with a long axon.

Cajal did not investigate the areas surrounding Area 17. In one short paragraph without illustrations he briefly summarizes his impressions of their differences from the visual cortex: (1) The number of large and small stellate cells in layers 4 and 5 is reduced while the number of pyramidal cells in these layers is increased, thus obliterating the difference between the visual and association cortex; (2) the layer of visual fibers is less well defined and their terminal ramifications form a looser plexus; (3) the number of small and medium-sized cells with an arcuate ascending axon in layers 6 and 7 is reduced while the number of medium-sized pyramidal cells of the usual type is increased.

When comparing the morphology of the visual cortex in man and animals, Cajal considers that there is almost complete agreement in the structure of the cells, variation occurring only in their number and the nature

---

* Brodmann's classification for the layers of the cortex used in this book and adopted at the Brain Institute, Academy of Medical Sciences of the U.S.S.R., does not coincide with Cajal's classification:

Layers of the Cortex (Area 17)

Brodmann	Cajal
I	*1*
II	*2*
III . . . . ⎫	*3*
IVa . . . . ⎭	
IVb	*4*
IVc ⎧	*5*
⎩	*6*
V	*7*
VI ⎧	*8*
⎩	*9*
VII	*9*

of their distribution. In man, for example, small cells with an arcuate axon form a special layer while in the cat they are scattered among the layers of stellate and giant pyramidal cells. Consequently, there is no true layer 6. Layers 4 and 5 do not exist separately in mammals, and the large and small stellate cells are intermingled. Cajal also stressed the fact that in the human cortex the pyramidal cells are more numerous and smaller in size than in cats and dogs.

Consequently, Cajal gave a careful description of Area 17 in man, but did not describe Areas 18 and 19; he gave no data for the visual cortex of other primates, no data on neurons in insectivores, and hardly any information and no illustrations of Area 17 in the dog. Apart from Cajal, only a few workers have studied the neurons of the visual cortex, and even then only in isolated mammals with no attempt at a systematic comparative anatomical survey. O'Leary and Bishop, for instance, investigated the neurons of the rabbit's visual cortex in conjunction with its electrophysiological properties. The neurons and cytoarchitectonics of Areas 17, 18, and 19 were carefully described by Conel (1939–1959) at various stages of development of the child. Neurons of the human visual cortex in ontogenesis, as well as neurons of other parts of the cortex, have also been studied by Polyakov (1949), who subdivided all cortical formations into primary projection areas (Area 17), secondary (Areas 18, 19), and tertiary areas. Neurons of Area 17 in the cat have often been the subject of study (O'Leary, 1941; Éntin, 1950; Sholl, 1953, 1955, 1956).

In his last investigations, Sholl approached the problems of cortical organization from the statistical point of view, but morphologically his studies of the cat cortex are somewhat schematic. Neurons of Area 17 in the monkey were described by von Bonin (1942) and Polyak (1957).

Unlike Cajal, Polyak emphasizes the large number of small stellate cells with a short axon in sublayer IVa (Polyak numbers the layers and sublayers after Brodmann, in agreement with my own observations made earlier, in 1955). Polyak describes sublayer IVc as a highly complex system in which axon endings of small granule cells unite sublayers IVb, IVc, and perhaps also IVa, but especially they join together the cells of sublayer IVc. Other cells of sublayer IVc give off axons in the form of narrow bands ascending vertically and merging sublayers IVa, b, and c, and layer V into a functional entity. Polyak mentions the lower layers only incidentally. In that part of the area striata representing the fovea centralis, the horizontal spread of a single afferent fiber may reach up to 100–300μ. Polyak assumes that synaptic contacts of the terminal loops and boutons of the afferent fibers evidently belong to the whole mass of nerve cells of sublayers IVa, b, c. The course of impulses in the area striata, according to Polyak, is hypothetically as follows: impulses from the lateral geniculate body are transmitted to sublayers IVa and IVc, where participation of the "granule" cells depends on the extent of the area stimulated. Excitation is transmitted from neuron to neuron and is exhausted in the labyrinth of innumerable synapses, so that these granule cells play the role of a functional barrier. Large neurons can transmit some impulses into other parts of Area 17 or into other cortical areas. The residue of this excitation can remain as a permanent memory trace. Even larger neurons can respond by automatic motor acts: rotation of the eyes, regulation of pupil size, and so on.

This brief description of the structure of Area 17 in some respects disagrees with my own observations (1954, 1955a). In Polyak's scheme of types of neurons and synaptic relationships in Area 17 in primates, first, there are no efferent cells with long axons in this part of the cortex; Meynert's cells and other pyramidal cells and Cajal's cells are drawn with short axons. The visual cortex thus does not possess its own efferent system, and Polyak mentioned this in the text. Second, afferent fibers are drawn as rising vertically and the large oblique afferent fibers whose presence was demonstrated by Cajal and confirmed by Polyak (1932) are completely absent. Third, it is uncertain from the diagram how binocular fusion of the visual image takes place. Fourth, the synaptic contacts drawn on the scheme are mainly shown as connections of visual afferents with small granule cells. However, as Éntin (1954) showed, the largest number of synapses in the visual cortex is found on the largest cells of layer IV. Again, Polyak mentions in the text that no horizontal fibers can be found running very far in Gennari's band. This observation is also in disagreement with my findings.

The numerous recent electrophysiological studies have shed new light on functional aspects of neurons of the visual system. On the basis of experimental findings, electrophysiologists have claimed that not only visual impulses, but others such as vestibular (Jung, 1958, 1961) and auditory (Skrebitskii and Voronin, 1965) impulses converge on the neurons of the visual cortex. It has further been shown that specific and nonspecific (from nuclei of the reticular formation) impulses converge on the same neuron (Creutzfeldt, Baumgartner, and Jung, 1956; Creutzfeldt and Akimoto, 1958).

The results of interesting investigations by Jung and his collaborators and also by Hubel and Wiesel (1963, 1965), demonstrating differences in the responses of visual cortical neurons to external stimuli and convergence of different impulses on the same neuron, have still not been explained from the point of view of fine morphology. Consequently, the discovery of even slight differences in types of neurons, and in the character of ramification of their dendrites and axons may be of vital importance to the understanding of recent electrophysiological discoveries.

In recent years neurons of the visual cortex have also been investigated histochemically. Stellate and pyramidal cells differ considerably in their distribution of amino acids and protein functional groups. In the stellate neurons they are distributed relatively uniformly; the pyramidal cells show their greatest concentration over the nucleus. The localization of the highest concentrations of tyrosine, tryptophan, and histidine, of the protein functional groups, is observed in the pyramidal neurons of layer IV and the lower level of the visual cortex (Svanidze, 1960, 1963).

Busnyuk (1963) found the highest succinate dehydrogenase activity in neurons of layer IV of the visual cortex and in the solitary pyramids of Meynert.

Many investigations have been made of the structure of the lateral geniculate body. Cytoarchitectonic and experimental studies have shown that the dorsal part of the lateral geniculate body is of decisive importance for the transmission of visual excitation to the cortex (Minkowski, 1911, 1913, 1920; Kononova, 1926; Brouwer, 1936; Polyak, 1933; Lashley, 1934; Pines and Prigonikov, 1936; Khananashvili, 1960). The dorsal part of the lateral geniculate body develops parallel to the cortex in phylogenesis (Poemnyi, 1940) and in ontogenesis (Preobrazhenskaya, 1955, 1966). The ventral part of the nucleus is well developed in rodents; in the higher mammals and man it is much smaller (Levin, 1953; Polyak, 1957). According to Levin (1953), the ventral part in primates develops from the subthalamic region and forms the nucleus praegeniculatus. According to Prigonikov (1949), the pregeniculate body is a transformed ventral part of the lateral geniculate body. Crossed and uncrossed fibers from each eye are represented in alternate layers of the lateral geniculate body. Crossed fibers are projected to layers 1, 4, and 6 and uncrossed to layers 2, 3, and 5. This was first shown by Minkowski (1911, 1913, 1920) by transneuronal atrophy, and later confirmed in monkeys by Le Gros Clark and Penman (1934) and in cats by Pines and Prigonikov (1936), by the Nauta method of studying degeneration of axons used by Silva (1956) and, finally, by Obukhova (1958, 1959) and Hayhow (1958). Polyak (1957), after removal of the eyes from monkeys, fully confirmed Minkowski's observations. Absence of fusion of the image in the lateral geniculate body has been demonstrated in man (Feigenberg, 1953).

Brouwer and Zeeman (1926), Le Gros Clark and Penman (1934), and Polyak (1957) destroyed very small areas of the retina in monkeys and demonstrated their precise projection to small zones of the lateral geniculate body. The presence of subsequent projection of the lateral geniculate body to the cortex was revealed by the work of Minkowski (1913), Polyak (1933), Lashley (1941), and Prigonikov and Pines (1936). Destruction of very small and distinctively shaped areas of the cortex of Area 17 in macaques (Polyak) led to the appearance of areas of degeneration of comparable shape in the lateral geniculate body.

/ Monakow (1889) raised the question of the role of individual types of cells in activity of the lateral geniculate body. According to his theory of transmission of visual stimulation, short-axon interneurons of the lateral geniculate body (*Schaltzellen*) play the leading role by transmitting visual stimulation from optic fibers to the principal large long-axon cells whose axons form the optic radiation. He regarded the whole group of small short-axon cells as the retinal part of the nucleus, the *Retinaanteil*. Monakow's main concepts were confirmed by Kononova (1926) and Pines and Prigonikov (1936). They found that after extirpation of the visual cortex in cats and dogs mainly the large cells of the lateral geniculate body degenerate, while after enucleation of the eyes it is mainly the small cells which degenerate. Directly opposite views were held by Polyak (1933) and Lashley (1941), who considered that complete death of all neurons of the lateral geniculate body after removal of Area 17 is conclusively proved. The experiments of Polyak described above confirmed that all the subcortical cells possess long axons. This view was subsequently maintained by Lashley, Le Gros Clark, and Hartridge. Evidence against Monakow's theory was also obtained by Obukhova, who demonstrated degeneration of synapses on all cells (both large and small) of the lateral geniculate body after division of the optic nerve.

An important fact was found by Matthews (1964) in experiments in macaques: When retrograde degeneration (small lesions of visual cortex) is combined with transneuronal degeneration (enucleation), the resulting changes in the neurons of the lateral geniculate nucleus are but little more severe than those caused by retrograde degeneration alone. There is no evidence of any widespread death of neurons. Shrinkage of neurons after enucleation appears to be less severe in the large-celled laminae than in the small-celled laminae.

However, none of the studies cited above investigated the neurons themselves. Koelliker (1896) made the first attempt to study the lateral geniculate body by Golgi's method. He described brushlike neurons with a round body and short dendrites in rabbits and cats. In man he also found brushlike cells and a dense plexus of afferent fibers. Tello (1904) observed endings of complex type of visual fibers in the lateral geniculate body (dorsal part) in cats corresponding to the three layers of the nucleus. He described two types of neurons, neither of which corresponded to Monakow's interneuron.

According to Cajal (1911), only neurons with a long axon are present in rodents, and Golgi type II cells were not found. Cajal distinguished between marginal and deep long-axon cells. The marginal cells lie between bundles of nerve fibers, they are fusiform and triangular in shape, and their dendrites run parallel to the white matter. Most of the cells are in the center of the nucleus, and are triangular, fusiform, and star-shaped. After turning, their long axons run into the central visual pathway and they give off a descending branch to some as yet unidentified structure. Schemes taken from other works published by Cajal (1911) suggest that these axons may run into the optic tract and to the retina.

Some interesting data on the neuronal structure of the lateral geniculate body were obtained by Henschen (1925, 1926). He described very intimate contact between crossed and uncrossed visual fibers with each other inside the layers themselves. Henschen distinguished nine varieties of cells in the human lateral geniculate body. The more important of these are: coronal cells, arranged in rows, principal cells *(Kranzhauptzellen)*, triangular, and cup-shaped or goblet-shaped cells, the marginal cells of Cajal, large tetragonal cells, small cells, and cells corresponding to Monakow's interneurons or Golgi type II cells. Henschen's main mistake, like that of Monakow, is that he regards the small neurons as possessing short axons. In my opinion (Shkol'nik-Yarros, 1959a, 1961b, 1962) the presence of small neurons with long axons is a typical and important feature of the lateral geniculate body in primates.

According to Taboada (1927, 1928), the structure of the layers in the lateral geniculate body of monkeys is isolated; dendrites of each neuron of the lateral geniculate body do not go outside the limits of their own layer. The cells are multipolar, each with 3–6 dendrites; they are joined together to form glomeruli of 12–15 cells in layers 1 and 2, 30–40 cells in the middle layers, and as many as 60–100 cells in layers 5–6.

O'Leary (1940) found that neurons of the lateral geniculate body of the cat are identical in size, shape, and distribution in layers A and A_1 (to use Thuma's classification). Medium-sized cells predominate in these layers although large and small cells also occur. O'Leary's principal cells are characterized by a long axon, entering the optic radiation. They are medium-sized or large, with an ovoid multipolar or bipolar body. Dendrites emerge as several trunks which ramify considerably. Small principal cells have dendrites with few branches. O'Leary saw few collaterals to the axons of the cells just described. He gives a detailed description of short-axon cells: they are multipolar or, more rarely, bipolar and fusiform. Their body is medium-sized or small, and their dendrites thin and with few branches. Their axons do not cross from one layer to another. The type of ramification of the axon is usually diffuse, and its diameter diminishes during successive dichotomous division. Some cells with short axons have basketlike terminal ramifications surrounding the principal cells.

In layer B of the dorsal part of the lateral geniculate body there are large principal cells with thick polar dendrites. Their axons enter the optic radiation without giving off substantial collaterals to the dorsal nucleus. The small cells sometimes give off collaterals to layer B. Axons from some cells can be traced toward the optic tract. Their ending could not be seen; they perhaps run medially toward the mesencephalon. Short-axon cells of layer B are indistinguishable from those in layers A and A_1. As a result of comparison of the morphology of the nucleus with physiological findings, O'Leary postulated that the short-axon cells have the role of synchronizers for groups of principal cells. Since presynaptic and postsynaptic delay lasts long enough to allow passage through only one synapse, no significant reactivation takes place in this nucleus. Anatomically this corresponds to absence of significant collateral ramification of axons running to the cortex.

No description of neurons of the lateral geniculate body of the dog could be found in the literature.

Polyak (1957) describes two types of neurons in the lateral geniculate body of the macaque. The principal cells are typical multipolars: their roundish body gives off six thick dendrites, in turn giving off secondary, tertiary, and later branches. These branches are about equal in length, and they diverge radially, so that the cells look like stars. The diameter of spread of the dendrites varies from 300 to 500 μ. Polyak observed overlapping of dendrites from neighboring cells. Their axons run into the visual cortex. He calls the cells of the second type association cells. They are considerably fewer in number. Their body is small, oval or circular, and their short axon forms axo-somatic synapses on 12 surrounding cells.

Polyak later makes a very interesting attempt to compare the endings of afferent branches which he found in the lateral geniculate body of monkeys with the varieties of ganglion cells which he described in 1941 in the retina of primates. The classical type of ending is exemplified by axons of "parasol" ganglion cells. A thick fiber runs from the hilus of the lateral geniculate body or from one of the partitions between its various layers, and divides into several dozens of short, winding branches, forming boutons. In the layers of small cells, endings of this type form axo-somatic contacts with approximately 24 cells. In layers 1 and 2, thicker afferent branches of the same type are present. Endings of axons of ganglion cells of a different type (shrub) have the appearance of long, thin fibrils stretching through all layers of the nucleus. Along their course the boutons form axo-somatic synapses with adjacent cells, thus uniting the different layers.

The third type of endings of axons belonging to individual midget ganglion cells of the retina form thinner, more delicate baskets for groups of cells. Unfortunately this state of affairs is not illustrated and it is not specified in the text in which layers endings of this type are mainly found. Finally, a description is given (but, again, not illustrated) of hypothetical endings of axons from the cortex. These are fairly thick fibers, entering the lateral geniculate body on its dorsal surface, not from the optic tract, dividing into several branches spreading over a territory with many cells. At the end of the chapter, Polyak concludes that the principal cells are approximately the same in appearance in all layers of the nucleus. The only difference lies in the size of these cells. On the basis of a study of the neurons of this nucleus in monkeys and man, I cannot agree with the conclusion drawn by Polyak concerning the neuronal structure of the lateral geniculate body in primates.

Despite numerous investigations, many problems concerned with the fine structure, interneuronal connections, and even the function of the lateral geniculate body still remain unsolved. The role of the subcortical center of vision has not yet been completely explained. The most widely different views are still held regarding the significance of this nucleus. Some workers claim that the lateral geniculate body is a relay station for visual impulses, and that only one synaptic interruption is present there (Chang, 1952a; Bishop and Clare, 1955). Conditions do not exist in the lateral geniculate body for comparison of fields of vision in binocular vision, the mechanism of which exists in the cortex (Cajal, 1911; Minkowski, 1920b; Feigenberg, 1953). Others however, ascribe more complex functions to the lateral geniculate body. In their opinion it is not simply a relay station, but a structure where neurons may exhibit a reciprocal influence (O'Leary, 1940; Bishop, Jeremy, and McLeod, 1953; Polyak, 1957). Fibers from both eyes are mixed in the lateral geniculate body (Henschen, 1926), and all the conditions are present for the combination of the fields of vision required in binocular vision (Balmasova, 1950). Finally, electrical interaction between fibers has been postulated on the basis of their simple contact in the layers of the nucleus (Silva, 1956). The latter confirmed the anatomical differentiation of layers reported by earlier workers, and in an attempt to elucidate communication between the layers taking place without the intervention of synapses, collaterals, and so on, he falls back on the theory of Arvanitaki (1942) and others to explain how excitation can pass from one fiber to another.

Comparison of the neuronal structure of the lateral geniculate body in members of different orders of mammals is thus interesting not merely from the purely morphological point of view, but also for correlation with physiological facts.

In my analysis of neuronal structure in the visual cortex and lateral geniculate body of certain mammals and man I paid particular attention, first, to the architectonics, then to the varieties of neurons present, the size of their body and processes, the number and length of the processes, which are connected with the size of the synaptic zone of the neuron in both its receptive and transmitting parts, and the character and direction of the

branches responsible for interneuronal connections. I attempted to correlate
the type of neuronal structure with physiological data.

The method chiefly used in this investigation was Golgi's bichromate–
silver impregnation. The methods of Nissl, Marchi, Nauta, and Glees were
also used. Altogether about 350 specimens from various mammals and
man and 42 retinas of rabbits and dogs were analyzed.

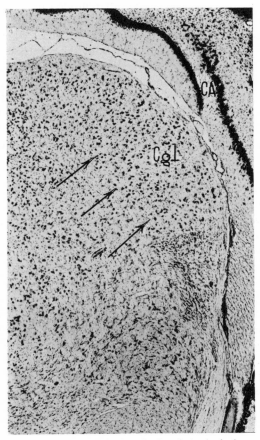

Fig. 2. Lateral geniculate body of the hedgehog.
Cgl, lateral geniculate body; Ca, cornu ammonis;
arrows indicate boundary of nucleus. Nissl stain;
30×.

NEURONAL STRUCTURE OF THE VISUAL CORTEX AND LATERAL GENICULATE BODY IN SOME MAMMALS

Visual System of the Hedgehog (Insectivora)

The hedgehog is a nocturnal animal and its retina consists almost entirely of rods, with only a few cones (Menner, 1929; Walls, 1942). The olfactory system plays a much more important role in the life of the hedgehog, and this is reflected in the highly differentiated structure of the olfactory cortex. Numerous fibers from the retina run toward the superior colliculi. They are of large size and are clearly differentiated into layers. The lateral geniculate body (Fig. 2) is poorly differentiated, indistinctly separated from the nuclei of the thalamus, and its layered structure is almost completely absent. Neurons of the lateral geniculate body are remarkably uniform, and only two varieties of large cells can be distinguished, although intermediate stages exist between them, and they differ only very slightly from each other. The first variety (Fig. 3) consists of triangular, polygonal, and semilunar cells with radially arranged dendrites. The second variety consists of pear-shaped, triangular, or fusiform cells (referring to the shape of their body) with a shrublike arrangement of their dendrites, in which several (as many as 15) thinner branches are given off by the main dendritic trunk. All the neurons of the hedgehog's lateral geniculate body are comparable in size and type of dendritic branching only with neurons of the magnocellular layers of this nucleus in primates. No cells similar to the principal or small (midget, i.e., possessing a few short dendrites) cells of the four dorsal layers of the nucleus in primates can be found in the hedgehog.*

The neocortex of the hedgehog possesses only a few cytoarchitectonic areas. The neurons of these areas are not clearly distinguished from each other. Differentiation of the archicortex and paleocortex, which are evidently connected with olfaction (Brodmann, 1909; Filimonov, 1949), is much more complex in the hedgehog. The typical higher mammalian features are completely absent from Area 17; there is no clearly defined system of horizontal layers, no subdivision of layer IV into sublayers, no special part of the layers in which the cells are particularly dense or small, and so on (Fig. 4). The upper layers in the hedgehog's cortex are not yet clearly differentiated from each other. Neurons very similar to the undifferentiated cells of this layer described by Zhukova (1953) in the motor cortex of the hedgehog are present in layer II. The cells are uniform in size, with none particularly large

---

* In this book I shall examine the neuronal structure of the dorsal part of the lateral geniculate body as the most important part for transmission of visual excitation to the cortex.

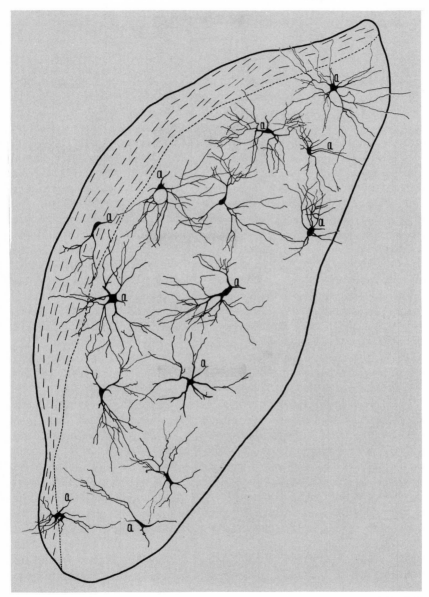

Fig. 3.   Neurons of lateral geniculate body of a hedgehog. a, axon; 100× (Shkol'nik-Yarros, 1962).

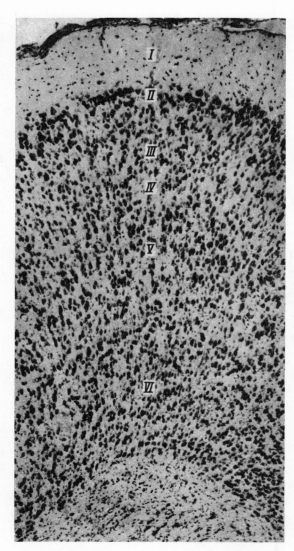

Fig. 4. Cytoarchitectonics of the visual cortex of the
hedgehog. Here and in subsequent figures layers of the
cortex are designated by Roman numerals. Nissl stain;
100×.

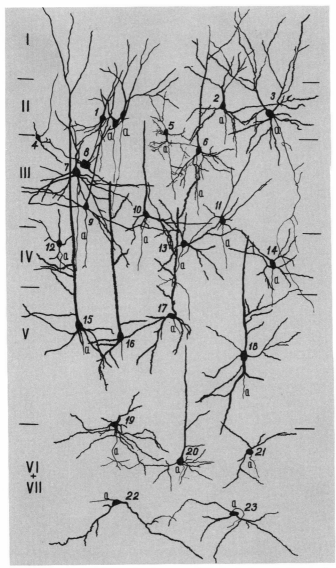

Fig. 5. Neurons of the visual cortex of the hedgehog. 1, 2, 3, cells of layer II; 4, 5, 8, short-axon cells of layers II and III; 6, 7, 9, 10, 11, pyramidal cells of layer III; 12, 13, 14, stellate cells with descending axon of layer IV; 15, 17, pyramidal cells of layer V; 16, 18, fusiform cells of layer V; 20, pyramidal cell of layer VI; 19, 21, cells of layer VI; 22, 23, cells of layer VII; a, axon. (Shkol'nik-Yarros, 1964.)

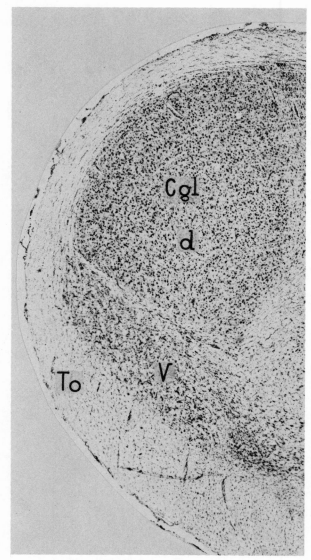

Fig. 6. Lateral geniculate body of the rabbit (Cgl). d, dorsal part; V, ventral part; To, optic tract. Nissl stain; 30×.

and none particularly small (Fig. 5). The pyramidal cells are rarely conical in shape and they give off few branches. The mean number of dendritic branches from one pyramidal cell is 15–20 (counting not only the large trunks but also small secondary ramifications). Many neurons appear somewhat out of proportion because their apical dendrites are not oriented vertically. The cortex as a whole is characterized by its poorly developed bundles of fibers entering and leaving the cortex, so that there is no regular vertical and horizontal striation. In layer IV, which is difficult to distinguish, stellate cells with a descending axon are present (Fig. 5; 12, 13, 14); these may

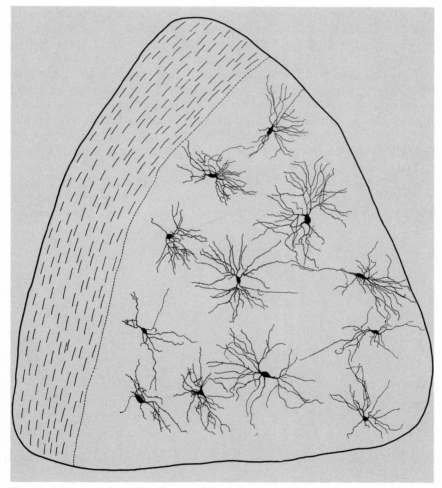

Fig. 7. Neurons of the dorsal part of the lateral geniculate body of the rabbit.

perhaps be the prototype of the large star cells of Cajal in layer IV of the primate visual cortex. There is no diversity of cell forms, the neurons are similar to each other; this is associated with the lack of variety in the ramifications of the dendrites and axons, which gives cells their different shapes. Unfortunately, the material at my disposal did not allow me to trace the final ramifications of the axons or to identify their connections.

Visual System of the Rabbit (Rodentia)

Vision is not the dominant feature of the sensory system of the rabbit, just as with other nocturnal animals (Menner, 1929). The olfactory and auditory systems play an important role in its life. In the rabbit the almost total decussation of the optic nerves, together with the lateral position of its eyes, correspond to the predominant role of monocular vision in this animal.

The first point to be noted in the rabbit retina is the relative thinness of the layers, particularly of the outer and inner nuclear layers, compared, for example, with the retina of birds. If the retinal neurons are impregnated by the bichromate-silver method, differences can be detected between the photoreceptors—the rods and cones; this is of interest in view of the absence of a definite answer to the question: Do cones exist in the rabbit's retina?

The subcortical visual centers of the rabbit differ essentially in their structure from those in carnivores and, in particular, in primates. The superior colliculi are large in volume and complex in structure, and they are still the main point for relaying of stimuli arriving in the central nervous

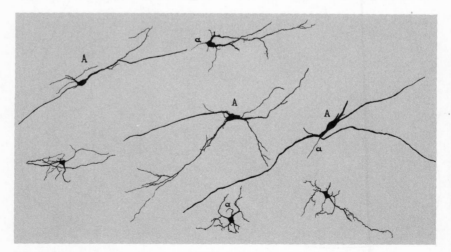

Fig. 8. Neurons of the ventral part of the lateral geniculate body of the rabbit. A, cells with few branches; a, axon.

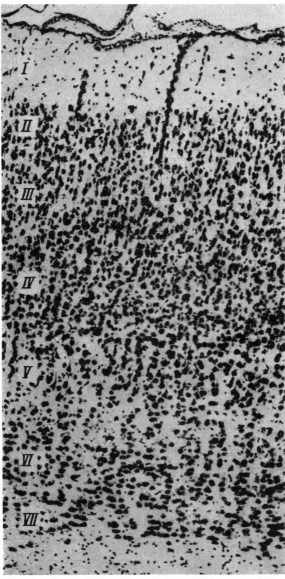

Fig. 9. Cytoarchitectonics of Area 17 in the rabbit. Nissl stain; 100×.

system from the retina. The precise projection of individual areas of the retina to the superior colliculi was investigated by Brouwer (1923). The lateral geniculate body of the rabbit is larger and more clearly defined than in the hedgehog (Fig. 6), but the obvious and clear subdivision into layers which is observed in primates and carnivores is absent.

My observations show that neurons of the lateral geniculate body of the rabbit can be subdivided into four main types depending on the ramification of their dendrites. Radial (Fig. 7) and shrublike cells, as well as cells with few branches, differ only slightly from each other. All neurons are

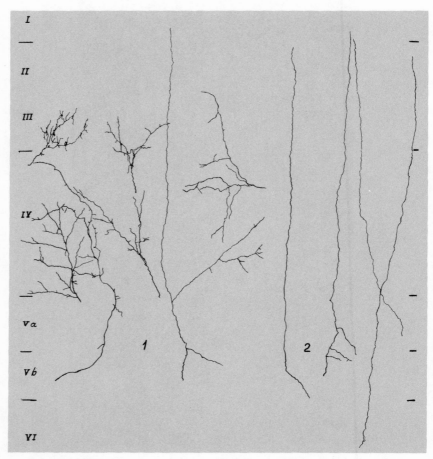

Fig. 10. Afferent branches in Area 17 of the rabbit. 1, afferent branches of specific type ramifying in layer IV and the lower part of layer III; 2, afferent branches of nonspecific association type, reaching to layer I and giving off few collaterals.

medium-sized and their dendrites ramify more freely than in the hedgehog. The cells with few branches, resembling neurons of the reticular formation, have three or four long, straight dendrites (Fig. 8). They are found mainly in the ventral part of the lateral geniculate body. Also in the ventral part

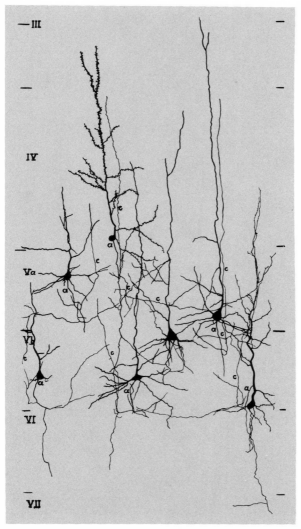

Fig. 11. Pyramidal cells of Area 17 of the rabbit. a, axon; c, axon collaterals.

are cells with a few short dendrites richly supplied with spines. The body of the radial and shrublike cells is mainly circular in shape.

Despite the primitive macroscopic structure of the rabbit's brain (absence of fissures and gyri), its cortex is much more complex than that of the hedgehog. Cytoarchitectonically this was clearly demonstrated many years ago by Brodmann. However, individual areas of the neocortex are

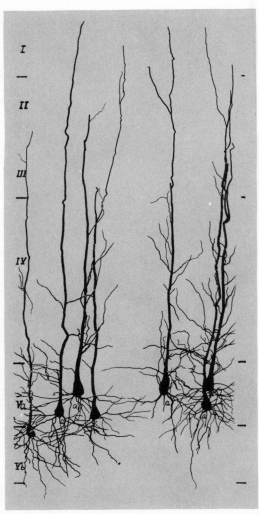

Fig. 12. Pyramidal cells of layer V of Area 17 of the rabbit. Drawing made from one section; 100×.

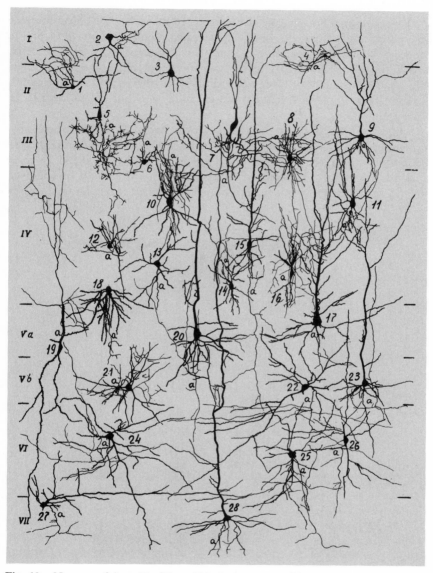

Fig. 13. Neurons of Area 17 of the rabbit. 2, 4, neurons of layer I; 3, pyramidal cell of layer II; 1, short-axon stellate cell of layer II; 5, 6, 7, 8, short-axon cells of layer III; 9, pyramidal cell of layer III; 10, 11, 12, 14, 15, stellate short-axon cells of layer IV; 15, pyramidal cell of layer IV; 13, 18, star cells with long descending axon (star cells of Cajal); 17, 20, 23, pyramidal cells of layer V; 19, cell with ascending axon of layer V; 22, 24, cells with basal dendrite directed downward; 21, 25, short-axon neurons of layers V and VI; 26, fusiform cell of layer VI; 27, cell with horizontal arrangement of basal dendrite in layer VII; 28, pyramidal cell of layer VII. (Shkol'nik-Yarros, 1954.)

small in size and not sharply demarcated from each other. Considerable differentiation is observed only in the retrosplenial region, possibly in connection with the special development of olfactory function. The dense distribution of cells in Area 17 can be seen in cytoarchitectonic preparations (Fig. 9). The structure of layer IV, with its three striae, typical of primates, is absent (Fig. 9). Translucency is present in layer V but not in layer IV in Nissl preparations.

Afferent branches of two types occur in Area 17. The first type corresponds to the specific afferents of Lorente de Nó (1938) and gives brush-like branches in layer IV and the lower part of layer III (Fig. 10, 1). In some cases the course of an obliquely running afferent fiber could be followed through several microscopic fields. Afferent fibers of the second type ascend

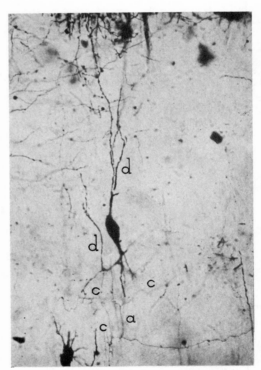

Fig. 13a. Short-axon cell of layer III in Area 17 of the rabbit's cortex. Photomicrograph. d, dendrite; a, axon; c, axon collateral. Marginal astrocytic glia visible in layer I. Note the fusiform body of the short-axon cell.

to the top without branching and sometimes give off collaterals in the lower layers (Fig. 10, 2).

The pyramidal cells in the rabbit's cortex have bodies of different shapes: round, oval, pear-shaped, triangular, tetragonal, or less commonly, conical (Figs. 11, 12, 13). Ramification of the dendrites is slight (compared with carnivores). The number of dendritic branches varies from 10 to 34, counting both large dendritic trunks and small secondary ramifications. The vertical orientation and regularity of the apical dendrites extending into layer I are much more pronounced than in the hedgehog (Figs. 11, 12, 13).

Since the pyramidal cells in the various layers of the cortex have been fully described by O'Leary and Bishop, I shall dwell only briefly on them.

In layer II the pyramidal cells are small in size and shape, and in the poor development of their processes they resemble immature neurons (Fig. 13, 3).

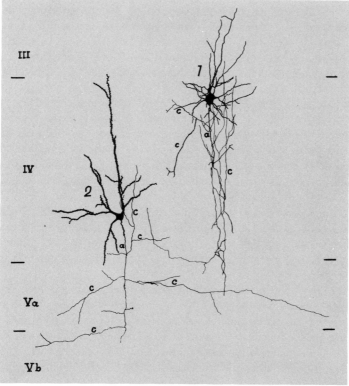

Fig. 14. Neurons of layer IV of Area 17 of the rabbit. 1, short-axon stellate cell; 2, intermediate form of neuron between pyramidal and stellate cell types: a, axon; c, axon collaterals.

Layer III contains orderly pyramidal cells whose dendrites are distinguished by their thinness (Fig. 13, 9).

Both small pyramidal cells and others larger than in layers II and III are present in layer IV and are often round or oval in shape (Fig. 13, 15); there are also others which are typically conical in shape.

The dendrites of pyramidal cells of layer IV of stellate type or transitional toward them often possess large numbers of spines (Fig. 14, 2). The axons of these atypical pyramidal cells ramify extremely liberally, giving up to 10 collaterals which run toward the upper layers and for a considerable distance horizontally in layer V (Fig. 14, 2).

The pyramidal cells in layer V are relatively larger than in the more superficial layers. However, they have no features in common with the solitary pyramidal cells of Meynert which are typical of layer V of the visual cortex in primates. The pyramidal cells of layer V in the rabbit are characterized, first, by the absence of a powerfully developed horizontal band of branches of the basal dendrites and, second, by their arrangement in groups. The basal dendrites of these cells are very small, short and thin (Fig. 13, 17, 20; Fig. 12).

In layers VI and VII the pyramidal cells differ from those described above in that their body is elongated transversely and their apical dendrite pursues a tortuous course (Fig. 13, 28).

The difference between the thin, regular pyramidal cell of layers II–III and the more massive, large pyramidal cell of layer V is clearly visible.

Some of the pyramidal cells of the lower layers give off an apical dendrite not in layer I, as described by Cajal (1911), but in layer V or VI (the short and medium-sized pyramidal cells described by Lorente de Nó, 1922). I have observed similar pyramidal cells in the rabbit's cortex, as well as in the cortex of dogs, monkeys, and man.

The most powerful and thick horizontal collaterals from axons of the pyramidal cells of layer IV extend into layer V. Intracortical association connections most probably correspond to the horizontal collaterals of axons of the large pyramidal cells of the upper layers, which are thus association collaterals.

The number of spines on dendrites of the pyramidal cells is highly variable, for sometimes the dendrites are covered with them, while at other times they are almost completely absent (for example, many spines can be seen in Fig. 11 on the cells of layers II and III, while few are seen in Fig. 12).

Area 17 in the rabbit contains many fusiform cells (not as regards the shape of their body, but of the type described by Cajal, 1900, 1911; Polyakov and Sarkisov, 1949). In my specimens they are found not only in the lower layers—VI, VII, but also in layers III, IV, and V (Fig. 15). Axons descending into the white matter give off numerous collaterals, ascending, horizontal,

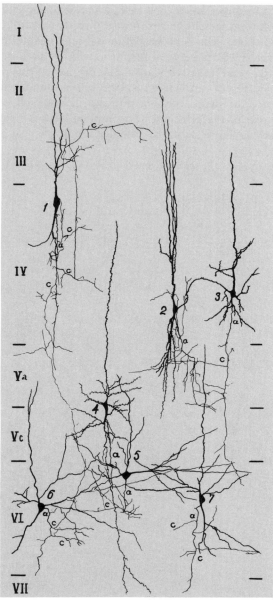

Fig. 15. Various neurons of Area 17 of the rabbit. 1, fusiform cell of layer IV with complex ramifications of its axon; 3, pyramidal neuron of layer IV; 5, short-axon neuron of layer VI; 2, 4, triangular cells of layers IV and V; 6, 7, fusiform cells of layer VI; a, axon; c, collateral.

and descending in direction. In one case, when dendritic trunks typical of the fusiform cell were present, the axon went directly upward. Consequently, not only intermediate cells between pyramidal and stellate may be found, but also cells intermediate between fusiform, with an axon descending into the white matter, and cells with an ascending axon, called Martinotti's cells. In layer IV a very distinctive fusiform cell is found, with a fully impregnated axon. The axon, running downward, gives off numerous collaterals; from one of the principal horizontal collaterals a large ascending collateral arises, giving a terminal ramification (a typical terminal with

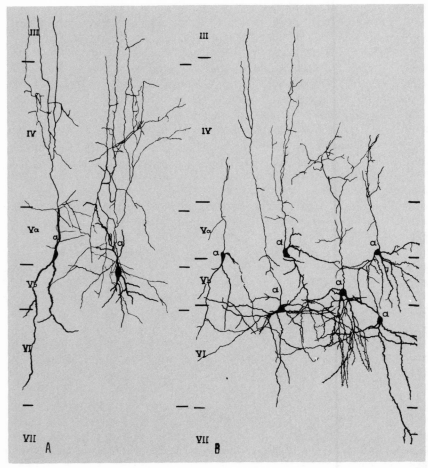

Fig. 16. Cells with ascending axon (Martinotti) in Area 17 of the rabbit. A: Cells of large caliber with complex ramification of their axon. B: Cells of small caliber. a, axon.

small branches, Fig. 15, 1) in the upper part of layer III. This was possibly a neuron transitional in type to the stellate neuron. Other fusiform cells whose dendrites are very densely covered with spines (Fig. 15, 2, 4) can be seen in the same figure, whereas the cell just described is poorly supplied with spines. Some of the fusiform cells are remarkable for the considerable extent of their dendrites in vertical sections, from the upper border of layer IV to the white matter. Absolutely typical fusiform cells can be seen in the upper part of layer IV. All these small details indicate the important role unquestionably played in the process of transmission of excitation by the fusiform cells, which in the rabbit cortex are not confined to the lower layers.

In Area 17 of the rabbit two varieties of Martinotti's cells are present: large and small (Fig. 16). The larger cells have more highly ramified axons, i.e., they form more contacts with the cells of the upper layers. Dendrites of these cells, nearly all of which descend directly or obliquely, in most cases are covered with many very long, thin spines. The body of these neurons is fusiform, semilunar, or turnip-shaped (Fig. 16). The dendrites of these cells presumably collect excitation in horizontal and vertical directions in layers V, VI, and VII for transmission upward to the neurons of the upper layers.

A few stellate cells of the rabbit visual cortex are illustrated in Figs. 17 and 18.

In layer I the axons and dendrites of the stellate cells tend to spread in a horizontal direction; not only do the Cajal–Retzius cells (Fig. 13, 2) typical of layer I give horizontal axons, but also stellate cells of medium and small caliber. The axon shown in Fig. 17 impregnated without the cell body is an example of such a spread.

In layer II the stellate cells often have dendrites reaching as far as layer I (Fig. 13, 5, 7) and, consequently, receive excitation from that layer. The terminal branches of axons of these cells are arranged as baskets or nests.

In both layer II and layer III axons of narrowly branching types are predominant, i.e., axons adapted for the formation of pericellular plexuses around adjacent cells of small size (Fig. 13, 5 and Fig. 17, 3). Widely branching axons are much less common. The diameter of the axons is very small. The dendrites of some stellate cells run obliquely. Some axons ascend and are connected to horizontal branches of the axons of layer I.

In layer III, besides stellate cells with a descending axon, cells with an ascending axon are found (Fig. 13, 6, 8; Fig. 17). Neurons described originally by Cajal, with descending and horizontal axon collaterals, are typical of Area 17 in the rabbit (Fig. 13, 7; Fig. 13a). In the shape of their body, stellate cells of the upper layers are more frequently oval or round, and bodies of angular shape are less common.

Besides stellate cells with complex ramification of their axon adapted

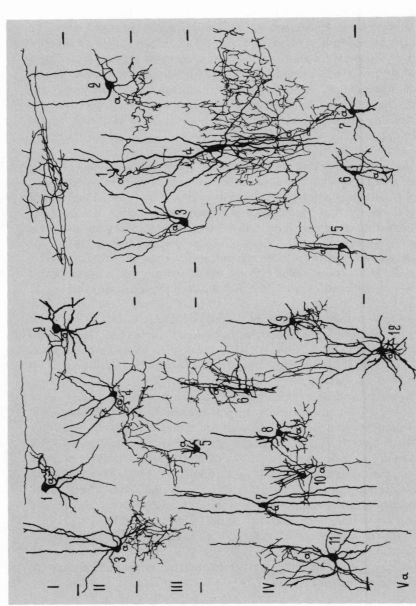

Fig. 17. Short-axon cells of the upper layers of Area 17 in the rabbit. A: 1, 2, Cajal–Retzius cells of layer I; 3, stellate cell with basket type of axon ramification; 4, 5, stellate cells of layer III; 6, 11, short-axon cells with ascending axons of layer IV; 7, short-axon cell with axon of concentrating type; 8, 9, 10, short-axon cells with descending axons of layer IV; 12, cell with ascending axon of layer V. B: In layer I the axon system has a mainly horizontal type of spread of its branches; 1, small stellate short-axon cell of layer II; 4, short-axon stellate cell of large

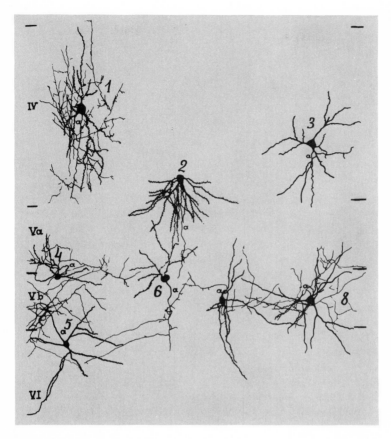

Fig. 18. Stellate cells of layers IV and V of Area 17 in the rabbit. 2, 3, semilunar and radial types of star cells with a long, descending axon; 1, 4–8, different varieties of short-axon cells; a, axon.

for the formation of pericellular plexuses around many neurons, layer IV also contains cells whose axon ends as a single branch or a group of three terminals, while the dendrites extend from layer III to layer V (Fig. 17, 6). Besides many cells with a short axon, star cells with a long axon, descending into the subcortex, characteristic of Area 17 are also found. Known as star cells of Cajal, they are located mainly in the lower part of layer IV and two varieties of them, semilunar and stellate, are present in the rabbit (Fig. 13, 13, 18).

In layer V the initial part of the axon of most of the short-axon neurons is arcuate; the subsequent direction of the axon may be ascending, descending, or horizontal (Fig. 13, 21). In the upper layers of the cortex the nest

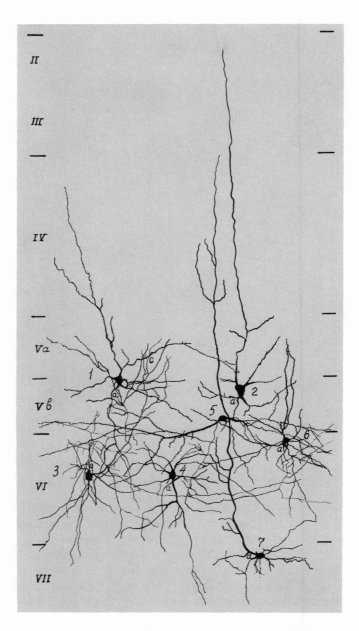

Fig. 19.   Neurons of the lower layers of Area 17 in the rabbit. Different types of cells can be seen: pyramidal, fusiform, stellate, and intermediate forms; a, axon; c, collateral.

type of axon distribution with the formation of narrow basketlike endings is more marked. In layers V and VI, just as in layer I, the horizontal type is more common, with the axon running parallel to the surface of the cortex. Martinotti's cells (with ascending axon) are commonly seen; the larger of them give off powerfully developed axons with numerous collaterals (Fig. 13, 19). Similar cells of smaller caliber have axons with fewer collaterals. Well-developed dendrites of cells with an ascending axon run downward and are usually thickly covered with spines of different shapes.

In layer VI, which is distinguished by its polymorphism, as well as pyramidal (Fig. 13, 24, 26; Fig. 19), fusiform, and inverted cells, the ordinary stellate short-axon cells are also found. Less frequently, impregnated neurons with a horizontal basal dendritic trunk, 0.7 mm in length, may also be seen (Fig. 13, 27).

The stellate cells may have not only ascending axonal systems, but also those of a locally spreading type. Some of the stellate cells give off well-developed horizontal axon collaterals, forming a complete system similar to the horizontal system in layer I.

The greatest variety of short-axon cells is found in the upper layers, where they differ considerably both in caliber (compare cells 4 and 1 in Fig. 17, B) and in the extent of spread and number of branches of the dendrites and axons. The body of the stellate neurons may be round, triangular, fusiform, or pear-shaped, depending on the direction of ramification of the dendrites from the body surface. The number of dendritic branches is small, and the dendrites sometimes have no spines, although others are richly covered with them (Fig. 18, 1). It is possible that short-axon cells with numerous spines on their dendrites are a special feature of Area 17 in the rabbit, because no such neurons are present in the primate cortex. Unusually varied forms of stellate short-axon cells, from a small granular cell to one of giant size, from the narrow type of the concentrating variety just described to the wide type with hundreds of synaptic endings, can be seen in a small area of the section.

Thus in the rabbit I identified three varieties of stellate cells. The first type is characterized by a dense ramification of its axon with numerous endings in contact with neighboring neurons; such cells are apparently dispersive. The second type has a completely different arrangement: the dendrites of these cells are spread over a wide area, collecting excitation from layer III to layer V, while their axon is in contact with a few neighboring neurons only. Stellate cells of this type can be called concentrating. The long axon of cells of the third type descends into the white matter.

In addition to the types of neurons which were studied, I also examined the isolated impregnated axonal systems, allowing a more detailed analysis to be made of the structure and direction of axons belonging to cells in

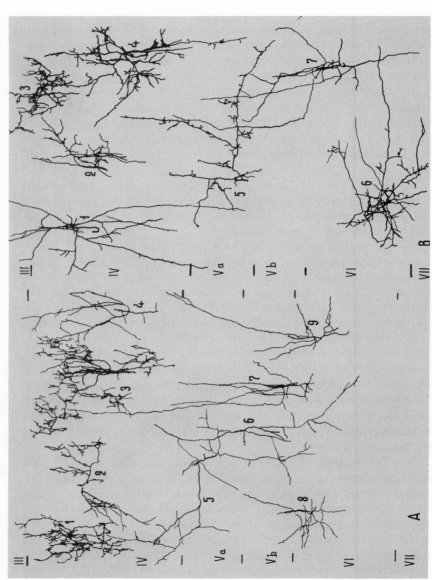

Fig. 20. Axonal systems of Area 17 in the rabbit. Ramification of axons in layers III and IV is mainly of the nest or basket type (A: 1, 2, 3; B: 2, 3, 4). In layers V and VI the axons are mainly ascending and horizontal in direction (A: 5, 6; B: 5, 6)

different layers. In layers III and IV the narrow type of ramification with highly complex and dense axonal systems was predominant (Fig. 20). Some axons give terminal branches resembling baskets described by Cajal. In the lower layers ascending and horizontal axons are predominant (Fig. 20). Ascending collaterals from different types of axons—from pyramidal, fusiform, triangular, and upturned cells—are present in large numbers. Axonal systems of narrowly branching type with large numbers of synaptic endings on their ramifications are much less numerous. Cells resembling those of layer IV could not be seen in the lower layers.

A drawing showing some of the varieties of the neurons present in Area 17 of the rabbit (Fig. 13) can give only an approximate idea of the variety found among cortical cells and of their qualitative differences.

Visual System of the Dog (Carnivora)

Olfaction and hearing are more highly developed than vision in dogs. However, vision in the dog has developed in a distinctive manner, discrimination of the intensity of light being superior and discrimination of color and shape being immeasurably inferior to that in primates (Pavlov, 1927, 1951; Frolov, 1918; Shenger-Krestovnikova, 1921). Doubts are still expressed on the question of whether dogs possess color vision. Some admit this possibility while others deny it completely (Orbeli, 1908, 1913; Walls, 1942).

The less complete decussation of the optic nerves than in insectivores and rodents and the less lateral position of the eyes correspond to an increased role of binocular vision in the dog.

My observations show that well-defined cones, differing sharply from rods, are present in the dog's retina. These differences are much clearer than in the rabbit. Horizontal and ganglion cells possess richly branching dendrites. Axons of the horizontal cells terminate in complex ramifications with thousands of synaptic endings. The more complex and more highly differentiated structure of the retina corresponds to a more complex system of layers in the structure of the lateral geniculate body. The relative volume of the superior colliculi is reduced. The lateral geniculate body is of considerable size and is clearly divided into four layers (Fig. 21). Only one of these layers is predominantly composed of small cells, another is filled with very large cells, and the remaining two layers are composed of neurons of different sizes, large neurons constituting more than half the total, and many of the cells being medium-sized.

The region of the small cells lies inferiorly, superiorly, and to some extent medially, and it is filled with small cells with medium-sized cells here and there among them.

The magnocellular region consists of less densely packed, large cells.

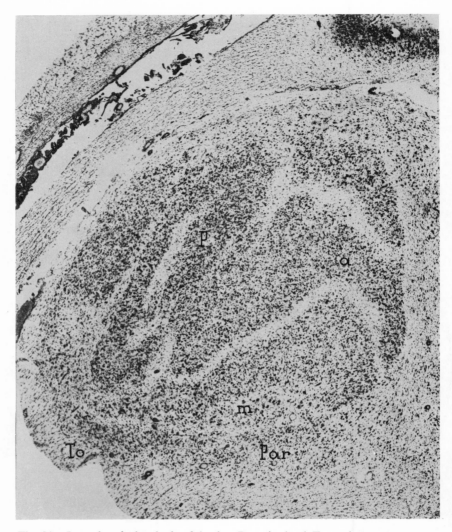

Fig. 21. Lateral geniculate body of the dog. Posterior level. To, optic tract; m, magnocellular layer; a, p, principal layers; Par, parvocellular layer. Myelin partitions can be seen (pale areas on the photograph). Nissl stain; photomicrograph; 45×.

In this part the nuclei contain no small cells whatever. The magnocellular region extends through all levels and forms a layer of irregular shape above the parvocellular part in the inferior portion of the nucleus and below the parvocellular part in its superior portion.

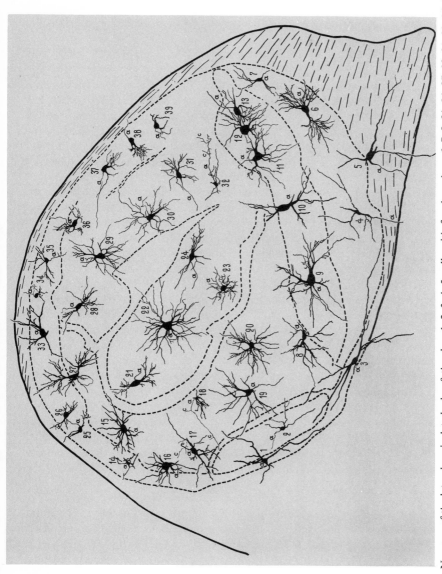

Fig. 22. Neurons of the lateral geniculate body of the dog. 1, 2, 3, 4, 5, cells with few branches; 6, 7, 8, 21, 24, 27, 28, 31, 33, 36, 37, 38, shrublike cells; 17, 18, 32, short-axon cells; 14, 25, 26, 34, 35, 39, midget cells; 12, 15, 16, 19, 20, 22, 23, 29, 30, radial cells; 9, 10, 11, 12, 13, large cells of the magnocellular sublayer of the nucleus; a, axon; c, collateral. (Shkol'nik-Yarros, 1958b.)

The middle portion, lying between the nuclei of large and small cells, is divided into compartments by myelin partitions. The compartments are arranged arcwise and are varied in composition: small, medium-sized, and large cells. The curious shapes of some areas of these nuclei must be studied in sagittal sections.

The subdivision of the nucleus proposed by Rioch (1929, 1930) must be accepted.

The lateral geniculate body of the dog (Fig. 22) contains five principal varieties of neurons: (1) those with long axons (radial, Fig. 22, 12, 22, 23); (2) shrublike (Fig. 22, 6, 21, 27); (3) marginal, with few branches (Fig. 22, 1, 2, 3, 4, 5); (4) midget (Fig. 22, 14, 34, 35); and (5) cells with short axons (Fig. 22, 17, 18, 32). Along the course of the fibers of the optic tract and along the medial border lie the marginal cells with few branches. They are fusiform or triangular, their dendrites are few in number, thick, straight, long, and they run along the course of the optic fibers. The cell bodies are mainly large in size. The axons are given off in different directions, but more frequently medially and they soon disappear from view. These cells are very similar to the neurons with few branches in other structures of the brain stem. No such cells have previously been described in the lateral geniculate body of the dog and man.

In the parvocellular layer of the nucleus the cell bodies are fusiform, round, or pear-shaped. Small cells are predominant, but medium-sized cells also are found. The distribution of the dendrites varies. Sometimes dendrites are given off as thick trunks from the cell poles and rapidly break up into numerous thin branches. More commonly, the small cells give off only a few dendritic trunks, although not less than three, and these subsequently ramify. The direction of the initial parts of the axon is mainly outward, toward the myelin capsule of the nucleus.

In the magnocellular layer of the nucleus the cell bodies are larger than in any other part of the nucleus. The bodies are fusiform or polygonal in shape. Dendrites are given off radially or from the poles; they are thick but not particularly long and they give rise to secondary branches. The initial segments of the axons are directed medially, laterally, and superiorly.

In the anterior layer of the nucleus the cells are medium-sized or large, and their bodies are fusiform or polygonal. The dendrites diverge radially or from the poles and the thick trunk breaks up into thin branches. The initial segments of the axons run in various directions, sometimes forming bends or loops before assuming their final direction.

In the posterior layer of the nucleus the cell bodies are small, medium-sized, and large. In shape they are bicornuate, oval, or round. The dendrites are given off radially or from the poles of the cell and they give rise to secondary branches. The initial segments of the axons run in various directions:

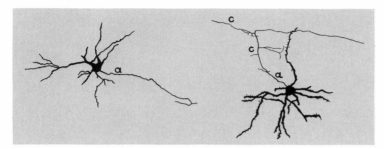

Fig. 23. Long-axon cells of the lateral geniculate body of the dog drawn from sagittal sections. Note bifurcation of the axon.

medially or laterally, sometimes giving loops and bends, and occasionally giving off collaterals initially. In this nucleus I found cells of very small size with small, winding dendrites, covered with long spines. The axon can be followed for a considerable distance and it gives off collaterals. In the character of their body, dendrites, and axon these cells bear the closest resemblance to the short-axon type.

Sections from the anterior part and sagittal sections (Fig. 23) also were used for examination of the details of the course followed by the axons. Some of them give off collaterals forming bends and loops. Sometimes axons in sagittal sections divide clearly into two principal branches. The course of one of the main branches is absolutely clear—it runs into the cortex. To determine the direction of the other branch, further investigations are necessary (for example, destruction of the lateral geniculate body followed by tracing of the degeneration). It can be postulated that the second branch runs toward the retina or the reticular formation. Some cells which I observed resemble short-axon cells in the nature of their processes. To verify the existence of these cells, an additional study was made of sections through the lateral geniculate body of the cat. Axons of some cells in the cat also resemble the short-axon type (Fig. 115). Consequently, O'Leary's results indicating the presence of Golgi type II cells in this subcortical nucleus were confirmed.

The study of visual afferent fibers reaching the lateral geniculate body reveals the following properties: first, the very wide area covered by an afferent fiber (Fig. 24). One visual fiber of large diameter gives off many branches forming pericellular networks around the cells of the lateral geniculate body. Second, overlapping of afferents is observed, i.e., cells of the lateral geniculate body receive afferent impulses from several optic fibers. Not all optic fibers are of the same caliber, but they may be thick, thin, or of medium caliber (Fig. 24).

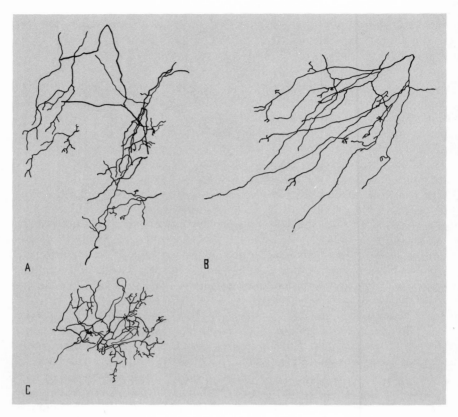

Fig. 24. Afferent branches in the lateral geniculate body of the dog. A: Axons and endings of different calibers. B: Extensive area of spread of an afferent fiber. C: Overlapping of afferent ramifications.

In carnivores (the dog) cortical differentiation is much more complex than in insectivores and rodents. The surface relief of the brain is complex and deep fissures are present. Variability of structure of the fissures and gyri have been demonstrated in different dogs (Filimonov, 1928). Even in the frontal region of the dog's cortex, five structurally different areas can be identified (Svetukhina, 1959). In the principal auditory projection zone of the dog four areas can be distinguished (Mering, 1951), and in the motor projection zone there are two areas (Adrianov, 1951; Adrianov and Mering, 1959). The dog's visual cortex, however, differs sharply from the cortex of primate type. No clear division of layer IV into three sublayers can be seen, and the typical Gennari's band (IVb) and sublayer IVc are absent. Horizontal and vertical striation is distinctly visible, but bears not the remotest resemblance to Area 17 in man (Fig. 25). Layer IV is uniformly filled by neurons of different shapes, some circular, others polygonal.

A study of afferent fibers in Area 17 reveals at least four different varieties (Fig. 26). The first is characterized by large, oblique fibers running from below upward, from right to left, or from left to right, into layer IV, where they form a large brush (Fig. 26). With good impregnation, the dense plexus formed principally by these fibers can be seen. The large oblique afferent fibers correspond to Lorente de Nó's (1938) "specific afferents." They differ from their equivalent in the rabbit: they are larger in the dog and their ramifications occupy a considerable area. Afferent fibers of the second type run vertically upward and give off branches which also proceed in an upward direction (Fig. 27). This type resembles the association afferent distinguished by Lorente de Nó in mice. The third type of afferent has its main axon running vertically, stretching in a straight line from the white matter up into layer IV, where it gives off large horizontal collaterals at right angles (Fig. 26). No account of afferent fibers of this type could be found in the literature. The fourth type (*cf.* Fig. 87, B) is a large, oblique fiber ending on a dendrite of a pyramidal neuron as a terminal "paw." Further studies will undoubtedly bring to light other varieties of afferent fibers in the visual cortex. The presence of cells of different types and size in the lateral geniculate body must correspond to the presence of several different types and calibers of afferent branches.

Pyramidal cells in the visual cortex of the dog vary in shape, size, and number of dendritic branches. In shape, they are conical, triangular, or pear-shaped. In size they vary from very large to very small (Figs. 27, 28).

The mean number of dendritic branches of the pyramidal cells in the dog varies from 17 to 80. The large size and abundance of branches of many pyramidal neurons in the dog cortex is very conspicuous, not only in Area 17, but also when other areas are examined.

Characteristics of the pyramidal cells vary considerably from layer to layer. In layer II the cells are small and have few branches.

In layer III large and regularly arranged pyramidal cells are frequently seen (Figs. 27, 28) along with small and medium-sized cells (Shkol'nik-Yarros, 1950b). The presence of a supplementary bunch of dendrites on the pyramidal cells of the upper layers must be emphasized in particular (Fig. 27). Usually the basal dendrites and apical bouquet form dendritic contact zones of the pyramidal cells, but for some pyramidal cells in the dog a third dendritic contact zone is outlined by ramifications of dendrites given off by the lower third of the ascending dendrite. Sometimes only two or three branches emerge at this level, but at others there are many such branches and

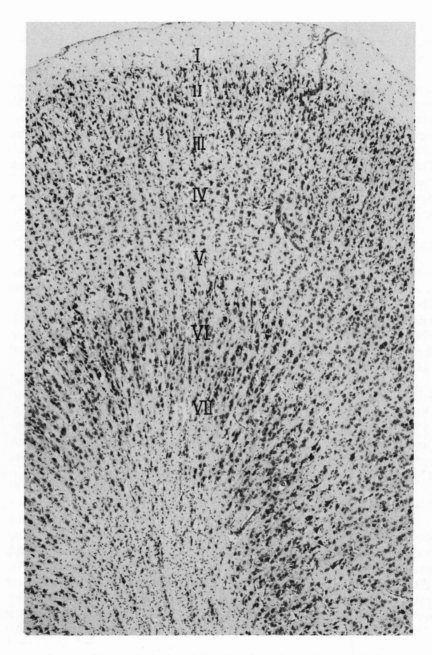

Fig. 25. Cytoarchitectonics of Area 17 of the dog. Nissl stain; 100×.

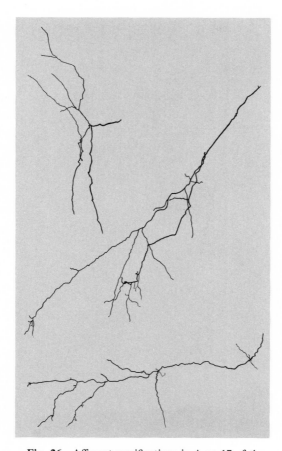

Fig. 26. Afferent ramifications in Area 17 of the dog. On the left: association afferent fiber with single collaterals; in the center: specific afferent fiber ascending obliquely and branching into a brush in layer IV; on the right: afferent fiber climbing vertically and giving off horizontal branches in layer IV.

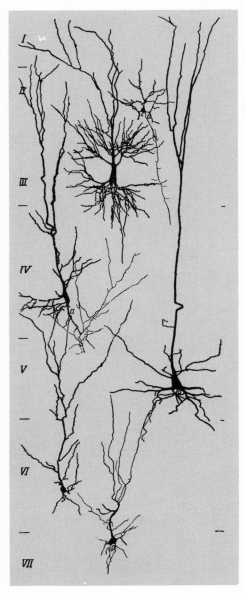

Fig. 27. Pyramidal cells of Area 17 of the dog. Differences in pyramidal cells of layers III and V; a, axon. The pyramidal cell of layer III is shown under high power in Fig. 91.

the outlines of the ramification are circular in shape. In these cases, besides the cell body and ascending dendrite, where the endings of numerous synapses are located, there are three well-defined dendritic synaptic zones. Ramifications of dendrites at the level of the lower third of the ascending dendrite were not found in such large numbers in the hedgehog and rabbit, and they were not so well marked in the cat. These branches found in the dog can be compared only with similar branches in the cortex of monkeys and man.

Many of the dendrites are intersected repeatedly in all directions by thin axon collaterals arising from other neurons. This pattern of surrounding and intersection of dendrites by innumerable fibers was most frequently observed in layer III, especially on large dendrites of the pyramidal cells.

The largest pyramidal cells and those with the most branches in layer III are located at the boundary between Areas 17 and 18 and they evidently correspond to the limes parastriatus gigantopyramidalis of Area 18 distinguished by von Economo and Koskinas (1925). The total number of branches of the dendrites of the pyramidal cells in the dog's cortex is very great (Shkol'nik-Yarros, 1950b). The views expressed by Kaplan (1952) on this question are surprising: it seems that the methods used did not reveal all branches of the dendrites. According to Sholl (1953), the number of dendritic branches of some neurons in the cat's visual cortex likewise exceeds 80.

Besides small pyramidal cells, medium-sized and larger cells also are found in layer IV, although they are smaller than the cells in layer III (Fig. 28, 7, 10, 14).

In layer V of the dog's cortex the large pyramidal cells are much closer in structure to the solitary pyramidal cells of Meynert as found in primates than the corresponding cells in the rabbit. The basal dendrites run in a horizontal direction and are of considerable thickness. These large cells are not grouped together as was observed in the rabbit (Fig. 28, 20; Fig. 29) and, consequently, they resemble the solitary pyramidal cells in their arrangement also.

Besides the ordinary pyramidal cells with dendrite ascending to layer I, small and medium-sized cells are also found in layer VI, giving a terminal ramification of bouquet type in layers IV and V. The pyramidal cells of the lower layers give off very long collaterals, running horizontally, which I regard as associative in character (Fig. 29). Pyramidal cells with an arcuate axon are present; their body is either triangular or circular and their axon makes a slight downward turn, then climbs upward without giving off collaterals downward into the white matter (Fig. 28). These neurons are appreciably fewer in number in the dog than in Area 17 of the primate. They can sometimes be seen in layers V and VII. Photomicrographs of the

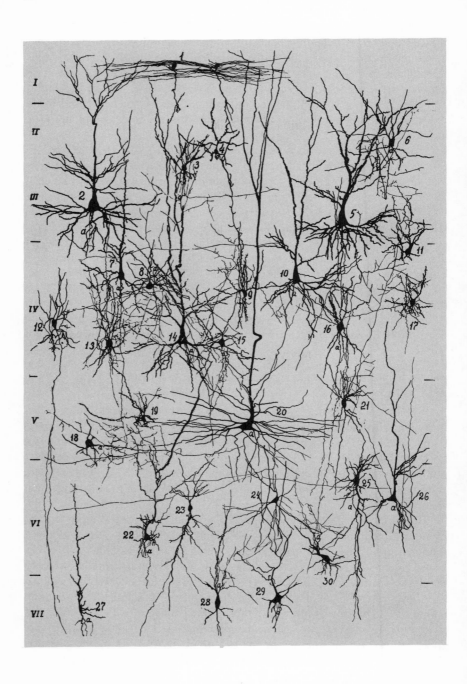

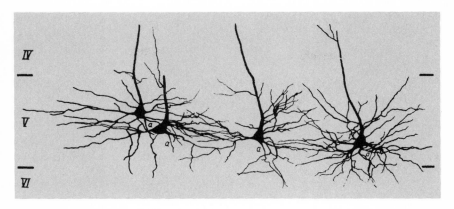

Fig. 29. Large pyramidal cells of layer V of Area 17 in the dog. Drawn from one section. a, axon.

pyramidal cells of the upper layers of the dog's cortex give a more accurate idea of the degree of ramification of the dendrites and their relative number (Fig. 30).

Fusiform cells (Fig. 31) are numerous in layers VI and VII, and are seen less frequently in layer V, where, on the other hand inverted pyramidal cells are frequently observed. Such a wide variety of fusiform neurons, and their presence in the upper layers as in the rabbit, cannot be seen in the dog. Martinotti's cells with ascending axon are observed in all layers of the visual cortex (Fig. 32). Sometimes the axons ascend as a single fiber, sometimes they give off numerous ascending and descending collaterals in contact with surrounding dendrites of the pyramidal cells. In typical cases the axon runs vertically upward, giving off numerous collaterals and ascending twigs along its course. Sometimes the ascending branch twists and turns repeatedly in a characteristic fashion and gives off numerous branches initially. Long spines are often seen on the dendrites of these cells.

Star cells with a long axon (Fig. 33), resembling Cajal's star type are found in the middle and lower part of layer IV. Their dendrites mainly

Fig. 28. Neurons of Area 17 of the dog. 1, Cajal–Retzius cell in layer I; 2, 5, large pyramidal cells of layer III; 3, 6, short-axon stellate cells of layers II and III; 4, small pyramidal cell of layer II; 8, 9, 11, 13, 15, 17, short-axon stellate cells of layer IV; 7, 10, 14, pyramidal cells of different calibers in layer IV; 12, 16, star cells with long axon in layer IV; 18, 19, 21, stellate short-axon cells in layer V; 20, large pyramidal cell of layer V (resembling the solitary pyramidal cells of Meynert); 22, small pyramidal cell of layer VI; 23, 25, inverted pyramidal cells of layer VI; 24, cell with widely branching horizontal axon in layer VI; 26, pyramidal cell with arcuate axon in layer VI; 27, fusiform cell of layer VII; 28, 30, cells with ascending axons in layers VI and VII; 29, pyramidal cell of layer VII with short dendrite; a, axon. (Shkol'nik-Yarros, 1959b.)

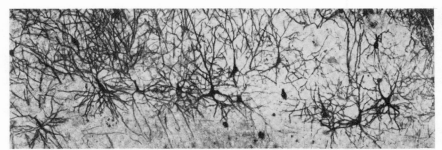

Fig. 30. Upper layers of Area 17 of the dog. A dendritic plexus in layers I–III can be seen. Photomicrograph; 100×.

emerge radially from the body, and no semilunar forms could be clearly distinguished. The body of the star cells is polygonal in shape, depending on the character of emergence of the dendrites. The axon descending into the white matter often bifurcates into branches of almost equal thickness (Fig. 33). This unique and as yet unexplained phenomenon was not observed in the visual cortex of other mammals or of man.

The dog's visual cortex is very rich in short-axon stellate cells. They can be seen in all layers. In layers II and III they are very polymorphic (Fig. 34). Cell forms are observed which are very similar to the types described in the visual cortex of rodents and man. In this case the axon at first runs downward, then bends in an arch and gives off branches running upward. The axons of other short-axon cells run upward or horizontally. The bodies of these cells are oval or angular in shape. The dendrites give off numerous branches and are frequently covered with spines (Figs. 34 and 35).

In layer IV (Figs. 34, 35), where these neurons are particularly numerous, they are clearly distinguishable into two different types. Some cells are circular or oval with a limited range of axonal branches, and the axons ramify close to the cell body. Other cells have axons which ramify widely (the distance between extreme branches of the axon may reach 1.4 mm) and they are of fairly large caliber. Such axons may spread horizontally, downward, upward, or in an arcuate manner. Their large caliber is clearly seen by comparison with the thin ramifications of axons belonging to cells of the upper layers in the rabbit cortex.

Dendrites of the stellate short-axon cells sometimes possess a few spines, but at other times, by contrast, their spines are relatively numerous (Figs. 34, 35). In this respect the stellate cells in the dog resemble some varieties of stellate neurons in the rabbit. Spines were also observed on the body of the short-axon cells, more especially in layers III and IV (Fig. 35, A). In layer V the small size of the stellate cells (Fig. 35, B), with axons of various forms, is a noticeable feature. In addition to small cells, there are

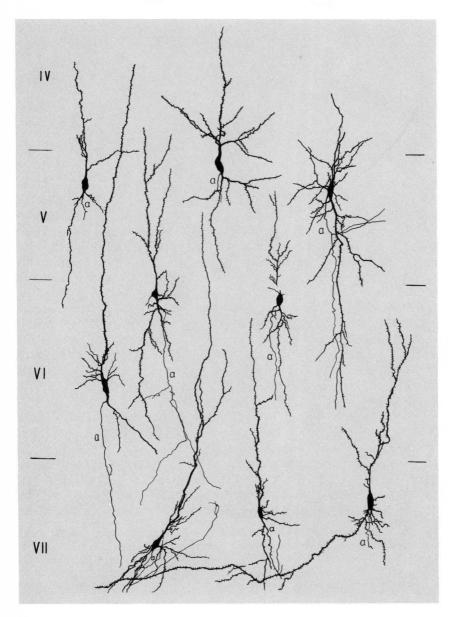

Fig. 31. Fusiform cells of the lower layers of Area 17 in the dog. Some cells have short and medium-sized dendrites; a, axon.

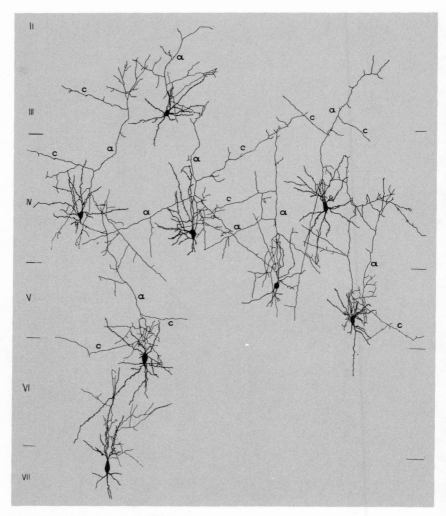

Fig. 32. Cells with ascending axons in Area 17 of the dog. a, axon; c, axon collateral. Cell bodies are located in all layers. Most axons have a wide range of distribution.

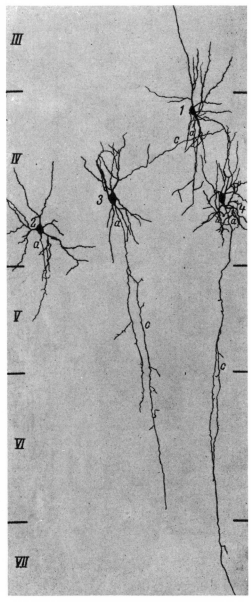

Fig. 33. Star cells with a long descending axon (star cells of Cajal) in layer IV of Area 17 of the dog. 3, 4, cells with bifurcating axon; a, axon; c, collateral.

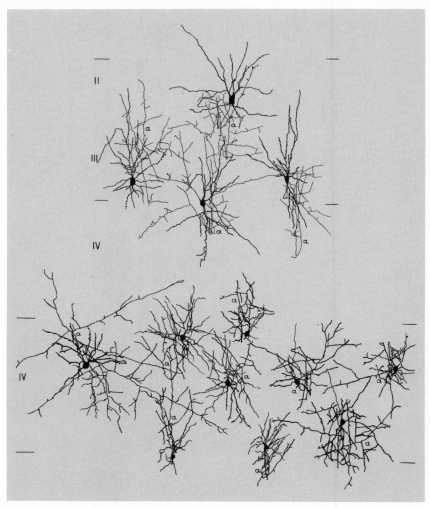

Fig. 34. Stellate short-axon cells of layers II, III, and IV of Area 17 of the dog. A cell with an extensive axonal system is seen below on the left in layer IV, other cells have narrowly branching axons.

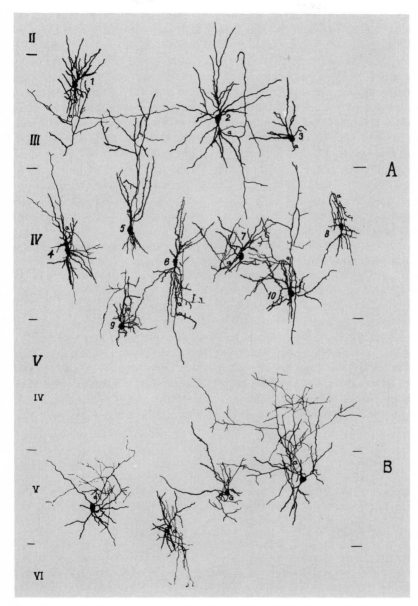

Fig. 35. A: Stellate short-axon cells of layers III and IV of Area 17 of the dog (1–10). Axons running in different directions can be seen. 6, 7, 8, 10, dendrites of these cells are covered with spines. Spines can also be seen on the cell bodies. B: Stellate short-axon cells of layer V (1–4).

others which are very large, with widely ramifying axonal systems. In layer V more frequently than in other layers, cells were observed with their axon running horizontally. Such a short-axon stellate cell in layer V, forming what amounts to nests for neighboring cells, can be seen in Fig. 36. The curious pattern of interweaving branches repeats the pattern of the bodies of neighboring neurons, with which terminal boutons are in contact along the course and at the ends of branches of the axon collaterals. Sometimes an extensive axon gives rise to a dense system of branches around a cell and at the same time sends collaterals with ramifications into more distant parts of the cortex (Fig. 37). The stellate short-axon cells of layer V have bodies of many different shapes—oval, circular, triangular, and polygonal. Stellate cells in layer VI also differ in the shape of their body and the direction of their axon. Most commonly the axon runs obliquely or directly upward, or it may have large horizontal branches which can be traced for a considerable distance (Fig. 28, 24).

Drawings and studies of successfully impregnated axons confirmed that widely ramifying axons, forming large pericellular nests for neighboring neurons (Fig. 37), and spreading over a wide area of the cortex in both horizontal and vertical directions, are very characteristic of the dog's cortex. In addition to these widely branching axons, others with narrower branches are present, but they never attain the same degree of concentration as axons of the stellate short-axon cells of sublayer IVc of the monkey's cortex.

In the lower layers of the cortex, the direction of the axons is mainly upward and horizontally, with the formation of nests in the horizontal plane. Area 17 is surrounded by Area 18, characterized by a less highly developed afferent plexus in layer IV. The next important and typical feature of this area is the large number of fusiform and triangular cells in its lower layers.

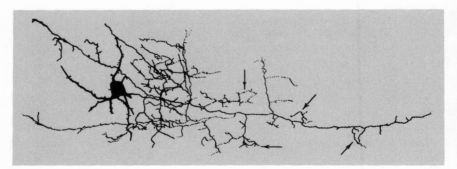

Fig. 36. Stellate short-axon cell of layer V in Area 17 of the dog. The axon forms what is virtually a nest for the bodies of neighboring cells. Numerous bouton endings of the axon can be seen. Drawing made from magnification of 600× with subsequent reduction. Arrows point to examples of "nests." (Shkol'nik-Yarros, 1963.)

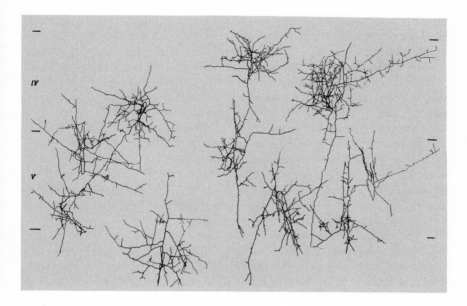

Fig. 37. Axonal systems of stellate short-axon cells of the upper layers of Area 17 of the dog. (Shkol'nik-Yarros, 1959b.)

Visual System of Monkeys (Primates)

Vision plays an important role in the life of monkeys, much more important than in the case of insectivores, rodents, or even carnivores. The well-developed vision, touch, and motor activity lie at the basis of that extraordinary development of the orienting, investigative reflex about which Pavlov wrote. His studies were carried out on the anthropoid apes. Many workers have described the importance of vision in the life of monkeys as well. Voitonis (1949) studied the effect of the increasing complexity of interaction with the external environment, with the development of improved organs of locomotion and sense organs (stereoscopic vision, and so on) on behavior of monkeys. He found that monkeys are attracted to objects by novelty, or changes in color, shape, and size. Their investigative reflex stems from direct subordination of their food-getting reflex and is connected with visual acuity and increasing perfection of the hand. Voitonis considers that interest in an object is one of the biological foundations of intellect formation.

A high level of activity of the visual receptor in monkeys is also reported by Tikh (1947). At the end of the first month of life, monkeys can distinguish between people from their external appearance. At the age of 6–9 months they recognize familiar people even after a separation of 2 months. This extremely interesting observation made by Tikh can only be explained by the ability of monkeys to retain traces of previous perceptions. Vatsuro (1948) demonstrated experimentally the ability of monkeys to retain traces of visual excitation. Roginskii (1947, 1948) concludes from his observations that monkeys may have visual illusions which are central in character. Color vision in monkeys was studied by Markova (1961).

Thus the highly developed vision of monkeys (stereoscopic and color vision) serves not only for direct perception of objects, but also for the formation of more permanent connections. Visual functions develop simultaneously with the development of movements, thereby ensuring a high level of perfection in the coordination between movements and vision during grasping of objects, or jumping, requiring precise coordination of vision with the timing and strength of muscular contraction.

The optical axes in monkeys are parallel, ensuring accuracy of binocular vision, and perception of depth and volume of objects. The ability to repeat movements of the hands with movements of the eyes appears only in monkeys (Sechenov, 1901). Decussation of the optic nerves in monkeys is partial. The fundus of the eye possesses a macula lutea. The retina in primates is a highly complex and differentiated organ. It is sharply divided into neurons of different types, not only ganglionic but also bipolar cells. The ganglion cells of the peripheral retina send their dendritic branches over a very extensive area and thus receive excitation from hundreds of bipolar cells and thousands of rods (Dogel', 1892; Polyak, 1941). The other extreme variety is the midget ganglion cells typical of the macula lutea (Polyak, 1941, 1957). They form contacts with only one bipolar cell, also a midget cell, and then with a single cone. However, this system can have collateral connections with other types of cells.

The number of fibers of the optic tract terminating in the superior colliculus is reduced. The relative volume of the superior colliculi is also reduced, although the neuronal structure of this formation points to the complexity and differentiation of its function (for a more detailed account of these neurons in different mammals, see Viktorov, 1965, 1968).

The lateral geniculate body of most primates leading a diurnal mode of life is highly differentiated and consists of sharply defined layers. The most typical form for diurnal monkeys is division of the nucleus into six layers, of which two are magnocellular and four parvocellular (Fig. 38). Cytoarchitectonically, the highest cell density is found in the parvocellular layers, and the individual cell layers are separated by clearly defined myelin interlayers (pale in specimens with Nissl stain), separating the cell layers from each other. The shape and size of the cells in the first two layers are very variable, but they are predominantly medium-sized and large, and small neurons are rare. In the upper four layers the commonest cells are small and round, or oval, but sometimes medium-sized or larger cells may be found.

Study of the neurons of the lateral geniculate body of monkeys shows the presence of complex differentiation. One type of neuron in layers 1–2 is a cell with long axon and medium-sized or large dendrites arranged radially or in the form of a shrub (the length of the dendrites may reach 725 μ). The dendrites give off branches of medium length, and the neuron as a whole is similar to the radial and shrublike neurons in the lateral geniculate body of the dog or in other structures of the thalamus. These neurons typical of thalamic nuclei are very numerous in the lower two layers and less numerous in the upper layers. The other extreme type consists of circular or oval or often fusiform neurons with very few and very short dendrites, giving off few branches (Fig. 39), traceable for up to 150–200 μ from the cell body. These neurons I have called midget cells. The name "midget" applies not only to

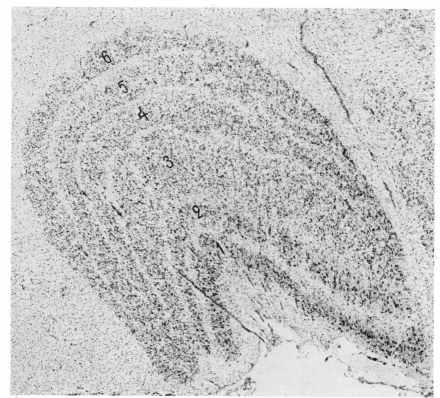

Fig. 38. Cytoarchitectonics of the lateral geniculate body of a monkey (*Macaca mulatta*). 1, 2, magnocellular layers; 3, 4, 5, 6, parvocellular layers. Nissl stain; 30×.

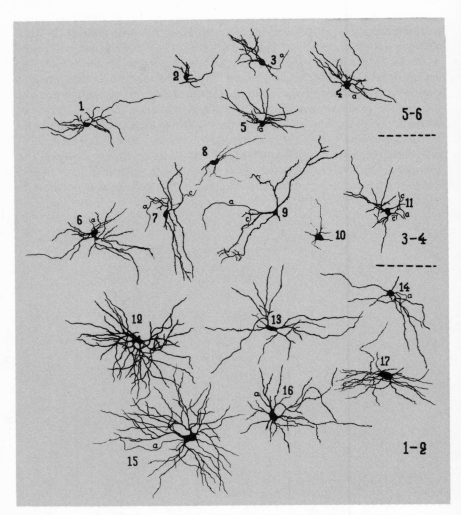

Fig. 39. Neurons of the lateral geniculate body of a macaque (*Macaca mulatta*). Layers are denoted by the large arabic numbers on the right. 1, 2, 3, 4, 5, midget neurons in layers 5–6; 8, 10, midget neurons in layers 3–4; 6, radial neuron of layer 3; 7, 11, short-axon neurons of layers 3 and 4; 9, neuron with few branches; 12–17, radial and shrub-like long-axon neurons of medium and large size in layers 1 and 2, with densely ramified and extensive dendritic systems.

the size of the cell body, which may sometimes be medium-sized, but more especially to the neuron as a whole, which with all its dendritic branches occupies a very small area, and it is this feature which distinguishes it sharply from all other neurons of the brain stem and thalamus. It is thus the area of its contact with the surrounding cells which is qualified by the word "midget." Midget cells are mainly located in layers 3, 4, 5, and 6, where a dense accumulation of them is present (Fig. 39, 1, 2, 3, 5, 8, 10). However, medium-sized radial and shrublike neurons are also found in these layers. In layers 3–4 I also found cells with dendrites characteristic of the neurons with few branches (Fig. 39, 7, 9) and short-axon neurons (Fig. 39, 11). Axons of neurons of the two last types give off collaterals along their course or form a bifurcation. Some afferents reaching the lateral geniculate body of *Macaca mulatta* terminate in a brush and are equipped with 25 or more synaptic

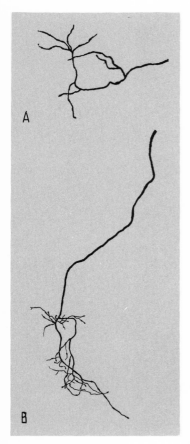

Fig. 40. Afferent fibers in the lateral geniculate body of the monkey. A: Fragment of afferent fiber demonstrating division into only five endings. B: More completely impregnated ramification with numerous endings.

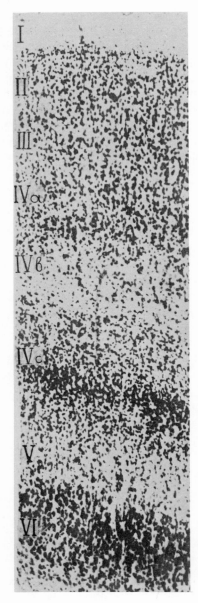

Fig. 41. Cytoarchitectonics of Area 17 of a macaque. Nissl stain; 100×.

endings (Fig. 40). The individual twigs of one of these complex afferents may resemble the pattern described by Glees and Le Gros Clark (1941); such endings cannot be the complete afferent fiber but only a small part of it. On the basis of a study of the structure of axonal ramifications passing into the lateral geniculate body of primates, I cannot therefore agree with the scheme for the transmission of visual impulses put forward by Glees and Le Gros Clark.

The cytoarchitectonics of Area 17 of the monkey is well known and has often been described. A conspicuous feature in the macaque is the small and densely packed arrangement of the cells in this area, together with the sharply contrasting bands of translucency in sublayer IVb (the stria of

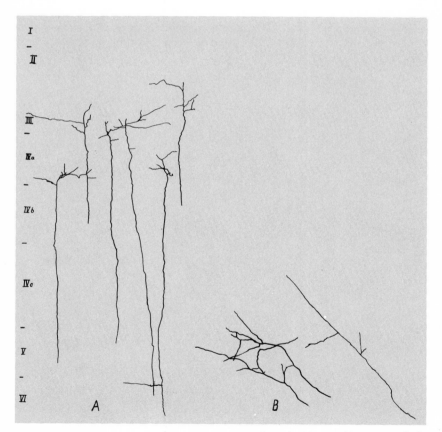

Fig. 42. Afferent branches in Area 17 of the monkey. A: Nonspecific or association afferents ramifying in layers III, IVa, and IVb. B: Afferent fibers ascending obliquely and giving off collaterals in layers V and VI (no plexus is shown in sublayer IVb).

Gennari or Vicq d'Azyr) and in layer V (Fig. 41). The density of the cells throughout this area and the width and density of sublayer IVc are greater than in man.

Afferent fibers entering Area 17 from other parts of the brain form powerful plexuses there. Most of these are oblique, thick afferent fibers, crossing the cortex obliquely from below upward, giving off collaterals to layers V and VI along their path to layer IV (Fig. 42). The terminal plexus formed by the endings of these fibers in layer IV could not be detected in my specimens. However, they are well known from the work of Cajal.

The second variety of afferent is a fiber rising vertically upward from the horizontal branches in sublayer IVc.

The third variety consists of fibers very similar to the last but climbing higher, into layer III and the sublayers of layer IV (IVa, IVb). Finally, brush endings from a large vertical afferent fiber, ramifying mainly in sublayer IVc, were found also in Area 17 of the cortex of the green monkey (*Cercopithecus sabaeus*) (Fig. 43).

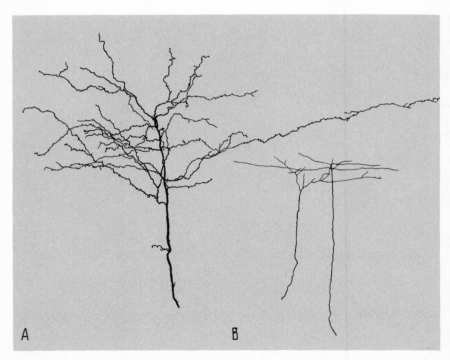

A   B

Fig. 43. A: Afferent fiber ramifying in sublayers IVb and IVc of layer IV in Area 17 of a monkey. B: Afferent fibers of sublayer IVc.

This type of afferent ramification, forming synaptic contacts with hundreds of surrounding small neurons in sublayer IVc, is apparently one of the principal elements in the system of transmission of visual excitation and its transformation into a visual image.

Layer I. This contains (Fig. 46, 1) small cells very similar in shape to those described by Cajal in this layer in man. The cell is small in size, round, and with a horizontal axon.

Layer II. Small, branching pyramidal cells with a well-developed system of axon collaterals, terminating not only in layer II, but also in layer I. Stellate cells of small size with an axon running both downward and upward, and to the side (Fig. 46, 3).

Layer III. Not clearly demarcated from layer II. Larger pyramidal cells. Here and there a well-marked bouquet can be seen in the ascending part of the apical dendrite, but not reaching the degree of development and extent observed in the dog. Among the pyramidal cells, the presence of elements with an arcuate axon must be emphasized.

Pyramids with an arcuate axon in the upper layers of the cerebral cortex are interesting for the reason that they may point to specialization of pyramidal cells for enabling excitation to follow a cyclic course in the upper layers also. Stellate cells of shrub type are also found (Fig. 46, 11, 12).

Very small pyramidal cells with a round body, and other larger and more regular pyramidal cells are observed in sublayer IVa. Sometimes arcuate axons are visible (Fig. 46, 18). Short-axon cells of varied character, some small and round, others larger and similar to the cells of layer III, and bearing only a slight resemblance to cells in sublayer IVc, are present.

In the upper part of sublayer IVb, large star cells of Cajal with a descending axon are found (Fig. 46, 21, 23, 27). The form of ramification of their dendrites often resembles the wings of a flying bird (Fig. 46, 23). These cells are sometimes found singly, sometimes in pairs (Fig. 47). They can sometimes be found also in the middle part of this sublayer. Pyramidal cells of the ordinary shape, and small stellate cells with ascending collaterals are also present; sometimes the descending branches change completely into ascending and horizontal branches (Fig. 46, 22, 26). In its lower part, sublayer IVb is filled with small short-axon cells, divided into the same type as the large stars, i.e., into stellate and semilunar. Their recurrent collaterals are powerfully developed and can be seen not only in layer IV, but also in layer III and also, perhaps, as far as layer I (Fig. 46, 22, 30). Small long-axon cells are also present, reduced copies of the true large star cells of Cajal. The results of a study of the neuronal structure fully confirm division of layer IV into IVbα and IVbβ suggested by O. and C. Vogt (1919) and Filimonov (1933) on the basis of cytoarchitectonics.

In some cases the main branch of the axon of the small stellate cells of

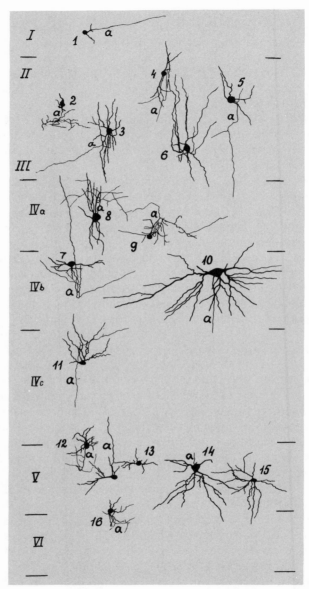

Fig. 44. Varieties of stellate cells in Area 17 of a monkey (the great contrast between the sizes of the cell bodies can be seen). 1, Cajal–Retzius cell in layer I; 10, Cajal's star cell with a long, descending axon; remaining cells with short axons.

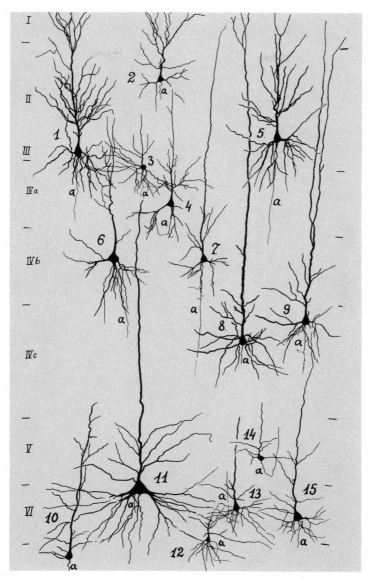

Fig. 45. Varieties of pyramidal cells in the cortex of Area 17 of a monkey. The contrast between the sizes of the cell bodies can be seen. a, axon; 2, small pyramidal cell in layer II; 1, 5, medium-sized pyramidal cells in layer III; 3, small pyramidal cell in layer IVa; 4, pyramidal cell with arcuate axon in layer IVa; 6, 7, pyramidal cells of different sizes in layer IVb; 8, 9, pyramidal cells in layer IVc; 11, solitary pyramidal cell of Meynert (apical dendrite not drawn) at border between layers V and VI; 10, 12, 15, small pyramidal cells in layers VI and VII; 13, 14, pyramidal cells with arcuate axon in layers V and VI. (Shkol'nik-Yarros, 1955b.)

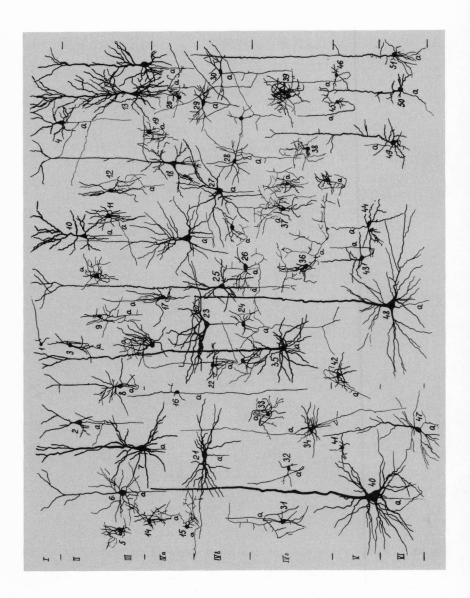

Fig. 46. Neurons in Area 17 of the green monkey (*Cercopithecus sabaeus*). a, axon; 1, cell with horizontal axon in layer I; 2, 4, 10, pyramidal cells of layer II; 3, 5, 9, stellate short-axon cells of layers II and III; 11, 12, stellate short-axon cells with shrublike ramification of dendrites in layer III; 6, 7, 13, pyramidal cells of layer III; 8, pyramidal cell with arcuate axon in layer III; 14, 15, 17, 19, 20, stellate short-axon cells of sublayer IVa; 16, granular pyramidal cell of sublayer IVa; 18, pyramidal cell with arcuate axon in sublayer IVa; 25, pyramidal cell of sublayer IVb; 21, 23, 27, large star cells of Cajal in sublayer IVb; 31, 32, 33, 34, 36, 37, 38, 39, varieties of short-axon stellate cells in sublayer IVc; 35, pyramidal cell of sublayer IVc; 40, 48, solitary pyramidal cells of Meynert (apical dendrites not drawn); 41, 42, 44, stellate cells of layer V; 43, 45, 46, cells with arcuate ascending axon; 49, pyramidal cell with ascending axon of layer VI with medium-sized apical dendrite; 50, pyramidal cell with long axon in layer VI with short apical dendrite; 47, 51, pyramidal cell in layers VI and VII. (Shkol'nik-Yarros, 1955a.)

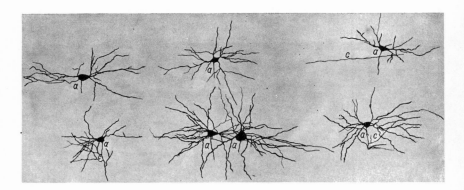

Fig. 47. Star cells of Cajal in layer IVb of Area 17 of the green monkey. Some axons give off collaterals. a, axon; c, axon collateral. (Shkol'nik-Yarros, 1955a.)

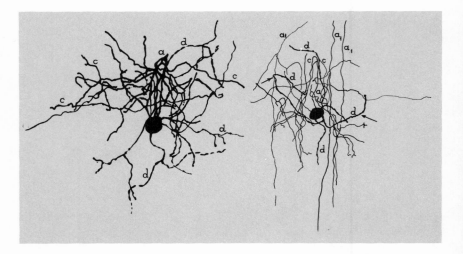

Fig. 48. Short-axon stellate cells in sublayer IVc of Area 17 of the green monkey. a, axon; d, dendrite, arrow indicates helical dendrites. On the left: cell with complex ramification of its axon, concentrated around the cell body in the region of branching of its dendrites. Dendrites shown by broken lines. (Shkol'nik-Yarros, 1955a.)

sublayer IVb descends into the white matter, thus acting as a connection over longer distances, while in other cases the axon has only a local distribution. The considerable difference in size of the cell bodies, and in the extent of development of the axon and, consequently, in the velocity of conduction of excitation suggest that the various stellate neurons of layer IV differ in their role in the act of vision.

Sometimes the axon from a star cell breaks up into two distinct branches, entering the white matter. This bifurcation of the axons of the star cells of Cajal is also found in the visual cortex of the dog.

Sublayer IVc is richly supplied with small stellate cells of a distinctive pattern; the axon first climbs upward, then gives off branches descending

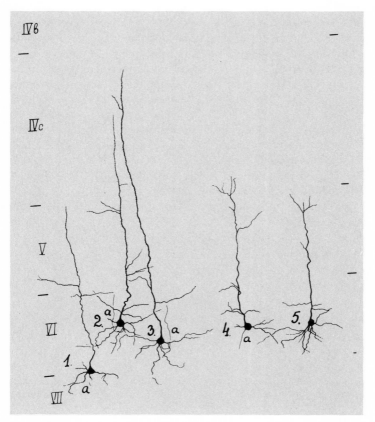

Fig. 48a. Small pyramidal cells of layer VI in Area 17 of the monkey. 1, 4, 5, pyramidal cells with a short apical dendrite; 2, 3, pyramidal cells with an ascending arcuate axon.

sideways, similar to the branches of a weeping willow. The dendrites of these cells usually have varicosities along their course and they twist spirally around the cells (Figs. 46 and 48).

Under high power it can be seen that the axon also carries boutonlike thickenings at its end, and these are also present occasionally along the branches (Fig. 48). Stellate cells of a different type have extensive vertical connections as far as layers III and IV or horizontal systems with numerous terminal ramifications (Fig. 46, 36). The stellate cells of sublayer IVc form circular groups, evidently joined by afferent fibers. Some idea of the complexity of the plexus around the neurons in sublayer IVc can be obtained from Fig. 48. Branches from different axonal systems, interweaving and forming pericellular plexuses (seen below in Fig. 48) are present around the cells. Dendrites winding spirally around the cell can be seen, and only a few of the fibers surrounding it are shown. The conditions created in sublayer IVc provide for very close interconnection between the cells with short axons. Division of sublayer IVc into three parts, revealed by cytoarchitectonic investigation, is also confirmed in the neuronal structure.

Layer V in its upper part is richly supplied with small pyramidal cells with an arcuate axon, forming what is essentially an independent sublayer (part of IVc). Besides their small size, these cells are characterized by the small number of their dendrites and the thinness of their ascending trunk, usually terminating in layer IV (Fig. 46, 43, 45, 46, 49). Cells of Martinotti with an ascending axon and small stellate cells with axons running in different directions (Fig. 44) are present. In the lower part of this layer giant solitary pyramids of Meynert may be found, and sometimes these are present in the upper part of layer VI. Their appearance is typical, and in the arrangement

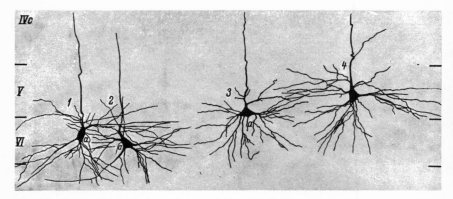

Fig. 49. Large cells in the lower layers of Area 17 of the green monkey. 1, 2, giant triangular and fusiform cells in layer VI; 3, 4, giant pyramidal cells of Meynert in layer V. (Shkol'nik-Yarros, 1955a.)

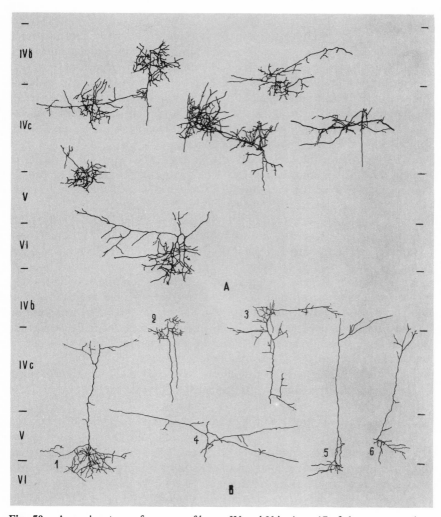

Fig. 50. Axonal systems of neurons of layers IV and V in Area 17 of the green monkey. A: Complex ramification of axons forming pericellular plexuses within the layer. B: 1, 5, 6, terminal ramification of axon in layer VI, origin of axon in sublayers IVb and IVc; 2, 3, 4, different types of ramification of axons in layers IV and V.

of their dendrites they show a much closer resemblance to the corresponding cells in the human cortex than in that of the carnivores (dog) (Fig. 46, 40, 48).

Layer VI is rich in pyramidal cells with an arcuate axon, and in simple pyramidal cells with an ordinary axon running into the white matter. The apical bouquet of these cells lies sometimes in IVb, sometimes in IVc, sometimes in layer V (Figs. 46, 48a). Layer VI is thus connected with excitation (visual) flowing in layers IV and V through the apical dendrites of the pyramidal cells. In the upper part of this layer cells are present with the appearance of giant spindles or giant triangular cells (Fig. 49). I also found similar cells in Area 17 of the human cortex.

Comparison of the stellate neurons in the various layers (Fig. 44) gives a clear idea of their contrasting sizes. The minute size of the stellate cells in layers I, II, and V and in the sublayers of layer IV is clearly visible by comparison with the giant star in sublayer IVb.

The very small pyramidal cells of sublayer IVa and IVb show the same degree of contrast with the solitary pyramidal cells of layer V. The largest pyramidal cells are located in the lower layers (Fig. 45). No such sharp differences in size could be found in the dog's cortex, where neurons as small as these were not present. I regard this as a sign of increasing specialization, where some neurons are adapted to the extremely rapid transmission of excitation into the subcortex (solitary pyramids of Meynert, star cells of Cajal), while others are adapted to ensuring the most perfect reflection of the external environment (the densely packed parvocellular layer IVc, where it appears that the visual image is mainly obtained).

The description given above reflects accurately the qualitative features of the cell varieties existing in the specimen but by no means does it do so exhaustively.

Axonal systems impregnated in isolation from the bodies of their neurons (Fig. 50) give a detailed idea of the types of connections in some layers. For example, an axon from layer IVa (the cell body was not impregnated) gives a dense ramification in layer VI. The large number of pyramidal cells with an arcuate axon located in these same layers may enable visual excitation to pass both from above downward, from layer IV into layer VI, and in the opposite direction, along axons of the arcuate pyramids, from below upward.

Sometimes the axonal system (Fig. 50) from one cell only may be highly complex and may form pericellular plexuses without the participation of other neurons.

Area 18 in monkeys differs essentially in its cytoarchitectonic features from Area 17 in that layer IV has no sublayers, there is no stria of Gennari and the cell density is lower in layers IV and VI (Fig. 51). Structural differences can be seen more clearly still when the neurons are studied. The

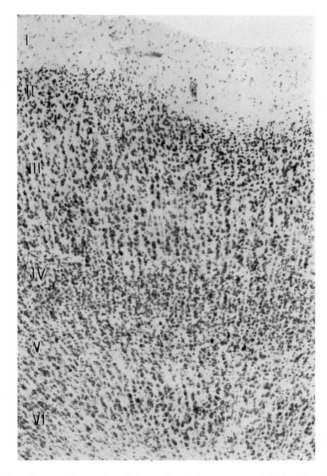

Fig. 51. Cytoarchitectonics of Area 18 of the macaque. Nissl stain; 100×.

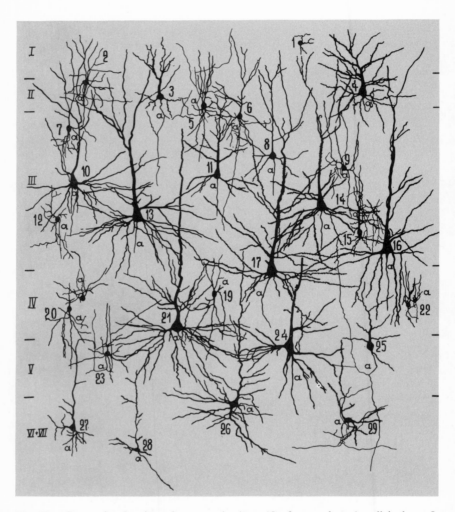

Fig. 52. Composite drawing of neurons in Area 18 of a monkey. 1, cell in layer I; 2, 5, stellate short-axon cells in layer II; 3, pyramidal cell in layer II; 4, pyramidal cell with arcuate axon in layer II; 6, 8, 10, 11, 13, 14, 16, pyramidal cells of various sizes in layer III; 7, 9, 12, 15, stellate short-axon cells in layer III; 18, 19, 20, 22, stellate short-axon cells of layer IV; 17, 21, pyramidal cells of layer IV; 23, pyramidal cell with arcuate axon in layer V; 24, triangular cell in layer V; 25, pyramidal cell in layer V; 26, 29, fusiform cells in layer VI; 27, 28, pyramidal cells with a short apical dendrite in layer III; a, axon.

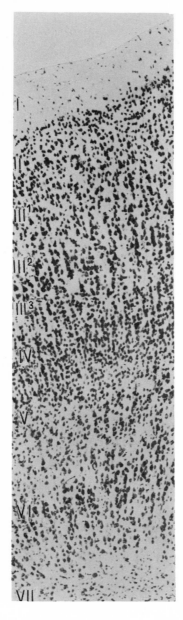

Fig. 53. Cytoarchitectonics of Area 19 of the macaque. Nissl stain; 100×.

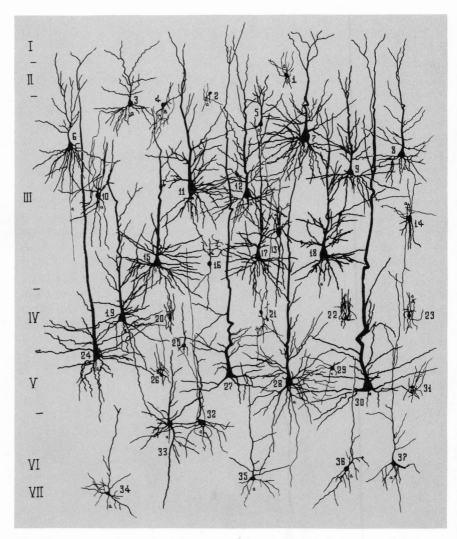

Fig. 54. Neurons of Area 19 of the green monkey. 1, 2, small short-axon cells in layer II; 3, 5, small pyramidal cells of sublayer III^1; 4, short-axon cell of sublayer III^1; 6, 8, 9, 12, medium-sized pyramidal cells of sublayers III^1 and III^2; 7, 11, large pyramidal cells of sublayers III^1 and III^2; 10, 13, bushlike cells of layer III; 15, 17, 18, pyramidal cells of sublayer III^3; 14, 16, short-axon cells of sublayer III^3; 19, medium-sized pyramidal cell of layer IV; 25, pyramidal cell of layer IV, small granular type; 20, 21, 22, 23, small stellate short-axon cells of layer IV; 24, 27, 28, 30, pyramidal cells of layer V; 26, 29, 31, stellate short-axon cells of layer V; 33, 34, 36, fusiform cells of layers VI and VII; 32, 35, 37, pyramidal cells of layers VI and VII.

most characteristic features are an increase in the degree of pyramidization of the cortex and the intensive branching of the dendrites (Fig. 52). Specialized forms of neurons—star cells of Cajal and solitary pyramids of Meynert —are absent. Cells with an arcuate axon were found in layers II and V (Fig. 52, 4, 23), but they do not form groups as in Area 17, and are appreciably fewer in number.

Many of the pyramidal cells in layer III are characterized by descending basal dendrites (Fig. 52, 13, 17). Triangular cells and fusiform cells are present not only in layers VI and VII, but also in layer V. In Area 18 of the human cortex, triangular cells of this type were even found in layer IV.

In Area 19 the radial structure is intensified and the width of the cortex as a whole and, in particular, of layer III is increased (Fig. 53). The cell density of the cortex is lower than in Area 18. The abundant ramifications of the neurons and an increase in the number of axons leaving the cortex grouped into bundles explain these cytoarchitectonic features. Regular rows of pyramidal cells giving off vertical trunks upward and axons downward (Fig. 54) fill layers III, IV, and V. The lower cell density of the cortex is due to the abundance of branches; the radial structure depends on an increase in the number of fibers entering and leaving the cortex grouped into bundles, of which the main components are axons of the pyramidal cells (as was shown by an investigation of material from the human cortex). Stellate short-axon cells are numerous and they are extremely varied both in Area 18 and in Area 19. In Area 17, however, they are more numerous, and more compactly arranged, especially in sublayer IV. Neither in Area 18 nor in Area 19 was there any resemblance to sublayer IVb of Area 17.

Visual System of Man

In man the central visual system is immeasurably more complex than in animals, including the other primates. This complexity reflects a new qualitative characteristic of the human brain alone, a quality connected with work and the appearance of what Pavlov has called the second signal system. Highly complex functions such as writing, reading, drawing, work of various types, arithmetical operations, playing musical instruments, and so on are inseparable from vision. Human vision is also inseparably connected with the functions of generalization and abstraction, with the intelligent perception of surrounding objects. The morphological characteristics of the structure of the visual system must evidently reflect functional complexity and, in conjunction with the specialized properties of other structures, they must provide the basis for performance of these highly complex acts. Comparison of structure in mammals and man readily reveals the morphological basis of the higher functions peculiar to man.

The human retina is morphologically very similar to the retina in monkeys (Kolmer, 1936; Polyak, 1941, 1957). The rods and cones are clearly differentiated structurally, and a well-marked fovea centralis and macula lutea are present. Some have even described a more highly developed retina in the monkey. According to Kolmer, for instance, the elements in the fovea centralis of certain monkeys are more densely arranged and are thinner than in man. This fact suggests their higher resolving power. The number of fibers of the optic nerve, according to Bruesch and Arey (1942) is 1,208,000 in monkeys and between 565,000 and 1,140,000 in man.

The human lateral geniculate body has the most distinct stratified structure in the whole of the central nervous system. The stratification appears by the sixth month of intrauterine life (Preobrazhenskaya, 1955). In the course of ontogenesis, stages of phylogenesis are reproduced during which the stratification is not present, as is the case, for example, in the insectivores. There is considerable variation in the outlines of the nucleus as a whole and the boundaries between its layers in different individuals (Polyak, 1957). A precise parallel can be seen between development of the visual cortex and development of the lateral geniculate body (Preobrazhenskaya, 1955).

The extent to which the first and second magnocellular layers differ from the parvocellular layers can be seen from the photograph (Fig. 55). In the two magnocellular layers, large, medium-sized, and, occasionally, small neurons of various shapes can be observed. In the upper four layers neurons are mainly small, frequently round and oval in shape; but triangular and polygonal bodies of cells of medium size or larger can also be seen.

Afferent fibers entering the human lateral geniculate body vary considerably in type. At least some of their forms can be distinguished, differing in their course, arrangement, and terminal ramification (Figs. 56, 57, 58). They also differ considerably in caliber. Most commonly a large fiber is seen to terminate in a typical, narrow brush (Fig. 57), with boutons on the ends of its branches. Next, most common are endings of more peculiar shape, giving off several terminal twigs at right angles to the main branch. The total number of boutons and of solitary and other endings and of boutons along its course may reach 20 or more for a single afferent fiber (Fig. 57, B). The most interesting fact from the point of view of the histology and physiology of the lateral geniculate body is the repeated dichotomous division of large afferent fibers as they ascend from the optic tract to the layers of the nucleus (Fig. 58). This repeated division of an afferent fiber from the retina indicates a connection between different parts of the same layer or simultaneous reception of excitation by different layers. Unfortunately I could not trace any of these dichotomously dividing fibers as far as their terminal twigs in order to ascertain to which layers they were proceeding. Besides afferent fibers forming obvious brushes, there are also long, thin

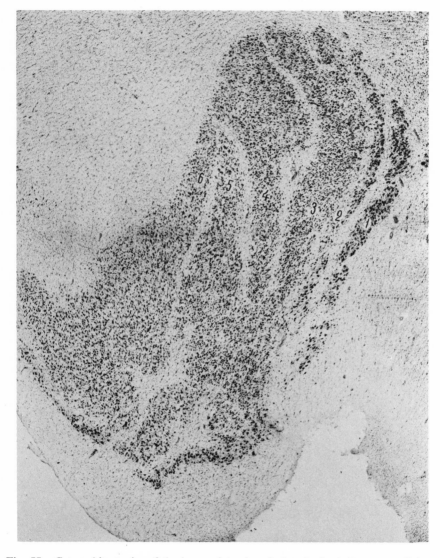

Fig. 55. Cytoarchitectonics of the human lateral geniculate body. 1, 2, magnocellular layers; 3, 4, 5, 6, parvocellular layers. Nissl stain; 40×.

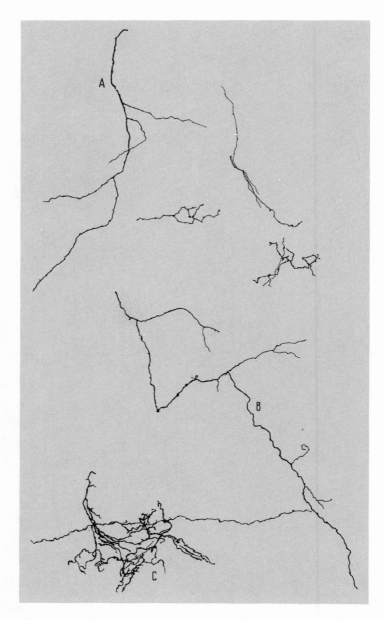

Fig. 56. Various forms of ramification of afferent fibers in the human lateral geniculate body. A, B: Axons possibly descending from the cortex. C: Brush ending from the retina.

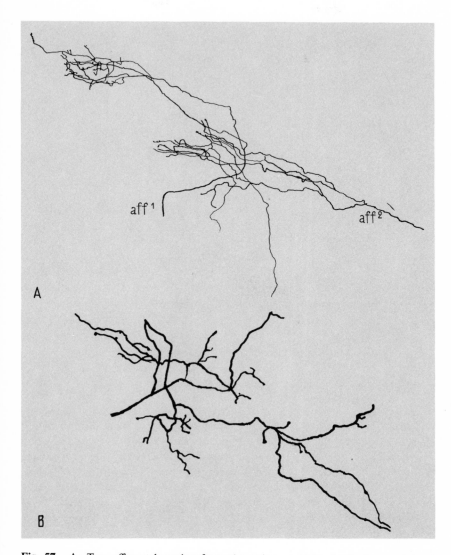

Fig. 57. A: Two afferent branches from the retina ramifying in the human lateral geniculate body as typical brushes. B: Ramification of an afferent axon typical of the human lateral geniculate body. Number of synapses (terminal boutons, boutons of passage) about 30; aff[1] and aff[2] represent afferents.

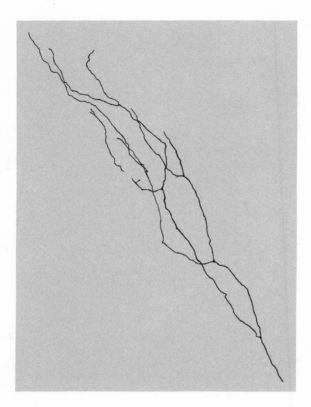

Fig. 58. Afferent axon of the human lateral geniculate
body dividing dichotomously.

axons not forming brushes. Such afferent fibers may cross several layers. It
can be postulated that they are fibers descending from the cortex (Fig. 56).

Neurons of the human lateral geniculate body vary considerably. In the
lower or first magnocellular layer, according to my observations, most cells
have a very distinctive appearance, best described by the term "fan-shaped"
(Figs. 59, 60). From one side of the long, stretched, fusiform cell body, three
or four main dendrites are given off, forming numerous secondary branches.
An axon emerges from the opposite side of the long cell body and runs
toward the lower periphery of the nucleus. Fan-shaped cells are a variant of
the shrublike cells but are adapted to form contacts on one side only.

The neurons in the second layer are more varied: (1) fan-shaped cells
are less typical in form and sometimes dendrites branch out from the lateral
surfaces of their body (Figs. 59, 60), and at other surfaces branches emerge
in a downward direction; (2) polygonal or triangular cells with a radial ar-

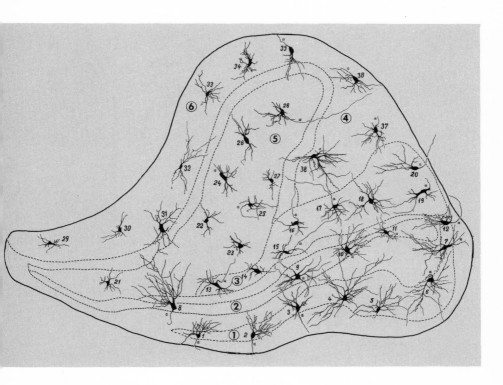

Fig. 59. Neurons of the human lateral geniculate body (frontal section). 1, 2, 3, 5, 7, 8, 12, fan-shaped cells of two magnocellular layers 1 and 2; 4, 9, 10, radial cells of the two magnocellular layers; 14, 15, 16, 21, 22, 23, 25, 27, 28, 29, 30, 33, 37, midget cells of the upper four layers 3, 4, 5, and 6; 13, 17, 18, 19, 20, 24, 26, 31, 32, 34, 35, 36, 38, shrublike and radial cells of medium size in the upper layers; 11, midget cell in layer 2; 6, midget cell in layer 1. Arabic numbers in circles denote layers.

rangement of their dendrites are often seen (Fig. 59; radial type); (3) cells are present with dendrites situated mainly on the inferior aspect of the cell body. The axon of radial cells situated near the lower border of the nucleus runs downward, while that of cells near its medial border runs toward the center of the nucleus; (4) neurons with few branches and with a fusiform cell body are observed; their axon often bifurcates (Fig. 60); (5) short-axon cells with a complex ramification of their axon are present (Fig. 60). None of the various types of long-axon neurons so far described give off collaterals from the initial segments of their axon. Neurons having several collaterals themselves giving off branches are seen very rarely.

Neurons of the four upper parvocellular layers have received very little study. The multipolar cells of Polyak (1957) and many of the cells described

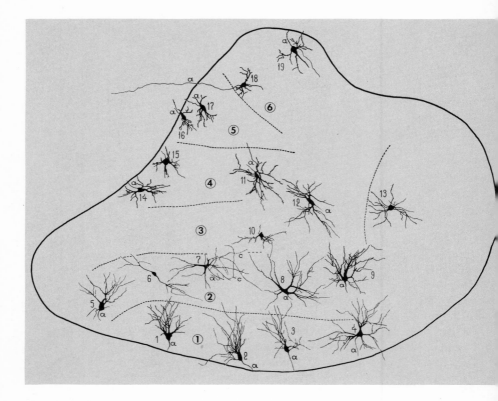

Fig. 60. Neurons of the human lateral geniculate body (sagittal section). 1, 2, 3, shrub-like (fan-shaped) cells of layer 1; 4, shrublike cell of layer 1; 6, cell with few branches; 7, short-axon cell; 5, 8, 9, large shrublike cells of layer 2; 16, 17, 18, long-axon midget cells with few short dendrites in layers 5 and 6. Arabic numbers in circles denote layers.

by Henschen (1925) evidently belong to the lower layers. These workers do not describe those neurons which, according to my observations, are the principal cells of the upper layers. I refer to the midget neuron, with a medium-sized or small, round, oval, or fusiform body and a few short dendrites giving off few branches. The difference between the midget neurons (Fig. 59, 15, 16, 27, 28) and the others (radial, shrublike, neurons with few branches) is great. Comparison clearly reveals not merely the large size of the body of the other neuron, which is not invariably present, but above all the much wider extent of the ramification of their dendrites. The charac-teristics of the midget neurons of the lateral geniculate body determine their connections which are bound to be far more individualized than those of the large and more expansive neurons.

It is strange that others have not described the midget neurons which I have found in the lateral geniculate body of primates. I can only explain this by assuming that the small neurons were usually taken for short-axon cells, particularly under the influence of Monakow's teaching.

In addition to the small cells, medium-sized neurons of the radial and shrublike types are also present in the upper layers (Figs. 59, 60). The course of the axons should be noted, for they run mainly toward the immediate periphery of the nucleus, although exceptions are sometimes seen. In the upper layers typical cells with few branches also appear. From time to time small neurons are encountered in the lower layers also, but their dendrites differ from those of the midget neurons of the upper layers described previously. No midget neurons of typical appearance are present in the lateral geniculate body of the hedgehog or rabbit and there are few of them in the dog, where they are mainly concentrated in the single parvocellular layer.

Area 17. The cytoarchitectonics of Area 17 changes sharply during ontogenesis, as Preobrazhenskaya (1939, 1948, 1955) clearly showed. The principal feature of the immature cortex is the dense arrangement and small size of its cells. In adult man the bodies of the nerve cells are much less densely distributed, and this is attributed to development of the processes of the cortical neurons themselves and of fibers arriving from other parts of the nervous system. However, in Area 17 of the adult human cortex, besides translucencies in sublayer IVb (Gennari's band) and layer V, layers VI and IVc remain densely packed with cells. The structure of the afferent plexus of fibers reaching Area 17 from the subcortex and other areas of the cortex is extremely complex and has been inadequately studied.

The afferent branches entering Area 17 from elsewhere in man are of widely different types (Fig. 61). Some fibers climb vertically upward in a straight line and then give off horizontal collaterals which can be followed for a considerable distance. No such long horizontal branches could be seen in the cortex of any of the mammals previously described. Since it is in man that the stria of Gennari is most sharply distinguishable, and it runs in a horizontal direction, this detail of the neuronal structure of the afferent branches corresponds completely to this situation. The other fibers make wide detours and then terminate in thinner branches. Sometimes a connection can be seen between afferent visual fibers and the bodies of stellate cells. Smaller branches depart from the large, horizontal fibers in upward and downward directions and terminate in typical brushes and boutons. The endings of axons of pyramidal cells with an arcuate axon were discovered in sublayer IVb or Area 17. The terminal branches of these axons, by virtue of the large number of such neurons, make an important contribution to Gennari's band. The afferent branches of layer IV differ considerably, depending on their depth. The network in sublayer IVa is looser, in sublayer

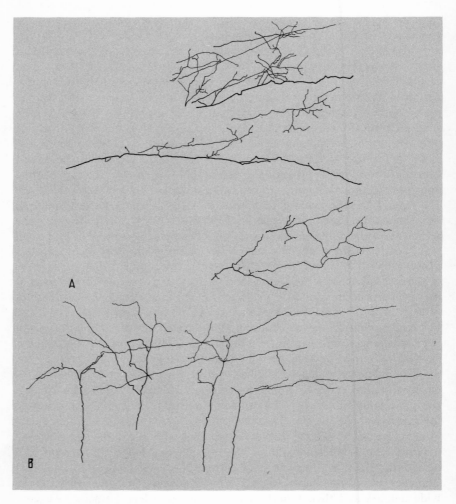

Fig. 61. Afferent branches in Gennari's band in Area 17 of man. A, Large horizontal afferents giving off thin terminal twigs with synaptic structures. Delicate terminals in sublayers IVb and IVc. B, Horizontal branches given off by the vertical trunk of an afferent in sublayer IVb (typical picture). The second afferent on the left differs in structure from the remaining connections which are more vertical. This afferent can provide a communication between the various levels of layer IV.

IVb the branches run mainly horizontally, and in sublayer IVc the network is very dense and consists of countless branches of different calibers, interweaving with each other in an intricate pattern and forming numerous connections with the neurons present in that sublayer.

The principal features of the neuronal structure of Area 17 of the human cortex are:*

1. The great concentration of stellate cells of various types in layer IV with its complex subdivisions.

Typical long-axon star cells of Cajal are present in sublayer IVb (Fig. 62, 11, 13). Their dendrites are widespread and often have the appearance of the wings of a bird in flight, as seen in the monkey's cortex. The long axons run into the white matter, and evidently into the subcortex. In the shape of their body, these neurons can be divided into two main groups: semilunar and triangular. The pattern of emergence of dendrites from the latter group is radial. The smaller cells are similar in character and their axon also runs into the white matter (Fig. 62, 12, 14, 16).

Sometimes a cell similar to a Cajal's cell as regards its dendrites has an axon of a completely different character, ramifying in sublayer IVb itself or giving off long branches upward and downward (Fig. 62, 15, 17).

Sublayer IVc is very rich in small, round, stellate cells with a short axon, forming complex branches (Fig. 62, 19, 20, 22). Sometimes their endings are of bouton type, and they can be seen to make contact with the bodies of neighboring neurons. In these cases the impregnated cell is an intense black color, whereas the bodies of other neurons appear as dark-yellow oval structures against a paler yellow background. Among these short-axon cells, several varieties can be distinguished: larger cells with widely spreading dendrites and an axon climbing upward; small, round cells with winding dendrites, sometimes curving around the cell body; and polygonal cells. Even in the adult, these small neurons remain minute in size (Fig. 62).

2. The second characteristic feature of Area 17 is the large number of pyramidal cells with an arcuate axon (Fig. 62, 21, 25, 27, 29, 32, 33). They are found in sublayer IVc and layers V, VI, and VII. The dendrites of these cells are few and the apical dendrite is more commonly short or of medium length (Fig. 63). The axons stretch upward without collaterals as far as sublayer IVb (according to Cajal, as far as layer III). The presence of cells with an arcuate axon is particularly interesting, because it shows yet another possible means of maintaining excitation within the area itself. The apical dendrite can receive excitation from afferents arriving from subcortical

---

* Cajal (1900, 1911) gave a full account of the neurons in Area 17 of the human cortex, and I shall therefore give only a short summary of my own findings for comparison with Areas 18 and 19 and with the structure of Area 17 in the other mammals which I studied.

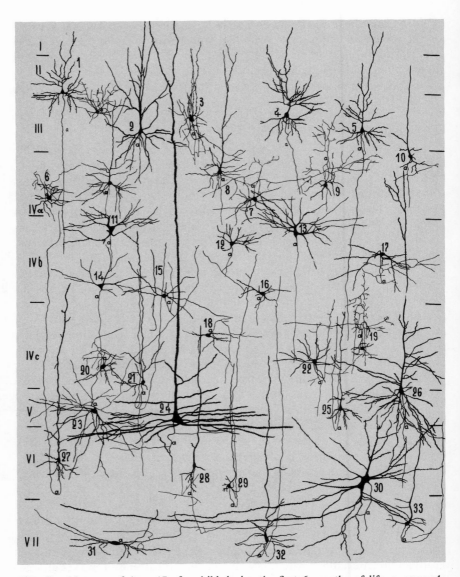

Fig. 62. Neurons of Area 17 of a child during the first 6 months of life. a, axon; 1, pyramidal cell of layer II; 2, 4, 5, pyramidal cells of layer III; 3, stellate short-axon cell of layer III; 6, 7, 9, stellate short-axon cells with ascending axons in sublayer IVa; 8, pyramidal cell in sublayer IVa; 10, fusiform cell in sublayer IVa; 11, 13, large star cells of Cajal in sublayer IVb; 12, 14, 15, 16, 17, small stellate cells in sublayer IVb with axons running in different directions; 18, 19, 20, 22, small stellate cells in sublayer IVc with axons running in different directions; 21, small pyramidal cell with arcuate axon in sublayer IVc; 23, large stellate cell in layer V; 24, solitary pyramidal cell of Meynert; 25, small pyramidal cell with arcuate axon in layer V; 26, medium-sized pyramidal cell

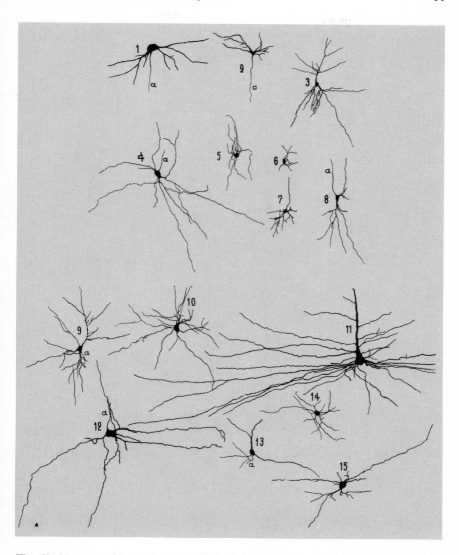

Fig. 63. Neurons of layers IV, V, and VI of Area 17 of the adult human cortex. 1, 2, long-axon star cells of Cajal; 3, pyramidal cell of sublayer IVb; 4, large cell with ascending axon in sublayer IVc; 5, 6, 8, short-axon cells in sublayer IVc; 7, small pyramidal cell of sublayer IVc; 9, small pyramidal cell of layer V; 10, 14, 15, short-axon cells of layers V and VI. The contrast between the sizes of the cell bodies and the extent of spread of their dendrites is clearly visible; 11, solitary pyramidal cell of Meynert; 12, very large cell with ascending axon; 13, cell with arcuate axon and short dendrite.

in layer V; 27, 29, small pyramidal cells with arcuate axon in layer VI; 28, fusiform cell in layer VI; 30, large fusiform cell in layer VI; 32, 33, pyramidal cells in layer VII with arcuate axon; 31, stellate cell in layer VII. (Shkol'nik-Yarros, 1960.)

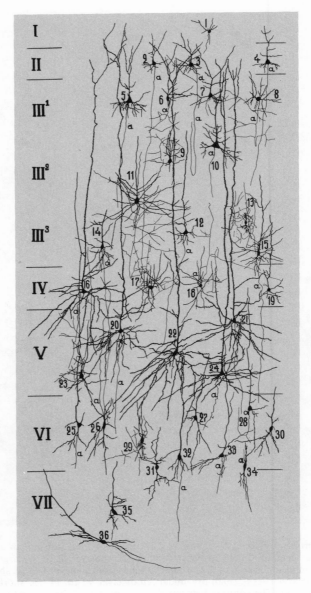

Fig. 64. Neurons in Area 18 of the cortex of a 2-month-old child. a, axon; 1, stellate cell in layer I; 2, 4, small pyramidal cells in layer II; 3, pyramidal cell with arcuate axon in layer II; 5, 7, pyramidal cells of sublayer III¹; 6, 8, stellate short-axon cells of sublayer III¹; 9, 11, stellate short-axon cells of sublayer III²; 10, pyramidal cell of sublayer III²; 12, 13, 15, pyramidal cells of sublayer III³; 14, stellate short-axon cell in

nuclei, and then transmit it to the cell body, so that the excitation can return again via the axon to the layers from which it arises. The cycles thus formed may be considered to provide a mechanism for the preservation of traces of visual excitation.

Solitary pyramidal cells of Meynert are particularly conspicuous in layer V because of the powerful development of the horizontal basal dendrites (Fig. 62). This latter feature was not so apparent in any of the species so far investigated, including the monkey. In this layer, in addition, I found small pyramidal cells, small and very large cells with an ascending axon, and stellate short-axon cells (Figs. 61 and 62).

Area 18. Area 18 of human cortex differs considerably from Area 17 cytoarchitectonically and in its neuronal composition. Mainly small pyramidal cells are observed in layer II. Occasionally pyramidal cells with an arcuate axon are found among them (Fig. 64, 3). The emerging axon first runs directly downward and at the level of sublayer III^2 it curves in an arch and turns upward. In sublayer III^1, as well as small pyramidal cells (Fig. 65, 5, 7) there are stellate cells whose axons mainly proceed downward (Fig. 64, 6, 8).

In sublayer III^2 the pyramidal cells are a little larger (Fig. 64, 10) and the stellate cells have a highly complex system of ramification of their axon (Fig. 64, 11). In sublayer III^3 richly branching medium-sized pyramidal cells are present (Fig. 64, 1, 2, 3). The region of the limes parastriatus gigantopyramidalis is characterized by large, branching pyramidal cells (Fig. 65). The stellate cells of this sublayer were seen to form complex contacts in the early stages with surrounding structures (Fig. 64, 14).

Various types of neurons are found in layer IV, which is narrower than sublayer IVc of Area 17. At least four varieties can be distinguished: (1) small pyramidal cells with a round body and a few dendrites giving off few branches (Fig. 64, 19). These pyramidal cells are similar to those in layer IV of Area 19; (2) medium-sized pyramidal cells more richly supplied with dendritic branches (Fig. 64, 16; Fig. 65, 1, 3). Cells of this type are found not only in the upper part of the layer, where they have also been observed cytoarchitectonically (Preobrazhenskaya and Filimonov, 1949), but also in the middle of the layer; (3) typical triangular cells, which in other areas are observed much more often in layers VI and VII; (4) stellate cells with axons running in different directions (Fig. 64, 17, 18).

sublayer III^3; 16, 19, medium-sized and small pyramidal cells in layer IV; 17, 18, stellate cells of layer IV; 21, 22, 23, 24, pyramidal cells of layer V; 20, 34, stellate cells with ascending axon in layers V and VI; 27, stellate short-axon cell of layer VI; 29, 31, 32, pyramidal cells of layer VI; 28, pyramidal cell with arcuate axon in layer VI; 25, 26, 30, 33, 36, fusiform cells in layers VI and VII; 35, pyramidal cell of layer VII. (Shkol'nik-Yarros, 1960.)

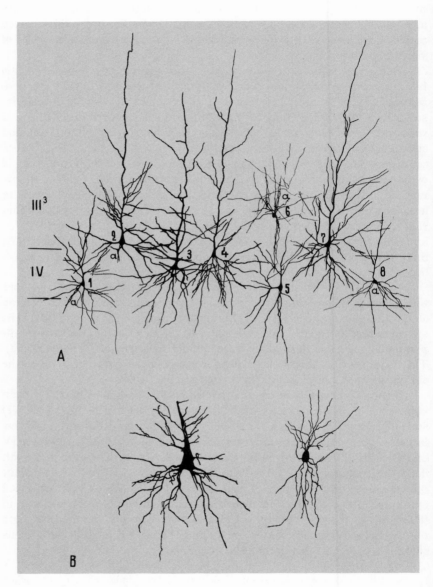

Fig. 65. Neurons of layers III³ and IV of Area 18 in man. A: Child aged 1 year 8 months; 2, 4, pyramidal cells of sublayer III³; 6, stellate cell of sublayer III³; 5, 7, triangular cells of layer III³ and IV; 1, 3, 8, pyramidal cells of layer IV. B: Adult. On the left, a large pyramidal cell of sublayer III³ of Area 18; on the right, a short-axon cell.

Hence, in layer IV of Area 18, the stellate neurons are joined by a large number of long-axon cells. Cajal (1911), when describing both types of cortex, drew attention to the presence of pyramidal cells in layer IV. They are also found in Area 17.

In layer V pyramidal cells of various shapes and sizes (Fig. 64, 21, 23, 24) are more numerous than the stellate cells, which usually resemble Martinotti's cells with an ascending axon (Fig. 64, 20).

Layer VI is rich in fusiform cells (Fig. 64, 25, 30, 33) and stellate cells with an ascending axon (Fig. 64, 26, 34). Besides the ordinary pyramidal cells with an axon descending into the white matter (Fig. 64, 31), other cells are sometimes seen with a curving, arcuate axon (Fig. 64, 32). This variety of neuron, a conspicuous feature of the structure of Area 17, is much less common in Areas 18 and 19. The pyramidal and fusiform cells in layer VII have a less regular appearance than those in layer VI (Fig. 64, 35, 36).

Area 19. Cytoarchitectonically, Area 19 has a less clearly defined radial striation than Areas 17 and 18. Cells are found in layer I with their dendrites arranged radially and covered with infrequent spines, and with a fairly thick axon emerging horizontally (Fig. 66, 1). Cells were also found with a thinner axon, the few collaterals of which also run horizontally (Fig. 66, 2).

In layer II, very small pyramidal cells (Fig. 66, 4) and round, stellate cells with dendrites branching in the same layer and also in layer I (Fig. 66, 3, 5) were seen. Unfortunately, complete impregnation of this layer could not be obtained.

The wide layer III is divided into sublayers. The pyramidal cells in sublayer III^1 are a little larger than in layer II, but still small (Fig. 66, 9). Stellate cells with bodies of different sizes and shapes, usually fusiform (Fig. 66, 7, 8, 10), are present. Numerous collaterals of an axon running at first upward, then curving downward in an arch could be seen, belonging to a small cell which was successfully impregnated (Fig. 66, 8). The collaterals run horizontally, some of them passing into the lower parts of the layer. Frequently the axon collaterals of stellate cells of this layer turn upward (Fig. 67, 1).

The pyramidal cells in sublayer III^2 are larger still (Fig. 66, 6, 11) and have highly ramified dendrites. The pyramidal cells in sublayer III^3 are very large, with numerous well-developed dendrites (Fig. 66, 12, 13, 14, 15). The number of dendritic branches from some of these cells reaches 65. Basal dendrites of the large pyramids frequently descend as far as layer IV. Stellate cells are usually small, mostly with an ascending axon (Fig. 67, 2, 3, 4). Axons of Golgi type II cells participate in the formation of vertical bundles (Fig. 67, 4; Fig. 68).

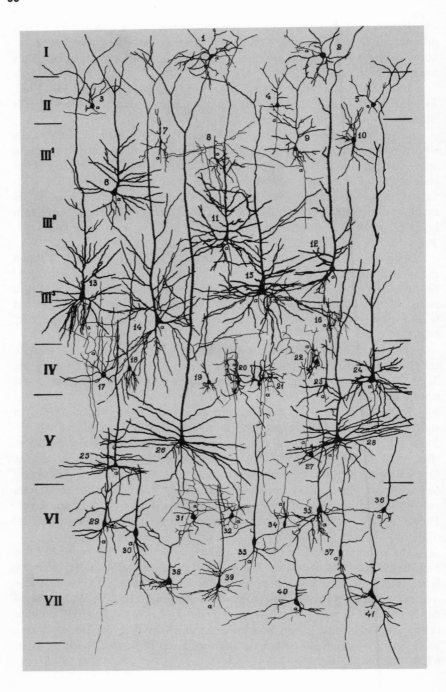

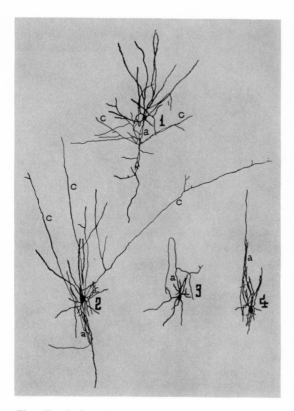

Fig. 67. Stellate short-axon cells of layer III in Area 19 of a 2-month-old child. 1, stellate short-axon cell of sublayer III^1; 2, 3, stellate cells of sublayer III^3; 4, stellate cell whose ascending axon participates in the formation of a bundle.

Fig. 66. Neurons in Area 19 of the cortex of a child aged 1 year 20 days. a, axon; 1, cell with horizontal axon in layer I; 2, cell with short axon in layer I; 3, 5, small stellate cells in layer II; 4, small pyramidal cell in layer II; 7, 8, 10, stellate short-axon cells in sublayer III^1; 9, pyramidal cell in sublayer III^1; 6, 11, pyramidal cells in sublayer III^2; 13, 14, 15, large pyramidal cells in sublayer III^3; 16, stellate cell in sublayer III^3; 12, small pyramidal cell in sublayer III^3; 17, 20, 21, 22, stellate cells in layer IV; 18, 19, 23, small pyramidal cells in layer IV; 24, medium-sized pyramidal cell in layer IV; 25, small pyramidal cell in layer V; 26, 28, small pyramidal cells in layer V; 27, small stellate cell with ascending axon in layer V; 30, 33, 37, fusiform cells in layer VI; 29, 35, pyramidal cells in layer VI; 36, pyramidal cell with arcuate axon in layer VI; 31, 32, 34, stellate cells with ascending axon in layer VI; 38, pyramidal cell (short) in layer VII; 39, pyramidal cell in layer VII; 40, 41, fusiform cells in layer VII. (Shkol'nik-Yarros, 1960.)

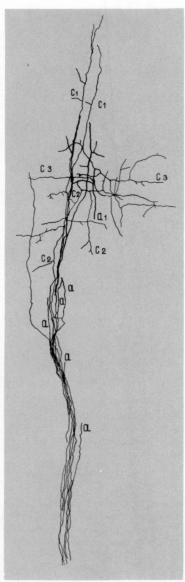

Fig. 68. Vertical bundle in Area 19 of the human cortex. a, axons of pyramidal cells joining a bundle at different levels; a_1, axon from a stellate short-axon cell whose collaterals also participate in the formation of the bundle; c_1, c_2, vertical and c_3, horizontal collaterals.

Layer IV is much narrower than sublayer IVc in Area 17 and is not divided into sublayers. The stellate cells are frequently supplied with beaded dendrites, with a tendency to turn around the body (Fig. 66, 20, 21, 22). They are grouped together in clusters of several cells. Only isolated examples are shown on the composite drawing. Spines are not present on the dendrites of these neurons. After curving upward in an arch, the axon turns downward, giving off in its course numerous short collaterals with boutons at their end or along their course. Twigs given off by the axons are distributed in layer IV itself, or they ascend to the lower part of sublayer III^3 and descend into layer V (Fig. 66, 21). The endings of the axon collaterals are sometimes single, sometimes bifurcations or more complex forms. The Golgi type II cells of layer IV in Area 19 are very similar to the cells of sublayer IVc of Area 17 of the human or monkey cortex. Besides stellate cells, very small and absolutely circular or rounded pear-shaped pyramidal cells are found in this layer (Fig. 66, 18, 19, 23), and their few short dendrites possess a small number of spines. Neurons of this type can easily be taken for stellate or granular cells in preparations with Nissl, a matter of considerable importance for cytoarchitectonic analysis. Besides small, round pyramids, larger pyramids with more richly branching dendrites are also found (Fig. 66, 24).

Layer V contains large pyramidal neurons, smaller than the pyramidal cells of Meynert in Area 17, and with much shorter basal dendrites running horizontally (Fig. 66, 26, 28). Their dendrites are covered with spines. Small pyramidal cells are also found in this layer (Fig. 66, 25). Axons of the stellate cells are mainly of the ascending type (Fig. 66, 27).

The pyramidal cells in layer VI are small (Fig. 66, 29) and round or fusiform in shape. Pyramidal cells with an ascending arcuate axon are rare (Fig. 66, 36). Fusiform cells are more common (Fig. 66, 30, 33, 37). The stellate cells of this layer usually have an ascending axon (Fig. 66, 31, 32, 34). The cells of layer VI are regular in shape and elongated vertically. The pyramidal and fusiform cells in layer VII are more stunted and awkwardly shaped (Fig. 66, 38, 39, 40, 41). Sometimes pyramidal cells with a short apical dendrite ramifying directly in layer VI can be seen (Fig. 66, 38). Together with pyramidal cells with an arcuate axon, these cells are of special interest because of the somewhat unusual shape of their connections. Pyramidal cells with a short or moderately long ascending dendrite were first described by Lorente de Nó in mice (1922). I found them in layer VI of the rabbit's cortex, in the lower layers of the dog's cortex, in layer VI of the monkey's cortex, and, finally, in Area 19 of the human cortex.

Vertical striation is clearly marked in Area 19. Fibers composing the vertical bundles mainly arise from axons of pyramidal cells (Fig. 68). They join the bundle at different levels (Fig. 68). They are later joined by collaterals of the short-axon cells (Fig. 68). The same pattern could also be seen with respect to the stellate cells of sublayers III^1 and III^3. Cells of Martinotti, whose ascending axons also merge into bundles, must be mentioned separately. Association and nonspecific afferent fibers also enter the radial bundles. These bundles show up as clear areas in Nissl-stained sections and

they account for the distinctive radial structure which is particularly conspicuous in the phylogenetically new areas of the human cerebral cortex.

Size of the Neurons and Density of Their Arrangement

In the long process of adaptation to the external environment, ap-
propriate sensory structures have developed and become perfected. For the
reception of visual stimuli, a complex central visual system has evolved,
differing in its structure from the corresponding auditory, olfactory, and
other systems. The specificity of the visual system and of its structure and
function is apparent from its peripheral to its central components. Areas of
the cortex in which association connections predominate possess the greatest
number of common features. However, a more specialized relationship to a
particular system is reflected in corresponding differences in architectonics
and, consequently, in connections.

Before examining in detail the distinguishing features of the visual
cortex of animals and man, a few remarks must be made on the size and
density of arrangement of the cortical neurons.

Pyramidal cells are of different sizes: small, medium, and large pyramidal
cells are present in the cortex of the dog, monkey, and man. However, careful
examination of the pattern of neurons in all representatives of the various
classes of mammals which I have studied reveals that they are larger and
more richly ramified in carnivores (in the dog). This curious fact was also
observed by Zhukova (1953) who studied neurons of the motor cortex and
by Zambrzhitskii (1959) who studied the limbic cortex in a series of mammals. The larger the pyramidal cell, the thicker its axon. The thickness of the
axon is directly related to the velocity of conduction of excitation along it.
This fact was demonstrated many years ago in the case of peripheral fibers
by Erlanger and Gasser (1937). It has recently been demonstrated once again
for fibers of different thickness in the optic tract, which is essentially a
projection bundle, one of the conducting tracts of the brain (Bishop and
Clare, 1955). These workers reached the interesting conclusion that thin
fibers are connected with old phylogenetic systems and thick fibers with new
phylogenetic systems. For instance, the group of fibers of the optic nerve
with the fastest conduction of excitation, $8-12\ \mu$ in thickness, activates the
dorsal nucleus of the lateral geniculate body and is then relayed to the
cortex. The group of fibers with the slowest conduction, $2\ \mu$ in thickness,
activates the superior colliculi. These observations formed important evidence in support of my claim made in 1954 that the size of the dog's pyramidal cell is related to the velocity of conduction of excitation along its
axon. Ecologically, this can be fully explained by the need for a rapid response of the carnivore to external stimuli.

Does this mean that the cortex of carnivores is more perfect than that of primates? If the cortex of Area 17 of monkeys is examined, the increased contrast between the size of the cell bodies will be apparent. There is a mass of small cells in sublayer IVc; very large stellate cells are present in sublayer IV and large pyramidal cells in layer V (solitary pyramidal cells of Meynert). They are not exceeded in size by the neurons of the dog. This contrast is evidently due to differences in the specialization of these layers. The large cells of sublayer IVb and layer V give off axons to subcortical structures. As Le Gros Clark (1942) showed, axons of the solitary pyramidal cells of Meynert run to the superior colliculi. Axons of the star cells of Cajal also apparently project subcortically. It may be assumed that rapid responses to visual stimuli, such as turning the head or the eyes, take place as a result of the rapid conduction of excitation along the thick axons of these large cells, and their subsequent relaying to the oculomotor nerve and tectospinal tract. Consequently, comparison of the cortex of the dog and monkey indicates that the monkey's cortex is most highly specialized for vision (the abundance of cells in sublayer IVc) and also for rapidity of its response as a result of the large cells in layers IVb and V.

Whereas the size of the efferent neuron unquestionably plays an important role in ensuring the rapid transmission of excitation to the periphery, a completely different role is played by the groups of small cells in various parts of the visual cortex. Concrete examples of the structure of the visual and other systems reveal a correlation between perfection of functions and density of receptor cells.

Zavarzin (1950) considered that cell density is the most important factor determining function: "in a structure such as a screen, the density of the dots must be of prime importance to function. An increase in the number of identical elements in a regularly organized stratified structure must increase its resolving power."*

On the question of cell density, Zavarzin cites a very interesting example concerned with the structure of the olfactory bulb. In macrosmatic animals the density of the mitral cells is considerably greater, and olfaction is more finely developed. In microsmatic animals the cells are larger and are more thinly distributed.

Many such examples can be given in connection with the structure of the visual cortex. Its density is least in the mole (Fig. 69), in whose behavior vision plays a subordinate role. A remarkable fact is the complete absence of concentration of neurons at the level of layer IV. In the hedgehog, with

---

* A. A. Zavarzin. *Selected Works. Essays on Evolutionary Histology of the Nervous System* [in Russian], Izd. Akad. Nauk SSSR, Vol. 3, Moscow (1950), p. 361.

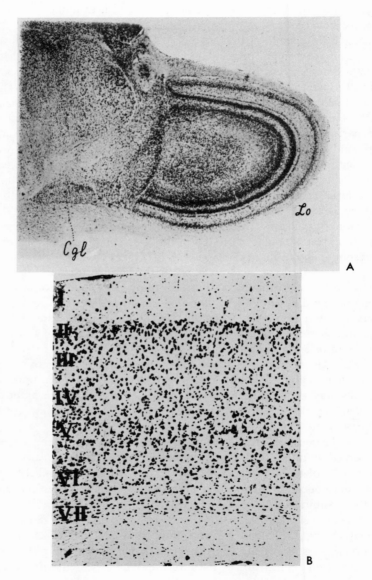

Fig. 69. A: Cytoarchitectonics of the optic tectum of a bird. B: Cytoarchitectonics of Area 17 in the mole; Lo, optic lobe; Cgl, lateral geniculate body. Nissl stain; 100×.

poorly developed vision, no concentration of cells can be found either in the cortex or in the subcortex (Figs. 2 and 4). In other vertebrates and mammals possessing highly developed vision, on the other hand, the distribution of cells receiving visual excitation is very dense. In birds, for example, there is

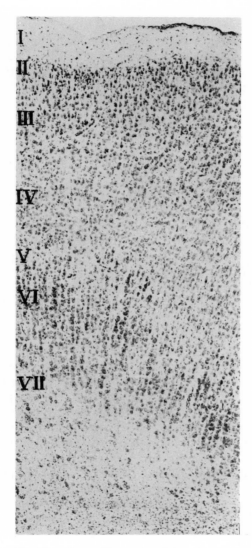

Fig. 70. Cytoarchitectonics of Area 17 of the cat. Nissl stain; 100×.

an enormous concentration of small, densely packed neurons in the retina. In the optic tectum the principal center receiving visual fibers, the striated neuronal structure is of extraordinary complexity (Cajal, 1909), and the bodies of its neurons are densely arranged (Fig. 69). In carnivores (the cat), with a wonderfully developed nocturnal vision (i.e., vision mainly of rod type) an enormous concentration of medium-sized round cells can be seen in the very wide layer IV (Fig. 70). However, despite the considerable width and density of this layer, it is not divided into sublayers, so that the concentration of cells of sharply contrasting sizes (very large and very small) is thus absent. In monkeys, with diurnal vision, layers in which the predominant cells belong to the cone-midget system to be described later, are particularly densely packed with cells. In the retina surrounding the fovea centralis, midget ganglion cells are extremely densely packed, forming as many as eight layers (Polyak, 1957). This part of the retina gives the most highly differentiated and fine reflection of the external environment. In the lateral geniculate body the upper layers, concerned with central vision, have the highest cell density. Finally, in the area striata the highest cell density is found in sublayer IVc (Fig. 41), which can be considered to be the natural continuation of this cone-midget system.

Comparison of layer IV of the visual cortex and the lateral geniculate body from the point of view of cell density in the series of mammals which I studied clearly demonstrates the correlation between a high concentration of cells and the finest and most highly developed vision. A correlation can also be seen between the number of cells at different levels of the central visual system (Lashley, 1934; Chow, Blum, and Blum, 1950).

Investigations have been carried out to show the relationship between the content and distribution of ribonucleic acid and the size of the cell body (Brodskii, 1956; Popova, 1959c). Using ultraviolet cytophotometry, Brodskii determined the RNA content in neurons of different sizes. He found that the RNA concentration is about equal in different neurons from the same part of the brain, so that the RNA content thus depends on the volume of the cell body. RNA is responsible for protein synthesis and associated with the specific function of the nerve cell; larger cells, with their more intense metabolism, are potentially more capable of constant renewal. In the pyramidal cortex of rats the pyramidal cells of layer V give the strongest reaction for RNA (Popova, 1959c). This cardinal fact illustrates the importance of size not only in connection with the speed of the reaction carried out, but also with the quality of metabolic processes in the particular neuron.

The synaptic surface area also depends on the size of the body and dendrites. The importance of the size and variety of synaptic surfaces has been demonstrated very clearly in the cerebellum by the work of Lavrent'ev and Plechkova (1955). My own findings with respect to the connections of pyramidal cells indicate that the length and degree of ramification of the dendrites are directly related to the number and variety of synapses terminating on them. It has also been found that there are just as many synapses on the end of the dendrites as at their origin (Kositsyn, 1962). Finally, electron microscopic investigations during recent years have shown that the surface of the neuron is completely covered by synaptic endings, as with a palisade (Palay, 1958), or synapses of many different types can be seen (Hamlyn, 1963).

Consequently, recent morphological, physiological, and cytochemical findings suggest that the large neuron responds faster, possesses a more intense metabolism, and receives the endings of a larger number of a greater variety, or of larger synapses than a small neuron. The size of the cell body and the length of its dendrites are interrelated with convergence of impulses on a particular neuron.

However, it is not always possible to compare the velocity of transmission of excitation directly with the size of a neuron. Despite the small or medium size of neurons in the upper four parvocellular layers of the lateral geniculate body of the diurnal primates, for instance, transmission of visual excitation to the cortex undoubtedly takes place very rapidly. In this case it is evident that the explanation must be sought in the properties of the synaptic connections, in their structure and organization. The range of neuron complexes covered by the afferent fiber, the area of the synaptic surfaces, and so on may play a role in such cases.

Characteristics of the Layers of the Visual Cortex

Most cortical areas which are primary projection zones (Area 4, the motor cortex; Area 17, the visual cortex; Area 3, for cutaneous sensation) are larger in absolute terms but smaller in relative size in man than in other animals (Filimonov, 1933; Poemnyi, 1940; Kukuev, 1953). The only exception to this pattern is the primary auditory cortex, Area 41, which according to Blinkov (1955) is relatively larger in man.

Can qualitative changes be found in the neuronal structure of areas most directly connected with the peripheral portions of sensory systems if they are compared in animals and man? Is there any question of a more perfect organization of areas which have become relatively smaller by comparison with other phylogenetically new cortical areas?

Statements in the literature to the effect that features distinguishing the human cortex from that of animals are difficult to detect or even are absent if the bichromate-silver impregnation technique of Golgi is used are not convincing. For instance, Lorente de Nó (1922, 1943) concluded from his meticulous studies of the mouse cortex that it is indistinguishable in its basic plan from the structure of the human cortex.

Lashley's opinion that no changes have taken place in the cortex during evolution coincides with that of Lorente de Nó. Lashley stated that the enormous range of visual memory in the rat makes it unlikely that any fundamental changes have taken place in primates compared with rodents.

A detailed study of the cortex reveals quite definite qualitative differences in the structure of the human brain. In a comparative study of the visual cortex of animals and man the most interesting features are the star cells of Cajal in layer IV of Area 17, the pyramidal cells of layer III, and the solitary cells of Meynert. Examination of changes in these neurons in different classes of mammals sheds light on the problem of their functional significance.

It is particularly important to compare areas of the visual cortex in monkey and man, in relation to the common morphological features observed in the series of primates.

The most conspicuous cells in the visual cortex are the star cells of Cajal, located in the center of layer IV of Area 17, within a dense afferent plexus of visual fibers whose course has been traced in the six classes of mammals which I studied (Fig. 71). The principal type of neuron remains the

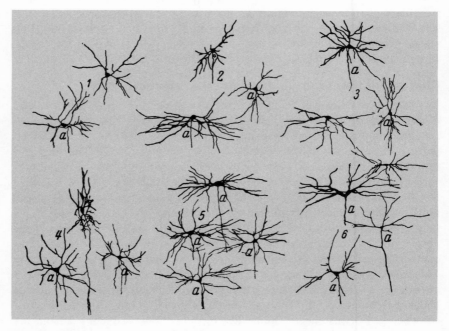

Fig. 71. Long-axon star cells of Cajal in layer IV of Area 17 in some mammals. 1, hedgehog; 2, rabbit; 3, cat; 4, dog; 5, monkey; 6, man. (Shkol'nik-Yarros, 1954.)

same in all species, i.e., it is stellate (radial) or semilunar in shape, with a long axon descending into the white matter. In mammals, however, variations of this type can be seen (Fig. 71).

In the hedgehog, for instance, they are difficult to detect, rare, and give off few branches; in the rabbit they are clearly divided into two varieties, radial and semilunar, and are much richer in dendritic branches than in the hedgehog. In the cat, the star cells of Cajal are particularly rich in dendritic branches, densely covered with spines. In the dog mainly the radial type of these neurons is found. Sometimes its axon divides into two equal branches. In monkeys (Cercopithecoidea) differentiation is observed: larger and sometimes giant cells are found in sublayer IVb, medium-sized cells may be found at a lower level in this sublayer. Ramification of the axon of this last group of cells may often be observed, which never happens with the largest stellate cells. The shape of the cells and, in particular, the character of distribution of their dendrites are very typical (Shkol'nik-Yarros, 1954, 1955a, 1960). Some single large star cells of Cajal in monkeys may actually be larger than the large star cells in man.

In layer IV of the human visual cortex the following features can be distinguished; (1) a very considerable increase in the number of Cajal's stars associated with an absolute increase in area of the cortex; (2) besides the large cells, a considerable number of delicate cells, similar to the large in shape but very small in size, are present. With this great increase in the number of neurons, the range of contrast between their sizes and between the fineness of structure of the small cells becomes apparent (Figs. 62 and 71). Just as in the monkey's cortex, the small stellate cells differ greatly in the direction of their axons. Some of them run toward the white matter, others remain in the cortex, sometimes climbing upward.

What is the interpretation of this steadfast persistence of Cajal's stars despite the great variation in structure of layer IV as a whole? It is undoubtedly concerned with the most constant function of visual reception in the cortex present in all species of animals studied. Cajal rightly considered that cells located in the center of the plexus of visual fibers must be directly concerned with the perception of visual impulses.

Changes in vision in different animals which depend on their relationships with the external environment lead to qualitative changes in the structure of the cortex as a whole and in the number, size, and shape of the bodies and dendrites of the neurons. An explanation of the structural features revealed by my investigations can therefore legitimately be sought in the peculiarities of vision.

The presence of Cajal's stars in all the animals studied indicates a function common to all. The long axon of these neurons, descending into the subcortex, conducts these visual impulses in the opposite direction, possibly playing a role in reflex eye movements. I thus include the star cells of Cajal in the visual efferent projection system (1954). An efferent role of these neurons is also accepted by Solnitzky and Harman (1946) and by Beritov (1960).

There is evidence for the projection of the star cells of Cajal. Retrograde changes have been found in them following subcortical destruction (Le Gros Clark and Sunderland, 1939), directly suggesting interruption of the axon and thus giving the most convincing proof. Second, the thickness of the axon is an important factor. Projection fibers are known to be the largest in diameter (Polyak, 1932; Polyakov, 1949; Shkol'nik-Yarros, 1958a). Typical star cells of Cajal have a thick axon descending directly downward (Fig. 71). As Leonova (1896) originally pointed out, when developmental anomalies of the eyes are present, the star cells of Cajal are particularly disturbed. More synapses terminate on them than on any other neurons of the visual cortex (Éntin, 1954a). Cajal's drawings (1900–1911) show that his star cells lie in the center of an afferent plexus. Indirect evidence also exists in the presence of many subcortical structures directly connected with the visual cortex. The more important of these structures are: the superior colliculi, pretectal nucleus, lateral geniculate body, the pulvinar, and the posterior nucleus of the thalamus. Axons of the solitary pyramidal cells of Meynert run toward the superior colliculi, and other descending tracts may originate in the star cells of Cajal. The latter neurons are characterized by a number of special morphological features. First and foremost is the complete absence of an apical dendrite although in all other respects they are similar to pyramidal cells (long axon, spines on their dendrites as typically found on pyramidal cells). It is the apical dendrite which, in my opinion, may play a special role in the voluntary regulation of neural activity. Its absence may indicate the involuntary nature of the processes subserved by these cells.

I found several axo-dendritic and axo-somatic connections of afferent branches and of other axons on these neurons (1961b).

There is thus morphological evidence of two afferent sources to Cajal's cells. Whether or not a more widespread convergence exists, corresponding to the findings of physiologists, remains an open question. I believe that the star cells of Cajal are one of the types of neurons which yield the responses to visual stimulation found in electrophysiological investigations.

The marked differentiation of the star cells of Cajal and the contrast in their sizes correspond to the complexity of visual function in primates. The largest cells presumably send excitation back into the subcortex the most rapidly. It is in this light that the larger size of some neurons in the cortex of monkeys as compared to man can be considered. Small neurons with a long axon will transmit excitation at a slower velocity; neurons

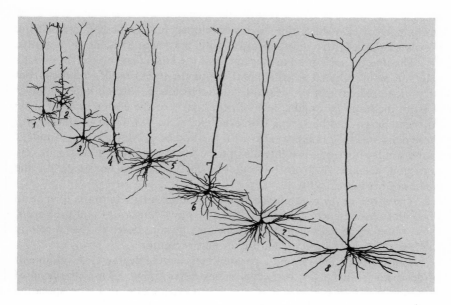

Fig. 72. Large pyramidal cells in layer V of Area 17. 1, hedgehog; 2, mouse; 3, guinea pig; 4, rabbit; 5, cat; 6, dog; 7, macaque; 8, solitary pyramidal cell of Meynert in man. (Shkol'nik-Yarros, 1960.)

exactly similar to the star cells of Cajal in the shape of their cell body and dendrites but with axons distributed only locally must be assigned to a completely different functional system. In primates, therefore, three varieties of star cells of Cajal can be identified.

I studied the structure of layer V and, in particular, the solitary pyramidal cells of Meynert, in eight different species of mammals (Fig. 72). In the mouse, rabbit, and guinea pig the large cells of layer V differ only slightly from the large cells of this layer in other areas; they are arranged in groups, and they cannot therefore be called solitary cells. It is only in carnivores and primates that the large cells of layer V attain a considerable size, acquire the specific features of the particular area, and are arranged singly in accordance with the name bestowed on them by Meynert.

The series shown in Fig. 72 gives some idea of the considerable changes expressed by the increase in size and development of the neurons in layer V, and the increase in number and length of their dendrites. In man they have a typical appearance, distinguishing them from all the cells of layer V in other areas. Characteristically, their cell body is elongated in the horizontal direction, and they have a powerful horizontal plexus of dendrites, forming a very distinct band in sections successfully impregnated by Golgi's method

(Figs. 62, 63, and 72). Consequently, the large cells of layer V in Area 17 of the human cortex possess more highly developed, long and compact dendritic plexuses adapted for communication with particular systems of neurons.

The unique horizontal arrangement of the basal dendrites of Meynert's cells can be interpreted as an adaptation for the reception of impulses from very wide areas. It can be assumed that horizontal collaterals entering layer V from the large pyramidal cells of other parts of the cortex or even from adjacent parts of other areas (for example, Area 18), form contacts with these dendrites (Fig. 128), as also with the bodies of Meynert's pyramids. I found similar horizontal collaterals in the cortex of the rabbit, dog, monkey, and man. Collaterals from afferent branches may also terminate on the bodies of Meynert's cells.

The axons of the pyramidal cells of Meynert contribute to the formation of the cortico-mesencephalic tract. The synaptic connections and the size of the surfaces of contact of these neurons may be considered to play a role in the formation of the specific nature of their excitation.

Krushinskii (1967) found a parallel between the degree of development of dendritic branches of the neurons illustrated in Fig. 72 and the level of development of reasoning activity (ability to extrapolate) in a corresponding series of animals.

A somewhat different picture was observed during the study of development of pyramidal cells in layer III of Area 17. I compared these also in eight species of mammals; the great abundance of branches of the pyramidal cell in the dog's cortex and the well-marked regularity and delicacy of the pyramidal cell in the human cortex were particularly noted. Consequently, fineness of structure was found both in layer III and in some of the neurons of layer IV, and large cells were found in layers IVb and V. It is very important to remember that the pyramidal cells of layer III[3] in Area 18 and, in particular, in Area 19 in primates are very large and highly ramified, the number of dendritic branches amounting to several dozens. Only a few of these cells are present in Area 17. The contrast in the sizes of neurons of the visual cortex in man compared with animals can be regarded as evidence of the higher development of the cortex in man, as an index of a qualitative difference observed in the primary visual projection area. The increase in size of the cells found in layers IVb and V can be associated with the primarily efferent function of these cortical cells. The upper layers, on the other hand, are predominantly sensory and perform associative functions.

A study of visual cortical neurons in various mammals thus reveals structural changes affecting the architectonics, size, and density of distribution of the neurons, the variability of their shapes and sizes, their range of contrast, the organization of connections of their dendritic and axonal branches, and their synapses.

The increase in complexity of neuronal structure is seen most clearly in the visual cortex.

In primates the number of neurons in the cortex reaches a maximum; the sharpest contrast is between concentration of cells in some layers and their low density in others; at the same time, the greatest contrast in their size is observed—from giant cells to very small, and also the most highly specialized synaptic surfaces; architectonic relationships reach an even higher level of complexity than in the subprimates. The increasingly complex development of the visual cortex is clearly reflected in the structure and connections of layer IV of Area 17, receiving the main mass of visual afferent fibers, and also in the progressive enlargement of the surface of contact of the pyramidal neurons in areas surrounding Area 17 (Areas 18 and 19). The visual cortex is particularly highly developed in man, with a higher proportion of pyramidal cells than in other mammals, and with a marked radial structure of the cortex in Areas 18 and 19. The fact that these features reach their highest development in man can be associated with the development of conditioned reflex activity.

Many features indicating an increase in the complexity of the neuronal structure of the lateral geniculate body are found to correspond to the increased complexity of the visual cortex.

Similarities and Differences Between Neurons of Monkey and Man

A study of the neuronal structure of the visual areas in monkeys and man is of interest in revealing common morphological features in the series of primates. Important work by physiologists and psychologists has shown that monkeys possess rudiments of the second signal system. Ignoring their desire to eat, monkeys may display a continual urge to investigate, and may spend hours solving problems presented to them (Pavlov, 1949). Monkeys also have some ability to communicate with each other through facial expressions and vocal signals connected with an emotional response (Tikh, 1947, 1949). Vatsuro (1948) considers that monkeys are at the stage of phylogenetic development corresponding to the early period of human post-natal development, with the characteristic contact orientation of that period.

Commonality in the visual system of man and monkey can be seen in the structure of many of its parts. For instance, the retina of both monkey and man has a macula lutea, which is absent in other mammals. From the similarity between retinal neurons in the primate series Polyak (1941) deduced certain conclusions regarding the human retina on the basis of its structure in monkeys. There is considerable similarity between the structure of the lateral geniculate body in primates, distinguishing it sharply from the structure of this nucleus in other orders of mammals. Its principal feature is its well-marked lamination, with a highly compact arrangement of cells in the parvocellular layers and well-defined myelinated partitions between them. Both in the diurnal monkeys and in man, as several workers have shown, the crossed visual fibers are connected with the second, third, and fifth layers and the uncrossed fibers with the first, fourth, and sixth layers of the lateral geniculate body. In carnivores the laminated structure is also well defined, but the magnocellular elements predominate.

Despite the great variability in the structure of the lateral geniculate body, with sometimes the parvocellular and sometimes the magnocellular layers being predominant, depending on the properties of vision (a mainly nocturnal or diurnal mode of life in different monkeys) and variations in the total number of layers, the well-defined lamination remains a constant feature. The myelinated partitions between the layers are formed by axons running from the lateral geniculate body to the cortex, constituting the beginning of the optic radiation, and also by reciprocal connections from the cortex. Consequently, the union of these axons into clearly defined bundles demonstrates their high concentration in the lateral geniculate body of primates. A contribution of retinal axons to the formation of this laminar pattern, however, cannot be ruled out.

Considerable similarity between the three areas of the occipital cortex in cercopithecoids, anthropoid apes, and man was demonstrated cytoarchitectonically by Filimonov (1932, 1933). This similarity is shown by the fact that they share the same fundamental architectonic features, so that all three areas can be distinguished as independent architectonic units in the species of primates which he described. In the visual cortex (in this case, Area 17), several workers have described considerable variation in the structure, striation, organization of the sublayers, and so on depending on the properties of vision (Henschen, 1930; Ozhigova, 1958, 1960), on the species of monkey (Bonin, 1942), or on the part of Area 17 chosen for investigation (central or peripheral sector; Solnitzky and Harman, 1946). However, the main characteristics of the primate type—the horizontal striation, division of layer IV into sublayers, the existence of other areas (18 and 19) around Area 17—remains constant in all species of primates (Brodmann, 1909; Filimonov, 1933).

My own investigations show that the neuronal structure of Area 17 in monkeys greatly resembles that of Area 17 in man. Accumulation of Cajal's stars principally in sublayer IVb, the presence of large fusiform or triangular neurons in layer VI, the small size of the pyramidal cells in layer III, the indistinct demarcation of this layer from layer II, and the presence of numerous pyramidal cells with an arcuate axon in the lower layers—all these features are similar in the cortical structure of monkeys and man, and they are interesting as an expression of the primate type.

Table I. Area of the Occipital Region in Primates[a]

	Area, mm^2			
Animal	Occipital region	Area 17	Area 18	Area 19
Man	10,490	2613 (25.45%)	3948 (37.7%)	3890 (36.9%)
Orangutang	4,740	1876 (39.6%)	1447 (30.5%)	1417 (29.9%)
Monkey	2,268	933 (41.1%)	725 (32.2%)	609 (26.7%)

[a] From Filimonov (1933).

A similarity can also be pointed out between the pattern of ramification of dendrites of the large star cells of Cajal in the monkey and man (Figs. 46 and 62), indicating a similar type of organization of their connections. A similarity is also found in the distribution of the principal types of neurons in all three areas.

What are the main features distinguishing the neurons of Areas 17, 18, and 19 in monkey and man? To answer this important question, Filimonov's observations must be consulted. The most important fact is an absolute increase in the extent of all three areas (Table I) despite their relative decrease compared with the area of the entire hemisphere.*

As these figures show, Area 17 in man is 2.8 times greater, Area 18 is 5.4 times greater, and Area 19 6.8 times greater in man than in monkey. How is this great increase in size of Area 19 brought about and what is the reason for it? As I have shown (Figs. 54 and 66), the principal characteristic of the structure of Area 19 in *Cercopithecus* and Area 19 in man distinguishing it from Area 17 is the presence of many branching pyramidal cells occupying the wide third layer which is divided into sublayers. Each pyramidal cell (Figs. 114 and 117) can receive excitation of different types, reaching it from different sources through a very large number (several thousands) of synapses. The increased width of layer III and the fact that Area 19 is 6.8 times larger in man must therefore increase by many times the possibility of interneuronal connections between this area and other cortical areas or, in general, between it and other structures of the central nervous system. This conclusion is in complete agreement with data indicating the more highly developed connections of this area with other cortical areas. The great similarity between Area 19, as regards its neuronal structure, not with Area 17, but with other cortical areas (not primary projection areas) must not be forgotten in this connection. The many millions of pyramidal cells added to the cortex in the human brain, besides its other morphological characteristics, may well be the structural basis for the differences between

* I. N. Filimonov (1933). Variability of Cortical Structure. 3. Regio occipitalis in higher and lower primates, *J. Psychol. Neurol.*, **45**, 2–3 (1933).

the human brain and the brain of the monkey, and they are therefore most probably connected with the appearance of specifically human features. These arguments apply also to Areas 18 and, to a lesser degree, to Area 17.

The second distinguishing feature is the much lower cell density in the human cortex compared with that of the monkey, resulting from greater development of the dendrites, axons, and afferent ramifications. A radial structure is conspicuous in Area 19 of the human cortex, due to the gathering of axons of the pyramidal cells together into bundles (Fig. 68).

The third distinguishing feature is the much greater length of the basal dendrites of the solitary pyramidal cells of Meynert in the human cortex. As pointed out above, large collaterals from axons of pyramidal projection cells run for great distances in a horizontal direction in layer V. Because of the enormous number of pyramidal cells in man, the number of horizontal collaterals also naturally increases. Correspondingly, the special length of the horizontal dendrites of Meynert's cells can be explained by specialization and adaptation to the reception of axo-dendritic synaptic collateral connections from the axon collaterals of the pyramidal cells just mentioned. Terminal synapses from collaterals of afferents from the lateral geniculate body or from other subcortical structures also probably occur. Since connections from the various cortical areas to the superior colliculi can be regarded as a final common path for the transmission of cortical impulses to the extraocular muscles, and also for the inhibition of the startle reflex, this property of the dendrites in Area 17 extends this system, especially in man.

Finally, it is an interesting fact that in Area 17 Gennari's band is much wider in man. This is connected with the greater development not only of the afferent plexus, but also of intracortical association connections in man.

More highly organized forms of neurons appear in the human cortex, particularly the shrublike neurons whose development is connected with the pyramidal cells of layer III. They are also observed in Area 19 of the monkey, but more commonly in the same area in man. The thin vertical axons of the shrublike cells evidently participate in the formation of the vertical striation and form contacts with neighboring dendrites. Important investigations by Polyakov (1953) showed the presence of short-axon stellate cells in the human cortex with a particularly selective distribution of their axonal branches. Neurons of this type may coordinate the activity of certain circumscribed groups of cells.

Distinctive Structural Features of Neurons in Areas 17, 18, and 19 of the Human Occipital Cortex

The distinguishing features of Areas 17, 18, and 19 of the human occipital cortex are of interest not only to the morphologist, but also to the physiologist and clinician. These differences are considerable and they can be considered from several points of view: development, structure, physiology, and clinical aspects.

In man the main features distinguishing the neuronal structure of Area 19 from Area 17 are the lower concentration of cells receiving excitation from specific visual afferents; the absence of special giant star cells in sublayer IVb whose axons evidently run into the subcortex; and the absence of small varieties of those neurons. Area 17, sublayer IVc contains far more short-axon stellate cells with their axon bending into an arch or radiating fanwise than layer IV of Areas 18 and 19.

The second distinguishing feature of these areas, especially Area 19, is the marked development of the pyramidal neurons in layer III, with highly ramified dendrites. As shown previously (Shkol'nik-Yarros, 1950b, 1958c, 1963), the pyramidal cell receives a wide variety of connections from all sides. Because of its structure, characterized by a particularly complex dendritic pattern, with its numerous ramifications and considerable length of the main dendrites, these neurons can receive excitation from many different sources.

Another important distinguishing feature of Area 19 is the increased vertical or radial striation. As cytoarchitectonic studies have shown, vertical striation is especially characteristic of most areas of the neocortex outside the koniocortex (to use von Economo's terminology) or what Pavlov called the central territories of the analyzers. In the cortex of other mammals, these vertical bundles and this radial striation are much less conspicuous and the cells are not arranged in beautifully straight chains. This important characteristic also reflects an increase in the number of connections between different parts of the cortex and between the cortex and subcortex. The increase in the number of pyramidal cells forming bundles with their axons which show up as clear areas in Nissl preparations, or as a radial bundle on sections stained to show fibers, is mainly responsible for this characteristic feature of certain areas of the human cortex. However, the bundles do not consist only of axons of pyramidal cells: they also contain collaterals of the short-axon cells (Fig. 68) and ascending axons of the cells of Martinotti.

Afferent fibers constitute another important element of the radial bundles. Experiments by Polyak (1932) on monkeys showed that specific afferent fibers run obliquely in the cortex whereas association afferent fibers run radially directly upward. I confirmed this observation in experiments on dogs. However, in Area 17 of the dog and monkey I found other large specific afferents with the main branch of their axon running vertically. Sholl calculated that three times as many axons leave the visual cortex of the cat as enter it (75,000 and 25,000/mm^2). These results are in agreement with my own observations on the composition of fiber bundles in the cortex.

As the structural differences between the neurons described above clearly demonstrate, connections between Area 17 and other parts of the brain must differ from such connections of Areas 18 and 19. These differences depend above all on the width of Area III on the cortex. The more pyramidal cells are present in this layer the more marked the radial striation, depending on the number of axons concentrated into bundles. Consequently, the width of layer III of Areas 17, 18, and 19 is related to the development of association connections, which are less numerous in the narrow layer III of Area 17 and more numerous in the wide layer III of Areas 18 and 19.

The differences in the structure of layer IV also shed light on differences in the character of the connections. For instance, the special sublayer IVb, which is completely absent in other areas, is responsible for connections specific for the visual system between the cortex and subcortical structures, both centrifugal and centripetal. The centrifugal connections originate in this layer from the star cells of Cajal, the centripetal from cells of the lateral geniculate body, most of whose axons ramify on neurons in sublayers IVb and IVc (Figs. 101 and 128).

Many investigations have shown that all parts of the retina, as well as of the lateral geniculate body, are accurately projected on the cortex of Area 17 (Polyak, 1957; Daniel and Whitteridge, 1962).

The connections of Areas 18 and 19 are completely different. Chow (1950) and Locke (1960) drew attention to a tract leading from the pulvinar to the temporal and occipital regions of the cortex, and the connection with the occipital cortex was predominantly with Area 19. Many investigators regard the pulvinar as a phylogenetically new subcortical correlation center, so that its development runs parallel to the development of phylogenetically new cortical areas. Reports have also appeared (Chusid, Sugar, and French, 1948) to indicate that the connections of Area 19 are much more extensive than those of Area 17 with other cortical areas. Special mention must be made of Area 18. According to Filimonov, this is intermediate in structure between Areas 17 and 19. Studies of the neurons have shown that numerous triangular and fusiform neurons are present in layers IV, V, and VI of Area 18. How can this predominance of fusiform cells be explained?

In the human cortex long-axon fusiform cells are much less common than pyramidal cells, and they occur mainly in the lower layers (Polyakov, 1956, quantitative data). They are particularly numerous in the limbic cortex (Cajal, 1911; Tsinda, 1959). Many investigators regard the limbic cortex as part of the central end of the interoceptive system.

In the cortex of the hedgehog, the lower layers, which contain numerous fusiform cells, are very wide, much wider than the upper layers. In rodents many fusiform cells are found in the upper layers also.

It follows from this description that these neurons are concerned with more primitive functions than the pyramidal cells, whose development takes place mainly in the upper layers of the cortex.

The fusiform neurons of the cortex are very similar to the cells with few branches typically found in the reticular formation. This similarity is manifested by the pattern of dendritic branching and sometimes by the shape of the body. Meanwhile, other workers at the Brain Institute have remarked on this similarity. Dzugaeva considers that the hippocampus contains scattered cells belonging to the reticular formation. Tsinda (1960) suggests that layer VI of the cortex is concerned with autonomic functions.

Cajal wrote many years ago that the structure of layer VI is the same throughout the cortex. Zhukova (1959) observed a similarity between neurons of the reticular formation and neurons of some parts of the visceral nuclei of the brain stem. These observations lead to the preliminary conclusion that the lower layers, which are particularly rich in fusiform cells, play an important role in the connections of the cortex with reticular neurons or with some parts of the visceral nuclei of the brain stem.* I found that fusiform and triangular cells are particularly numerous in Area 18 by comparison with Areas 17 and 19, so that there is reason to consider that Area 18 is the part of the visual cortex where autonomic functions are more strongly represented than in other areas.

---

* The existence of scattered reticular cells in layer VI of the cortex is also mentioned in a new paper by Zhukova and Leontovich (1964).

Chapter 2

CONNECTIONS BETWEEN NEURONS AND DETAILS OF THEIR STRUCTURE

Study of neurons of the visual system and the attempt to schematize the manner in which excitation propagates through its various components inevitably brings up the complex problem of interneuronal connections. This problem has particularly interested me because the method used in the present investigation is so far the only means for obtaining a complete picture of the neuron with all its dendrites and sometimes with its axon and collaterals; and more rarely, if the impregnation is wholly successful, a variety of connections can also be distinguished.

ENDINGS AND BRANCHES OF AXONS

The best-known terminal structures, which have often been described, are synaptic boutons and loops. A detailed account of these structures is given by Hoff (1932), Bodian (1940), Zurabashvili (1947, 1951), Éntin (1954a, 1960, 1966), Polyakov (1961a), Gray (1959, 1961) and others who have described these structures in the cortex and other parts of the nervous system.

The possibility of observing terminal branches in a more natural state by impregnating the neuron as a whole is less well known. By using Golgi's method, Cajal (1900–1935), Lorente de Nó (1922, 1938), O'Leary (1940, 1941), Polyak (1941, 1957), Polyakov (1949–1968), Shkol'nik-Yarros (1950–1968), and others have observed endings given off by an axon impregnated along with the body of a neuron.

Studies of different parts of the visual system have revealed a great structural diversity in axonal endings.

In the rabbit's cortex, the main differences between the upper and lower layers were judged on the basis of distribution of the axons. For instance, while the predominantly nest-and-basket type of ramification of the axons is found in the upper layers (Figs. 17 and 20), in the lower layers the branches run mainly horizontally and in an upward direction (Fig. 20).

Under high power, details of the ramifications and endings of axons can be distinguished.

As an example, a completely impregnated axon belonging to a cell in layer III of Area 18 is illustrated in Fig. 73. One axon ramifies to give a large number of endings of different types: hooks, arrows, bifurcations, forks, and triple endings. Boutons can be seen on the ends of these structures, through which the axon makes contact with a dendrite or cell body, and if these are

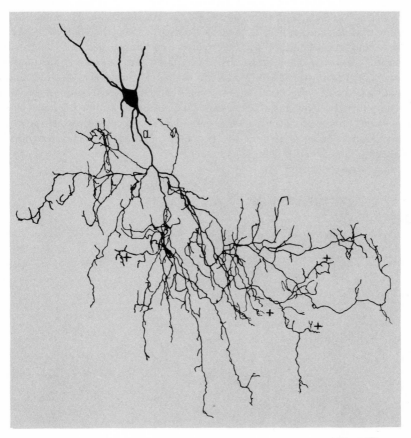

Fig. 73. Short-axon stellate cell of layer III of Area 18 of the rabbit. Different types of terminal ramifications of the axon are visible. Drawn from a specimen magnified 600×, with subsequent reduction; single, double, and more complex endings are denoted by (+). The formation of pericellular plexuses can be seen.

cut through in thin sections, rings and loops can be demonstrated by neuro-fibrillary methods. The formation of baskets for bodies of neighboring neurons is demonstrated in Figs. 36 and 73. Nests can be seen even better in sections stained by Glee's method, because under these circumstances fragments of several axons are revealed simultaneously.

In the dog's cortex the pericellular plexuses formed by axons of the stellate cells are more complex still. Besides dense concentrations of axon collaterals, more extensive axons can be seen whose individual collaterals run far from the original cell (Figs. 37 and 116). In layer V a horizontal axon gives off collaterals upward and downward, forming nests for the bodies of surrounding neurons (Fig. 36).

A photomicrograph (Fig. 74) made under high power shows an axonal ending and its ramification in the dog's cortex; synaptic structures along the course and at the end of this axon differ in shape, size, and number of synaptic boutons. Sometimes the patterns formed by ramification of an axon may be seen to be similar to the shapes of the bodies of surrounding neurons (Fig. 75), the bends and curves of the axon reproducing the shape of the cell body. Boutons are also observed along the course of the axon and at its end. In the monkey's cortex, the highest concentration of axon collaterals was observed around the bodies of the original and neighboring neurons.

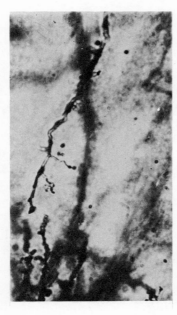

Fig. 74. Terminal ramification of an axon in the dog's visual cortex. Three varieties of endings from the same axon can be noted. Other varieties of endings can be seen in Fig. 73. Immersion; 1500×.

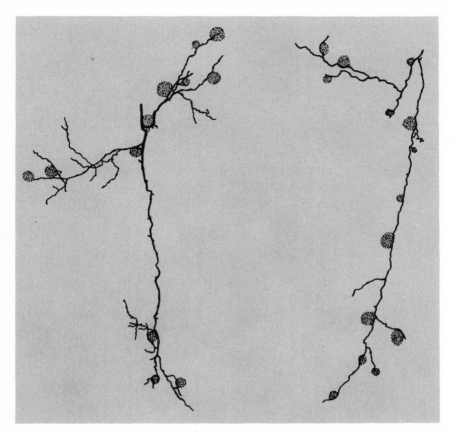

Fig. 75. Axons of short-axon stellate cells from the cortex of the green monkey (*Cercopithecus sabaeus*). Contacts between boutons along the course of the axon and bodies of neighboring cells, represented by stippling, can be seen.

Axon terminals are highly varied and finely differentiated in their structure. For example, the axons of cells of the lateral geniculate body arriving in the cortex are of various types: sometimes they are coarse, oblique fibers, terminating in brushes (Fig. 26), at other times they are delicate and intricately ramified structures given off by a vertical fiber (Fig. 43).

Endings of axons of the ganglion cells of the retina in the lateral geniculate body also vary in type: pincers, clusters, and simpler ramification (Figs. 24, 57, and 107). The number of neighboring neurons with which contact is made also differs greatly, from a few to many hundreds. The caliber of axons found in different parts of the system varies correspondingly.

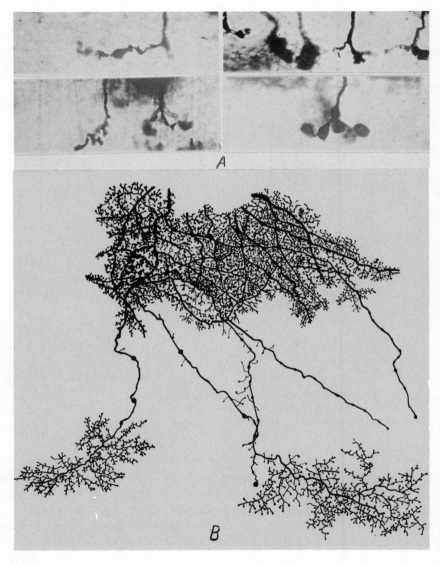

Fig. 76. A: Axonal endings of bipolar cells of the rabbit's retina forming large bulbous swellings. Photomicrograph, oil immersion. B: Axonal endings of horizontal cells in the dog's retina. (Shkol'nik-Yarros, 1958b.)

Neurons with a highly complex yet delicate structure of their axonal endings are found in the retina along with others of a coarser nature. The largest bulbous endings of axons are found on the amacrine and bipolar cells of the retina (Fig. 76, A). Terminal synaptic boutons in contact with photoreceptors are very numerous on axons of the horizontal cells (Fig. 76, B).

Along the course of the axons, thickenings resembling fusiform swelling are frequently seen a uniform distance apart (Fig. 77). These varicose swellings along the course of the axon are synaptic structures (Fig. 77) and are found under normal conditions. A more dense distribution of boutons on the axon of neurons of the visual cortex is seen in the dog than in the

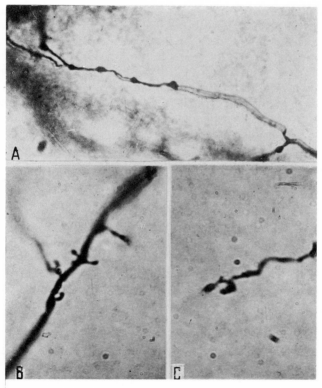

Fig. 77. A: Fusiform thickenings along the course of an axon in the rabbit's cortex, at equidistant intervals. B: Small branches with synaptic boutons along the course of an axon. C: Fork-shaped endings with synaptic boutons at their ends. Photomicrograph, oil immersion.

rabbit. Polyakov found them to be extremely numerous in the human cortex. The axons not only have well-developed collaterals with secondary and tertiary branches, but also short outgrowths very similar to the spines on the dendrites (Figs. 77 and 93). These short outgrowths frequently terminate in boutonlike thickenings. The synaptic nature of these thickenings along the course of the axons is clear from the fact that they can form contacts "*en passant*" with the body, the dendrite, or the spine on the dendrite of a neighboring neuron. Relationships of this type are visible both in the cortex and in the subcortex (Figs. 95 and 96).*

DENDRITES, THEIR ENDINGS AND RAMIFICATIONS

The literature on dendrites and the spines with which they are covered is very extensive. Lateral appendages on the dendrites were first described by Cajal in 1891 and were called spines. Bekhterev (1896a) studied the ontogenesis of the spines. He found that after a period of complete absence they appear initially on the apical processes of pyramidal cells. Stefanovskaya (1897, 1898, 1900, 1901, 1906) studied the morphology of these structures, their development in the embryonic period and their changes under physiological and pathological conditions. She demonstrated pear-shaped appendages by five different methods, ruling out any possibility that they were artifacts. Interesting data on the structure of these spines were also obtained; their role as contact structures was postulated, although not confirmed by documentary evidence. Stefanovskaya was one of the first supporters of the neuron theory, defending it against many attacks by its opponents and by supporters of the reticular theory.

An important contribution to knowledge concerning the neuron and its dendrites was made by Sukhanov (1898, 1899, 1903). He paid particular attention to the pathology of dendrites. In his excellent monograph (1899) he shows how the varicose state of protoplasmic processes given off by neurons is dependent on nutritional disturbances of brain tissue, on the pathological process in which there is a reduction in the number or the total disappearance of the lateral appendages which, under normal conditions, serve in Sukhanov's opinion for the formation of contacts between cells. Sukhanov and his followers established the role of dendrites and spines in the system of interneuronal relations. Geier (1904) for instance, stated that the lateral appendages by increasing the volume of neuronal protoplasm make it more capable of holding, preserving, and accumulating excitation which

---

* Confirmation of the synaptic role of boutons occurring along the course of an axon has also been obtained by neurofibrillar (Éntin, 1954a) and electron microscopic (Gay, 1961) methods.

is received from other nerve cells, and of transmitting this excitation in a transformed state.

Although concerned with the morphology of dendrites in the spinal cord, Geier's doctoral dissertation (1904) nevertheless contains valuable conclusions for an understanding of general principles characteristic of the central nervous system. The demonstration that processes and lateral appendages of various types exist on dendrites of cells in the anterior and posterior horns was particularly important. As Geier showed, the dendrites of most anterior horn cells typically possess a very few lateral appendages of uniform type, while dendrites of most posterior horn cells possess numerous lateral appendages of various shapes and sizes. The number and shape of the lateral appendages correspond to activity of the nerve cell whose dendrites they cover. Ivanov (1901), followed by Sukhanov, Geier, and Gurevich, (1904), demonstrated lateral appendages by intravital staining with methylene blue. Taken in conjunction with the findings of Cajal (1896) and Stefanovskaya (1897), reliable evidence was thus obtained that these structures really exist.

In several publications (1891, 1909–1911, 1935) Cajal discussed dendritic spines and their role and devoted one special investigation to them (1896). He accepted the view that the spines have the function of increasing the receptor surface of the dendrite.

Bodian (1940) considered that the spines are axonal endings. In his opinion they are separated from the dendrite by a distinct membrane and are completely identical with the terminal pedicles (measuring 0.5 μ).

After a long period of inactivity in studies of the dendrites and their lateral appendages, a series of investigations of these matters and of contact relationships between neurons was published. This work was carried out at the Brain Institute, Academy of Medical Sciences of the U.S.S.R.

Sarkisov (1948) continued work along the lines started by Sukhanov. He considers that spines of extremely varied shape and size are a constant and important element of the dendrites. Spines are related to the receptor organization of the cortex. Sarkisov suggested two possible ways in which spines may perform receptor functions. In the first of these, endings of afferent fibers and intracortical axons, directly transmitting impulses, run toward vast number of spines. In the second, neural excitation is spread diffusely and transmitted in the cortex by physicochemical and humoral means. Sarkisov confirmed the observations of Sukhanov and Stefanovskaya concerning the very high lability of the spines under pathological conditions.

A particularly detailed study was made of the ontogenesis of neurons, dendrites, and spines of the human cortex (Polyakov and Sarkisov, 1949; Polyakov, 1951, 1953, 1954, 1955). Polyakov showed that the nerve cells of the lower layers of the cortex attain their fullest development first. By the age of 4.5 lunar months, before fissures and gyri appear on the brain surface, differentiation into areas and preferential development of neurons in the lower layers of the cortex can be observed. Development of the spines takes place in the same order. They appear first on dendrites of large cells in the lower layers, and later in the upper layers. Polyakov (1953) divides the spines into two main groups: short spines with a head, belonging to pyramidal cells of the cortex, and long spines with a thin head, belonging to short-axon cortical cells. Polyakov divided neurons into two groups depending on the nature of their lateral appendages on the dendrites: efferent neurons have many short lateral appendages with a thin pedicle and spherical head, while interneurons have a few long lateral appendages with a thick pedicle and a long head. Polyakov (1955, 1965) considers that interneurons, in contrast to efferent, form more circumscribed and more strictly selective, specialized connective systems.

Zhukova (1950, 1953) and Shkol'nik-Yarros (1950b, 1954, 1959b, 1961b) studied the characteristics of dendritic branches of cortical neurons and the spines covering them in members of various orders of mammals. These investigations showed that spines are constantly present on dendrites in insectivores, rodents, carnivores, and primates.

Leontovich (1952, 1954, 1958, 1959) investigated neurons of the striopallidum in several mammals and also the structure and distribution of spines on dendrites of neurons of the corpus striatum and globus pallidus, and later of the reticular formation. She showed that spines on neurons of the corpus striatum have the same structure and distribution as those in the cortex: Golgi type I neurons have numerous thin short spines with heads, while Golgi type II neurons have very long, infrequent, rodlike spines.

Zhukova (1959, 1960, 1961) revealed considerable differences in both the dendrites and spines of three types of neurons (motor, sensory, and reticular) in the spinal cord and brain stem. In sensory structures the lateral appendages of the dendrites vary in their density of distribution, while on motor neurons they are absent or very rare. Fewer lateral appendages are found on neurons of the reticular formation than in sensory structures.

Mokhova, Popova, and Sarkisov (1960) studied changes in the structure and function of neurons in the visual and sensorimotor cortex of albino rats under the influence of sodium bromide and caffeine sodium benzoate. They found that, besides changes in the electroencephalogram, appreciable changes took place also in the morphology of the neurons, especially of the spines on the dendrites.

Changes in the dendrites and in the spines on them were also observed as a result of the action of eserine on the brain (Sarkisov and Mokhova, 1958). The fact that their structure can be changed even in pathological states of negligible severity is evidence of the high sensitivity of neuronal contact structures.

Changes occurring in synapses, dendrites, and spines in pathological states before the appearance of clinical manifestations were observed also by Tolgskaya (1954, 1957). Many new discoveries of the effects of neurotropic drugs on dendrites, spines, and synapses have been reported by Popova (1968).

Gray (1959, 1961) demonstrated by means of the electron microscope that spines actually exist on the dendrites, and thus confirmed by the most up-to-date and technically refined method the results of all the investigations undertaken at the Brain Institute on dendrites and contacts during the last 10–15 years. According to Gray, the dendritic spines are sites of synaptic contact with the presynaptic ending. The cytoplasm of the spine contains a special structure which he calls the "spine apparatus," consisting of a group of sacs separated by bands of dense material. The work of Gray was later confirmed by electron microscopic investigations of Hamlyn (1962, 1963), Davydova and D'yachkova (1962), and Bogolepov (1964). These workers also showed that spines are present on the dendrites in the cerebral cortex of many animals.

In a paper by Chang (1952b) mention is also made of the role of dendrites and spines. In his opinion, the spines are a receptor apparatus for presynaptic impulses. They are most densely arranged on the apical dendrites and are absent on the cell body. Functionally the spines constitute a mechanical barrier preventing contact between synaptic boutons and dendrites, and they thus act as a limiting factor for synaptic conduction. They also hold up and weaken synaptic excitation because of the high resistance of the thin pedicles of the spine.

A quantitative analysis of the spines and their relationship to afferent fibers was made by Fox and Barnard (1957). Admittedly, they studied the Purkinje cells of the cerebellum, although their arguments, literature citations, conclusions, and methods have a direct bearing on the present theme. They consider that although it has not yet been precisely established whether spines are synaptic endings on dendrites or a means of increasing the synaptic surface of the dendrites in order to create more intimate connections, whatever the case, their number gives a good indication of the number of fibers converging on branches of the Purkinje cells. They suggest that the spines are dendritic collaterals and that they are found where dendrites are in contact with oblique or arcuate afferent fibers.

Because of the lack of comparative data in the literature, I have studied spines at different levels of the visual system.

Endings of dendrites in the cortex are very similar to axonal endings.

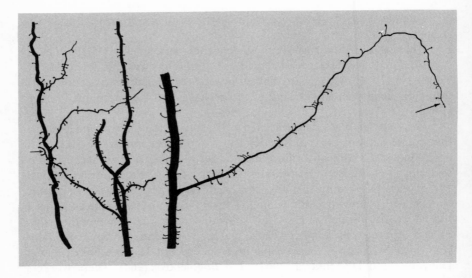

Fig. 78. Dendritic branches of a pyramidal cell in the rabbit's cortex. Thin endings of branches, very similar to axonal endings carrying boutons, can be seen. Drawn at a magnification of 900×. Differences in the shape and direction of the spines on the dendrites can be noted.

They are frequently shaped like forks with boutons at their ends (Fig. 78), and are evidently synaptic. Their morphological picture suggests that the terminal ramifications of the dendrites also play a synaptic role.

Dendrites of cortical neurons of the hedgehog are few in number and they give off few branches. Because of the presence of cells with an oblique apical dendrite, the vertical striation is ill defined in the hedgehog cortex. Dendrites of the pyramidal cells of the hedgehog in successfully impregnated sections are literally bristling with spines. However, the relative number of spines, depending on the number and the degree of ramification of the dendrites, is much smaller than in higher mammals.

Dendrites of the neurons of the lateral geniculate body of the hedgehog also are few in number, give off few branches, and are shorter than those of typical cortical pyramidal cells. The spines on the dendrites do not form a brush and they are less densely distributed than in the cortex.

Dendrites of the cortical neurons of the rabbit differ considerably with different types of neurons. The pyramidal cells of the rabbit not only have typical dendrites, with an apical trunk reaching as far as layer I, but also medium-sized and small dendrites, with an apical trunk, reaching as far as layer IV. The number of dendritic branches of the pyramidal cells varies on the average from 8 to 30. The basal dendrites do not extend over a wide area, and none are found in layer V with very long horizontal branches. Branches in the lower third of the ascending dendrite of pyramidal cells in layer III are solitary and are not present in great numbers. The apical bouquet in layer I has no horizontal branches stretching out far and wide.

Dendrites of the fusiform neurons have few branches and their lower trunk can be traced downward for a considerable distance, sometimes into the white matter. The apical dendrite trunk reaches into the upper layers, but occasionally in sections it can be seen to end in layer I.

Dendrites of the stellate neurons also differ in character. In some cases they are thick, short, few in number, and located mainly at the poles of the cells, while in other cases they are radial in their arrangement. Dendrites of some cells with a short axon extend over a wide area from layer III to layer VI, with a considerable vertical range. Dendrites of the star cells of Cajal with a long axon are distributed in a manner corresponding to the two types of cells, either radially or, in the case of semilunar cells, spreading out from the lateral surfaces of the bodies.

Dendrites of the neurons of the lateral geniculate body in the rabbit are less varied than in the cortex. In the dorsal portion of the nucleus they are mainly radial in distribution, around the body of the cells, and in some cases they give off numerous branches. At the edge of the nucleus the neurons have dendrites which follow the course of fibers of the optic tract and optic radiation. In the ventral part of the nucleus the dendrites are very long, straight, and few in number when arising from neurons with few branches, and short and winding when arising from cells of another type.

Dendritic spines in the rabbit's cortex are highly variable (Fig. 79). They are longest and most complex on dendrites of some cells of Martinotti in layer VI. Some spines have two or even three boutons along their course, while others terminate in double prongs with boutons at their ends. The direction of the spines on dendrites of the cells in the lower layers of the rabbit's cortex is also variable, for they may be perpendicular to the dendrite or at any angle whatever to it. Densely distributed spines, not very long, are most typical of the pyramidal cells. Many short-axon stellate cells either have no spines or very few. However, some short-axon cells are richly supplied with spines. I counted the spines on dendrites of several types of neurons. On a pyramidal cell in layer III the number of spines does not exceed 1000. On a short-axon stellate cell, with spines on its dendrite, their number may reach 700. Such neurons were particularly numerous in layer IV of the rabbit's cortex (Fig. 80).

In some cases in the same section dendrites with numerous spines could be seen lying alongside neurons without spines. In this latter case the dendrites could be either smooth, fragmented, or with varicose thickenings.

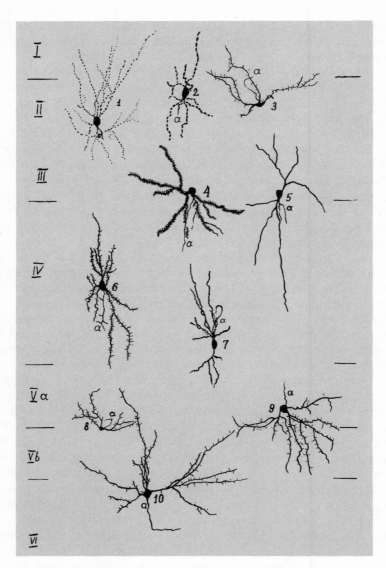

Fig. 79. Various types of stellate cells from the rabbit's cortex. 1, stellate cell with varicose dendrites in layer II; 2, stellate cell in layer II with necklacelike dendrites; 4, stellate cell with long, descending axon, and numerous spines on dendrites forming "brushes"; 5, stellate cell with long, descending axon and smooth dendrites; 3, 6, numerous spines on dendrites; 8, 9, 10, stellate cells in lower layers with longer and thinner spines. To give better visibility of the dendrites the axons of these cells are not drawn.

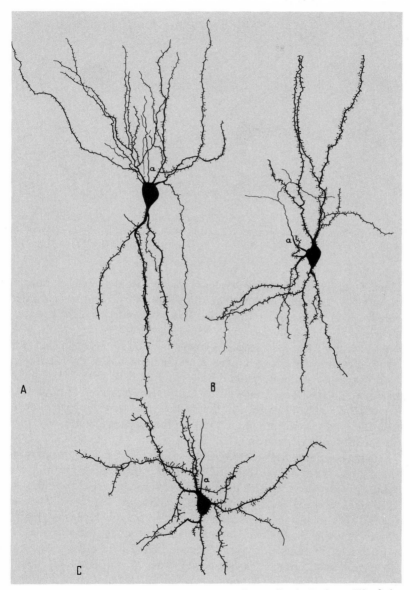

Fig. 80. Spines on dendrites of short-axon stellate cells. A: In layer IV of the rabbit cortex. Drawn at a magnification of 600× with subsequent reduction. To give better visibility of the dendrites axons are not drawn. Number of spines on dendrites of cells in A are 675, and in B are 677. C: Layer IV of the dog's cortex. Number of spines on dendrites is 460.

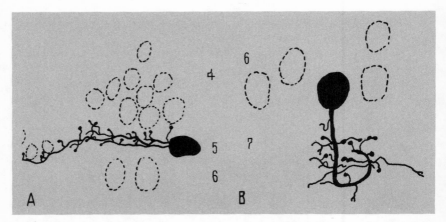

Fig. 81. A: Spines on dendrites of a horizontal cell of the rabbit's retina. B: Amacrine cell of the rabbit's retina. Drawn at a magnification of 900×. 4, 5, 6, 7, layers of the retina.

There are fewer spines on dendrites in the lateral geniculate body than on those of the cortical neurons. The spines are shorter and more numerous on dendrites of long-axon radial cells than on dendrites of cells with few branches.

Very clear pictures of dendritic spines may be obtained in the rabbit's retina. Spines are very clearly observed on the dendrites of the bipolar cells, and on dendrites of the horizontal and ganglion cells (Fig. 81). They have clearly distinguished heads, and often fairly long pedicles. The number of spines on the dendrites of cells in the retina, just as in the cortex, depends first on the type of neuron, and second on the number, length, and degree of ramification of the dendrites.

Dendrites in the dog's cortex differ even more sharply on neurons of different types than in the rabbit. Not only are typical pyramidal cells present, but also short and medium-sized pyramidal cells. The number of dendritic branches of the pyramidal cells averages 30–50, while on some particularly highly branched neurons in layer III their number may reach 80. The basal dendrites extend over a longer distance than in the rabbit, and they have horizontal branches in layer V. Some of the pyramidal cells in layer III have numerous branches in the lower third of the ascending dendrite, forming a special additional contact zone. The apical bouquet in layer I gives off more clearly defined horizontal dendritic branches than in the rabbit's cortex.

Dendrites of the fusiform cells ramify to a lesser degree than those of the pyramidal cell. They form powerful trunks which can be followed from the lower and upper poles of the cell toward the white matter and the upper layers. Dendrites of neurons of the stellate cells are higher variable. On some neurons they are short, few in number, and arranged radially, while in other cases they have a shrublike distribution. Dendrites of the star cells of Cajal with a long axon are mainly radial and give off more branches than in the rabbit's cortex.

Great variety of types of dendritic branches is also observed in the lateral geniculate body of the dog. In this case the distribution of the dendrites may be radial, shrublike, or fanwise, in which case the bouquet of dendrites emerges from only one pole of the cell body. The neurons with few branches give off only three or four, long, straight dendrites, whose branches are distributed along the course of fibers of the optic tract.

Dendritic spines in the dog's cortex are extremely variable. On large pyramidal neurons in layer III their number may reach 2600 in a particularly well-impregnated section (Shkol'nik-Yarros, 1950b). The spines most typical of the pyramidal neurons are densely arranged but not particularly long. Some short-axon stellate cells have almost no spines on their dendrites, while the dendrites of other neurons are richly supplied with spines. The number of spines on some of these neurons may reach 500. Similar neurons are found particularly frequently in layer IV of the dog's cortex (Fig. 80).

In the lateral geniculate body of the dog, the number of spines on the dendrite is very small. The spines on dendrites of long-axon radial and shrublike cells are shorter and more numerous than on dendrites of cells

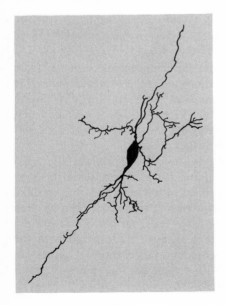

Fig. 82. Neuron from the lateral geniculate body of a dog, with long spines of different shapes on its dendrites.

with few branches. Spines on some neurons are infrequent and similar to appendages of the dendrites (Fig. 82). The typical picture of spines is less frequently obtained in sections through the lateral geniculate body than in the cortex.

In the dog's retina, dendrites of the ganglion and horizontal cells are more richly branched than in the rabbit's retina. Consequently the number of spines is greater. The spines have a typical appearance of pedicles with heads.

Dendrites of neurons in Area 17 of the monkey have still more obvious differences. This can be seen clearly by comparing neurons of layer III and layer V. In layer V the large dendrites run either horizontally or obliquely downward. Apical dendrites of large pyramidal cells as a rule give off no branches along their course but only an apical bouquet in layer I. The pyramidal neurons of layer III are distinguished by the development of a more luxurious ramification of the dendrites along the course of the ascending trunk. Dendrites of pyramidal cells with an arcuate axon are short or of medium length.

The structure of the dendrites in Area 18 is different, and the basal branches of the pyramidal cells in layer III as a rule are descending. In layer V the horizontal direction of the branches is ill defined. As a rule the dendritic trunks of fusiform and triangular neurons radiate from the poles. In Area 19 dendrites of the pyramidal neurons ramify to a greater degree than in Areas 17 or 18. The number of dendritic branches (in a child's brain) may reach 65.

Dendrites of stellate neurons of Area 17 vary considerably in structure depending on the type of cell. Dendrites belonging to star cells of Cajal of large caliber cover a wide area, give off many branches, and are of considerable diameter. They may be radial in their arrangement or emerge from the lateral surfaces of the cell body. The diameter of the dendrites belonging to star cells of Cajal is of small caliber and the area of their distribution is smaller. Short-axon stellate cells of layer IVc have a few short dendrites, frequently winding spirally around the cell body. Sometimes these dendrites have varicosities along their course and at their ends.

The neurons of Area 17 of monkeys have fewer spines. The great variety of their forms is very clearly seen. Sometimes on one dendrite intermediate forms between a typical short pedicle with a head and thin, rodlike spines is apparent. Often dendrites thickly covered with spines can be seen in the same sections side by side with dendrites free from spines and covered with varicosities. This phenomenon cannot always be connected with the type of cell. Sometimes pyramidal cells with dendrites covered in spines are observed in Area 18, while in Area 19 in the same section spines are completely absent on dendrites of the pyramidal cells.

VARIETIES OF CONNECTIONS BETWEEN NEURONS
IN THE CORTICAL AND SUBCORTICAL PARTS
OF THE VISUAL SYSTEM

The complexity of this problem of the morphological basis for the transmission of excitation is obvious. Lavdovskii (1879, 1888, 1889, 1902), one of the founders of the neuron theory, considered that neurons are interconnected not by a continuous bridge of neurofibrils but by contact between processes. Excitation is conducted not only by the axon, but also by dendrites of the nerve cell. Contacts provide the best transmission of excitation from one nerve cell to another. Bekhterev (1896b, c, 1898) stated that endings of axons of some neurons lie close to dendrites and bodies of other neurons. He considered that contact may take place in plexuses of dendrites, between dendrites of cells such as, for example, between the pyramidal cells of the cortex.

Detailed accounts of synaptic endings in the cortex and of their various forms were also given at the beginning of this century by Cajal (1903) and Larionov (1907).

The most penetrating and important generalization of the facts concerning interneuronal connections in the cortex and subcortex obtained by Golgi's method was that given by Cajal (1935) in his book on the neuron theory. Cajal considered that the problem of axo-dendritic and axo-somatic connections is one of the most important to have arisen in the study of the histology of the nervous system. He distinguished 11 different groups of mutual contacts between neurons: six groups were classed as axo-somatic connections, as for example, connections formed by nests rich in fibers, by baskets and cups, with few fibers, by terminal bulbs or by wide nests, from which terminal pedicles and so on arise; Cajal classed five groups of interneuronal connections as axo-dendritic contacts: through climbing fibers or long, transverse, and oblique fibers, through diffuse plexuses, and so on.

Cajal paid most attention to contacts between neurons in the cortex, where the most constant synapses are: (1) synapses formed by long, ascending, oblique, or descending collateral fibers (he was unable to state precisely how this connection takes place); (2) a dense and diffuse plexus, occurring mainly at the level of the layer of granules in the visual and auditory cortex, receiving fibers from the thalamus and other parts of the brain; (3) endings such as nests formed by branches of axons of Golgi type II cells, surrounding the bodies of pyramidal and other cortical cells (according to Cajal, this type of synapse is rare); (4) axonal endings of Martinotti's cells consisting of terminal fibrils resembling nests, surrounding cells with a short axon in layer I. The same type of contact through diffuse ramifications is also possessed by axons from other cells of the lower layers of the cortex, and also by descending axons not reaching the white matter.

Later classifications of synapses also were based on acceptance of two principal types. For example, Lorente de Nó (1933) described two types of synapses in the cortex, arguing that collateral axo-dendritic synapses are formed by a short, lateral branch or by the simple thickening of a fiber in contact with a dendrite. One axon may form many collateral contacts. Each dendrite has several hundreds of these collateral synapses. Synapses on the cell body (axo-somatic) are usually terminal; one, two, or three endings are applied to the body of the neuron. As Cajal originally showed, the cell body and the initial part of the dendrite, which have no spines, are covered with terminal pedicles. Most cortical cells have terminal synapses on their bodies, but other types of cell also exist with a short axon, apparently forming only collateral synapses, for spines are found on their body.

Bodian (1940) paid considerable attention to synapses; he claimed that axonal endings are practically identical in most vertebrates. He divides all the endings into two types: end plates and bulb endings. They vary in size from 0.5 to 5 μ. They are much larger on the cell body than on the proximal part of the dendrite, and they are also found at the axon hillock.

Sarkisov (1948) reached the important conclusion that axo-dendritic connections are particularly prominent in the cortex, in contrast to lower levels of the central nervous system. Spines are much more numerous in the cortex than in the brain stem or spinal cord. Axo-dendritic connections are particularly vulnerable; changes in them are reversible, and they may lie at the basis of neuroses.

Sepp (1949) drew a sharp distinction between the function of axo-dendritic and axo-somatic connections. He considered the basket plexuses around nerve cell bodies, i.e., what Cajal describes as axo-somatic contacts, to be an inhibitory apparatus. In the cortex, where inhibitory reactions reach their highest development, in his opinion pericellular plexuses are most powerfully represented.

Zurabashvili (1947, 1951) studied synapses by a modification of Hoff's method in various parts of the central nervous system and introduced the concept of synapse architectonics. He observed differences in the distribution of synapses not only between the layers and areas of the cortex, but also on the same neuron. Some large neurons are distinguished by the presence of synaptic zones or concentrations of groups of synapses at particular sites.

A close study of synapses was made by Grashchenkov (1948). When generalizing collective work carried out on this subject, he demonstrated the importance of synaptic conduction in clinical practice and stressed, in particular, the importance of neostigmine therapy as a means of stimulating and facilitating this process.

Snesarev (1950), in support of Cajal's opinions, considered that the transmission of excitation in the cortex takes place mainly through nests, baskets, and diffuse plexuses, not necessarily with the participation of specialized apparatuses (such as synapses of the loop type).

According to Chang (1952b), synapses in the cortex are divided into pericorpuscular and paradendritic. Pericorpuscular synapses are most active during postsynaptic discharges, whereas paradendritic synapses under normal conditions can give rise only to electrotonic changes and can only change the level of excitation of the neuron. The large pyramidal cells are connected by paradendritic synaptic boutons with commissural afferent fibers, association fibers, descending collaterals of pyramidal cells, and so on. The pyramidal cells receive pericorpuscular synaptic boutons from short-axon cells of the adjacent part of the cortex. Consequently, the large pyramidal cells of layer V probably cannot be activated directly by afferent fibers without the aid of interneurons.

Polyakov (1953, 1963) divides all contacts in the cerebral cortex into two main groups: terminal and tangential. The body of the neuron and the initial segments of the dendrites are adapted for the formation of terminal contacts. In Polyakov's opinion, terminal contacts are the main mechanism for the transmission of excitation in the central nervous system. It is by means of this mechanism that a relatively limited number of particular neurons is joined together into unified functional groups.

In contrast to terminal contacts, tangential contacts are formed either along the course of the dendrites or where they are intersected by axons. Stimuli of various types can be received "*en passant*" by such a connecting system, and it can act therefore as a regulatory mechanism modifying the functional state of a particular neuron. This mechanism of connections is additional to the main mechanism and is responsible for regulating and adjusting the functional relationships between neurons.

Polyakov* (1955, 1961b) and Shkol'nik-Yarros (1950a, 1955a, 1956, 1961b, 1963) observed what were unquestionably axo-dendritic contacts in the cortex of man and animals. These contacts were photographed for the first time, whereas all previous workers had simply drawn them in their actual form, or schematically, or had simply put forward hypotheses.

---

* The axo-dendritic contacts were found at the same time (1950) in the cortex of human brain (Polyakov) and in the cortex of other mammals (Shkol'nik-Yarros). I am grateful to G. I. Polyakov for the photograph of an axo-dendritic connection which he kindly furnished for publication (Shkol'nik-Yarros, 1950a).

Polyakov (1955) not merely subdivides all contacts into terminal and tangential, but also demonstrates in the human cortex just how these connections are brought about.

Axo-dendritic contacts were demonstrated by Leontovich (1952, 1958) in subcortical structures. She also concluded that spines are synaptic structures and for the striopallidum produced evidence in support of this conclusion. Zhukova (1960, 1961) also observed axo-dendritic contacts in the motor cortex of animals, and later in the spinal cord.

Gray (1959, 1961), in his studies of synapses, frequently saw the membranes of two processes lying opposite one another, with thickened edges and clusters of vesicles near the thickened membrane of one of the processes. These structures are synaptic contacts, because the presynaptic process containing vesicles arises from a medullated axon. The other postsynaptic process was identified either as the body of a nerve cell or the trunk or spine of a dendrite. Gray described two main categories of synapses: (1) type 1, found on trunks of dendrites and on spines; (2) type 2, found on bodies of neurons and on trunks of dendrites. Type 1 is characterized by a great length of opposed and thickened, dense membranes. The postsynaptic thickening of the membrane is more marked than the presynaptic. The thickened parts of the membranes lie further apart than the unthickened. Synapses of type 2 are characterized by shorter lengths of their opposed thickened membranes, and the pre- and postsynaptic thickenings are of similar dimension.

Using isolated pieces of the cerebral cortex, Szentágothai (1960) showed that the specific and nonspecific afferent fibers, and also other (commissural) fibers are very sparsely represented in layer I. Synapses with apical trunks of pyramidal cells, resembling pericellular baskets and parallel contacts, are mainly of intracortical origin. Spines on the dendrites in isolated cortex are extremely well preserved. Szentágothai (1960) concludes that axo-somatic synapses of pyramidal cells in the cortex are formed almost entirely by short-axon cells, producing inhibition.

The existence of a wide variety of axo-somatic and, in particular, of axo-dendritic synapses on pyramidal neurons in the cortex has been demonstrated (Shkol'nik-Yarros, 1956, 1961b, 1963). No fewer than 11 different types of contacts on the body and dendrites of these neurons were demonstrated in Golgi preparations.

Different types of synapses have also been revealed with the electron microscope (Hamlyn, 1963). Six ultrastructural variants of synapses were found on pyramidal neurons of the hippocampus.

Colonnier (1968) studied the varieties of synapses in the cat visual cortex and distinguishes two types: asymmetrical, with round synaptic vesicles, and symmetrical, with flattened synaptic vesicles. Most synapses of asymmetrical type on the pyramidal cells of layer II are observed on the spines of the dendrites; synapses on the bodies are of symmetrical type. Stellate cells of layers I and IV have synapses of both types, which are present both on the bodies and on the dendrites.

Besides the two principal and widely known groups of synapses—axo-somatic and axo-dendritic—a number of workers recognize the existence of dendro-dendritic (Kaplan, 1958; van der Loos, 1959, 1964), axo-vasal (Dolgo-Saburov, 1956; Dolgo-Saburov *et al.*, 1958), and axo-axonal synapses in the central nervous system. Axo-axonal synapses have been studied most convincingly and have been demonstrated with the electron microscope (Kidd, 1962; Gray, 1962, 1963; Szentágothai, 1963b). I found similar synapses in my own investigations (Shkol'nik-Yarros, 1961b, 1965). In particular, I found them not only in the lateral geniculate body, but also in the cortex. Axo-axonal synapses have been interpreted as a special arrangement for inhibition (Eccles, 1961; Gray, 1962). However, according to other findings (Szentágothai, 1968), the morphology of axo-axonal synapses is incompatible with the theory of presynaptic inhibition. In axo-axonal synapses between the endings of optic fibers and axonal endings of short-axon cells in the lateral geniculate body, for instance, the collection of synaptic vesicles is always in the large ending formed by the optic fiber.

Some writers, notably Estable (1961), consider that the concept of synapses and the neuron theory as a whole must be reexamined. Estable considers that any contact between axons and dendrites, even without the formation of specialized synaptic membranes and including contacts of dendrites and axons with each other, is a synapse.

This view cannot be accepted. The term synapse must be confined to connections in which specialized membranes are formed between the connecting units. There is a good case at the present time for supplementing the list of basic characteristics of interneuronal connections with yet another criterion: the extent of the contacts between two neurons and the number of synaptic endings.

Éntin (1950, 1952, 1954a, 1956, 1959, 1960) made a special study of interneuronal connections in the visual cortex along three lines: (1) the architectonics and structure of synapses, (2) the development of synapses, (3) the systems as revealed by studies of degeneration connections between neurons in the visual cortical and subcortical. She found that contacts between neurons in the cortex are provided mainly by synapses of loop type. The loop synapses are circular, oval, and triangular and vary in size from points to 2–2.5 μ. Synapses are most numerous in the middle and deep layers from III to VI inclusive; the upper layers contain few synapses. The largest number of synapses is found on large star cells of Cajal. They vary in size and are found on the body and processes of the cell. Sometimes in the same section several dozens of synapses can be seen on a number of cells.

Some pyramidal cells in layers III and V are almost completely covered with synapses, located on the body and dendrites.

According to Éntin's observations, development of the synaptic apparatus in the visual cortex of the cat takes place mainly during the postembryonic period of life, as the structure of the nerve cells is increasing in complexity. Solitary loop synapses are present in kittens during the first 2 days of life. In kittens 9–10 days old, with their eyes open, synapses are found in all layers of the cortex as far as the boundary between layers I and II. In 3-month-old cats synapses are numerous. In the adult cat still more synapses are present in the cortex.

The object of Éntin's investigation was to determine where afferent fibers end in the visual cortex and also to discover whether loop synapses are afferent endings. The occipital cortex was isolated in adult cats, i.e., all the afferent pathways leading to the cortex were divided. From 1 to 5 days later, degenerated synapses were demonstrated by the Golgi–Deineka method: swollen and fragmented synapses, and later synapses showing granular degeneration in all the layers, especially from III to VI were found. Degenerated synapses could be seen on the bodies and dendrites of all types of cells; although 5 days later normal synapses could be found in all layers. Éntin concluded that the great majority of synapses are endings of afferent fibers.

After Éntin's first investigations, Yuvchenko (1954) published his dissertation on synapses of the occipital cortex of the dog. He concluded that a specific feature of the cortex is the small number of loop or bouton synapses and that basket plexuses are totally absent from the occipital cortex. Éntin's preparations do not support this view that few such synapses are present in the visual cortex. Moreover, other recent work demonstrates the existence of a very large number of bouton-type synapses in the cortex (Armstrong and Young, 1957; Young, 1958; Polyakov, 1961a), a valuable contribution, especially in view of the fact that a number of investigators still remain sceptical about the number of such synapses in the cortex.

Yuvchenko's view that basket plexuses around the bodies of neurons are completely absent in the dog's cortex also cannot be accepted. Golgi preparations clearly reveal the basketlike character of plexuses which I described in the visual cortex of rabbits and dogs (Shkol'nik-Yarros, 1959b, 1961b). Basket ramifications of axons around the bodies of neurons were described previously by Cajal (1911) and O'Leary (1941) in the visual cortex, and also by Polyakov (1955).

Axo-dendritic Contacts of Cortical Pyramidal Cells

Axo-dendritic connections of cortical pyramidal cells are present at all levels of ramification of their dendrites. The large pyramidal cell can be

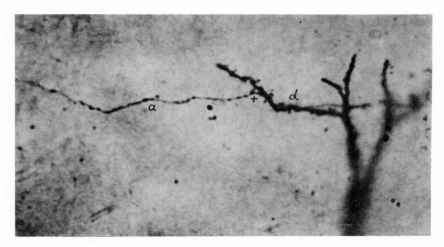

Fig. 83. Contact formed by the apical dendrite of a pyramidal cell in layer III with the tangential branch of an axon in layer I of the dog's cortex. Contact of double type, formed by bouton of the axon and tip of the spine. a, axon; d, dendrite; arrow indicates position of contact. Photomicrograph; 750×.

divided into five parts (excluding its axon): the apical bouquet, the apical trunk, branches of the dendrites in the lower third of the trunk, the cell body, and the basal dendrites. I have observed synapses on all parts of the pyramidal neuron.

The apical bouquet of the pyramidal cell, which ramifies in layer I, forms many contacts with fibers running tangentially. Despite the many descriptions of the structures present in layer I (Cajal, 1900, 1911; Retzius, 1894) no photographs or drawings of these contacts under high power could be discovered in the literature. It is shown in Fig. 83 that an axon collateral in layer I running tangentially forms a contact with the head of a spine on a branch of the apical dendrite of a pyramidal cell in layer III. A very large number of axons spreading along the surface of the cortex may come into contact in this way along its course with bouquets of dendrites from all layers, thus modifying the level of excitation of numerous cells simultaneously.

The apical dendrite of the pyramidal cell possesses contacts not only on its own thin dendritic ramifications, but also on its main trunk. Contacts between the apical trunk and surrounding fibers may be of several different types:

1. Tangential contacts at the tips of spines with surrounding axonal branches. An example of this type of contact in the rabbit's visual cortex can

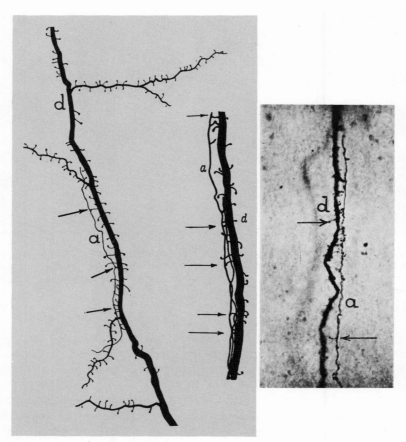

Fig. 84. Contacts (indicated by arrows) between apical dendrites of pyramidal cells and surrounding axons. An axon collateral touches the tips of the spines. Drawn under magnification of 600×. On the right: photomicrograph. Arrows on photomicrograph show similarity between spine on dendrite and branch of axon.

be seen in Fig. 84. The axon collateral appears to run directly along the tip of the spines. Some neighboring spines remain free, presumably being in contact with other axon branches which were not impregnated in the section. Sometimes tangential contacts of considerable extent can be seen when axons of pyramidal cells lying above drop down into the white matter along the course of apical dendrites of pyramidal cells in the lower layers (Fig. 84a).

2. A contact or winding type (Fig. 85; Shkol'nik-Yarros, 1956), in which an axon collateral winds around a dendrite, returning to it repeatedly.

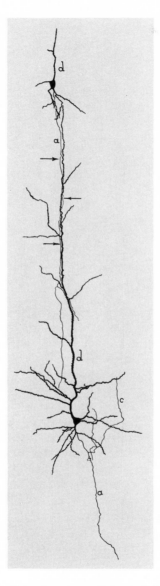

Fig. 84a. Extensive tangential contact between axon of a pyramidal cell in layer III and apical dendrite of a pyramidal cell in layer V of Area 17 of the rabbit. d, dendrite; a, axon; c, axon collateral.

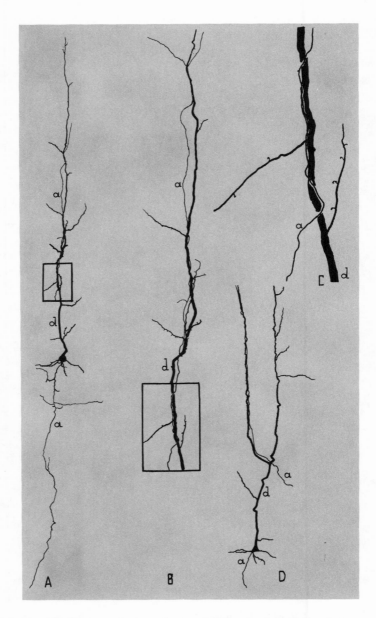

Fig. 85. Winding type of contact in the rabbit's cortex. A: Axon winds around an ascending dendrite of a pyramidal cell in layer V; 100×. B: The same dendrite, 175×. C: The same dendrite, 600×. D: Axon follows the dendrite as far as the upper layers of the cortex. a, axon; d, dendrite.

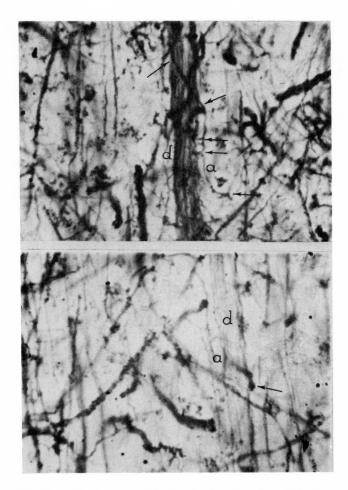

Fig. 85a. Winding contact in the visual cortex of a rabbit. The axon (a) winds around a dendrite (d). Photomicrograph; Golgi–Deineka. (Shkol'nik-Yarros, 1965.)

Whereas other techniques reveal only a small segment of an axon with a dendrite, the method which I used made it possible to see an entire pyramidal cell in layer V with its axon running into the white matter. The axon of another neuron approaches the apical dendrite in its lower third, winds around it, moves a short distance away, and then winds around it again. This pattern is sometimes repeated four times. Under high power (Fig. 85), the close contact between axon and dendrite where this winding takes place can be demonstrated. By the use of another technique I was able to observe contact between the winding branch and the dendrite through large synaptic boutons (Fig. 85a). The picture as a whole bears an extraordinarily close resemblance to a creeper winding around a tree or to the climbing fibers on the Purkinje cells of the cerebellum.

3. An axon collateral follows a dendrite, taking the same path but not winding around it (Fig. 85). I also saw this type of connection in the rabbit cortex. In this case the axon branch resembles an afferent fiber climbing to layer I.

4. Terminal contacts of axon collaterals on the apical dendrite (Fig. 86). These are also of several types: the bouton is in contact either with the dendrite or with the tip of a spine. Frequently only fragments of axons and segments of a dendrite can be seen, but sometimes these processes can be

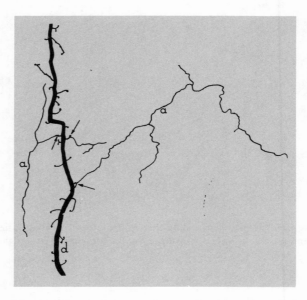

Fig. 86. Terminal contact of axon collaterals on the apical dendrite of a pyramidal cell.

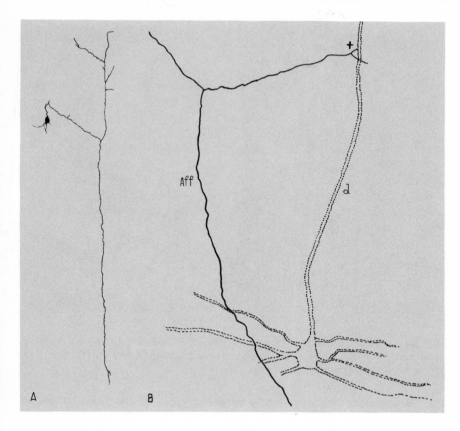

Fig. 87. A: Contact between ascending axon, evidently of a cell of Martinotti, with the apical dendrite of a small pyramidal cell in layer II of a monkey's cortex. B: Contact between a specific afferent and the ascending dendritic trunk (within layer IV) of a pyramidal cell of layer V of the dog's cortex. The pyramidal cell itself was incompletely stained. Aff, afferent fiber; (+) ending of afferent fiber on dendrite (d).

followed for a considerable distance. Contact was frequently observed between an ascending axon (resembling the axon of a cell of Martinotti) and apical dendrites of small pyramidal cells in layer II (Fig. 87) or larger pyramidal neurons of layer III (Fig. 88).

    5. The apical dendrite forms synapses with specific (Fig. 87) and nonspecific afferents. In some cases a large branch rises from the white matter and one of its endings in layer IV forms a contact with the dendritic trunk of a large pyramidal cell of layer V (Fig. 87). In other cases, a thin afferent branch in its upward course gives off collaterals terminating on the apical dendrite of a pyramidal cell situated alongside.

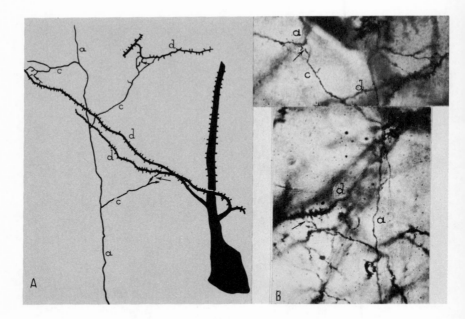

Fig. 88. Contact formed by an ascending axon with spines on dendrites of two pyramidal neurons in the rabbit's cortex. A: Drawn under magnification of 600×. B: Photograph from the same specimen.

Branches of the dendrite in the lower third of the apical trunk are connected synaptically with axon collaterals of stellate short-axon cells and with fibers arising from other parts of the brain. In Fig. 88 the same axon, as it climbs upward, forms contacts simultaneously from two of its collaterals with dendrites of one large pyramidal cell in layer III, while the third collateral is connected with the dendrite of another, neighboring pyramidal cell lying above it. In all these cases contacts are formed on the spines of the dendrites, and sometimes no direct connection with the spine can be seen, while at other times, on the contrary, no gap can be detected between the spine and the axonal ending (Fig. 88, indicated by an arrow). In the last case only the magnification provided by the electron microscope would be sufficient to demonstrate a small space between the two processes.

Contacts of the axon of a typical short-axon stellate cell of layer IV with branches of a dendrite, and also with the apical trunk of a pyramidal cell of layer III of the human cortex are shown in Fig. 89. Communication with the dendritic branch of the main trunk is effected through boutons.

A terminal contact of an axon collateral arising at some distance was observed on the end of a dendrite of a pyramidal cell in layer III of the dog's

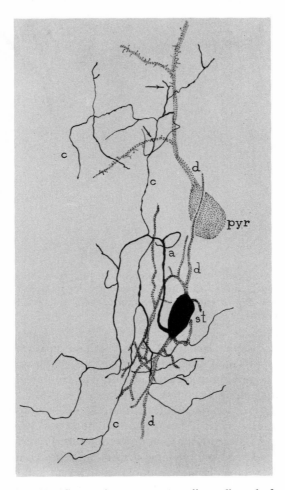

Fig. 89. Contact between an ascending collateral of the axon of a short-axon stellate cell of layer IV and dendrites of a pyramidal cell in Area 19 of man. Only part of the axon is drawn under magnification of 600×, with subsequent reduction. a, axon; d, dendrite; pyr, pyramidal cell; st, stellate cell; c, axon collateral; arrows indicate sites of contacts.

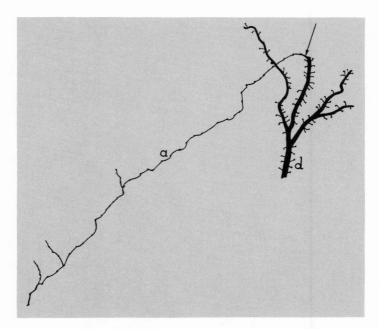

Fig. 90. Axo-dendritic terminal contact of an axon branch with branches of the apical dendrite of a pyramidal cell in layer III of the dog's cortex. Drawn under magnification of 600× followed by reduction. Legend as in Fig. 89.

cortex (Fig. 90). The thin axon collateral, climbing obliquely upward from layer IV into layer III, and supplied with numerous boutons along its course, terminates in a large bouton on the dendrite. The climbing collateral, with numerous boutons along its course, is similar to the short axons of stellate cells although its direction may indicate that it is a collateral of the axon of a pyramidal cell. This particular pyramidal cell possesses clear evidence that it is supplied from different sources at different levels. Figures 83 and 90, for instance, were obtained from the same neuron, and they consequently show that the dendritic bouquet of the pyramidal cell in layer I and branches of the dendritic trunk are connected with different systems of neurons (Fig. 90a).

The basal dendrites of the pyramidal cells form connections with axons of short-axon stellate cells and with specific afferent branches. Most of the fibers drawn in Fig. 91 are axon endings of short-axon stellate cells. Their thin terminal collaterals come into contact with dendrites forming terminal contacts or contacts *"en passant."* A brushlike ramification, similar in shape to an afferent fiber, likewise forms a synapse with the basal dendrites. Terminal contacts on the apical bouquet and tangential contacts with the

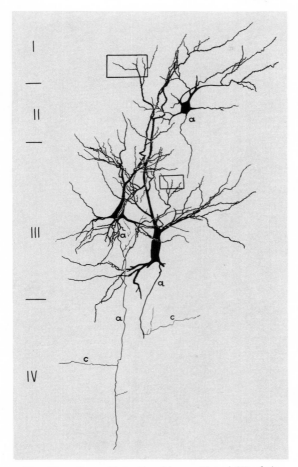

Fig. 90a. Pyramidal cells of layers II and III of the visual cortex of a dog. a, axon; c, axon collateral. Rectangles show areas where dendrites form synapses with axons (Figs. 83 and 90).

trunk along its course and with the branches of the dendrite in the lower third of its trunk were impregnated on this same pyramidal cell. The connection between axon collaterals of a short-axon stellate cell and the basal dendrite of a pyramidal cell can be seen clearly in Fig. 92. The photograph demonstrates numerous axon collaterals and a synaptic contact with the tip of a spine. Terminal contacts on basal dendrites of pyramidal cells also were frequently observed.

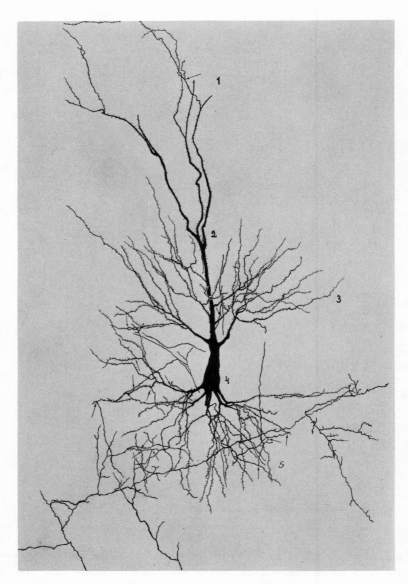

Fig. 91. Large pyramidal cell of layer III of the dog's cortex with surrounding axons. Division into five parts can be seen: 1, apical bouquet; 2, trunk; 3, branches of dendrite in lower third of trunk; 4, cell body; 5, basal dendrites. Arrows indicate positions of contacts between axons and dendrites or their spines. Number of spines on dendrites is 2600. Drawn under magnification of 600× with subsequent reduction. (Shkol'nik-Yarros, 1963.)

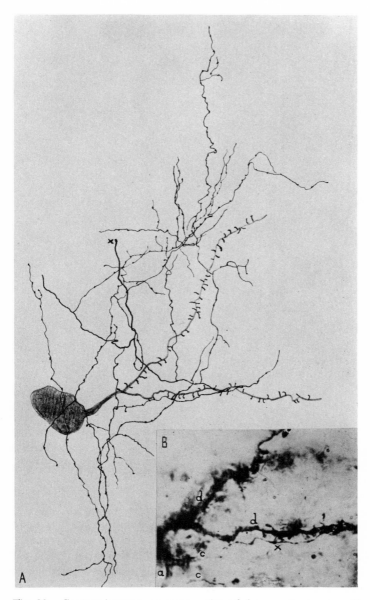

Fig. 92. Contact between an axon collateral from a short-axon cell and dendritic spines of a stellate pyramidal cell of layer IV of the rabbit's cortex. A: Drawing. B: Photomicrograph of the site of contact. Immersion. In A, × denotes the origin of the axon from a short-axon cell whose body is not drawn. (Shkol'nik-Yarros, 1950a.)

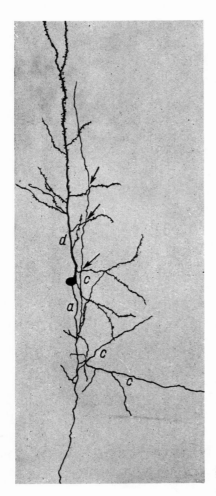

Fig. 93. Contact of the axon of a pyramidal cell "with itself" in the rabbit's cortex. a, axon; c, collateral; d, dendrite; arrows denote points of contact.

One of the various types of synapses on pyramidal cells is that known as the contact with itself. One of these "self" contacts of a pyramidal cell in the visual cortex of a rabbit is shown in Fig. 93. A recurrent axon collateral, as it runs upward, forms three contacts with dendrites, given off from the main trunk at different levels. A contact "with itself" in the cortex of a dog is shown in Fig. 94, where the connection also is formed by a recurrent collateral, but this time it does not proceed further but terminates on that dendrite so that a terminal connection is thus formed.

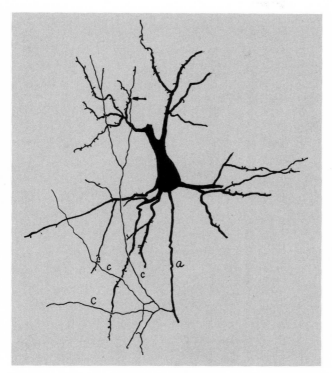

Fig. 94. Contact formed by a pyramidal cell in the dog's cortex "with itself." The axon gives off an ascending collateral which ends on the dendrite of the same cell. Drawn under magnification of 600×; a, axon; c, collateral; arrow denotes point of contact.

Axo-somatic Connections of Cortical Pyramidal Cells

I found several different types of axo-somatic connections with the bodies of pyramidal cells. To begin with, I confirmed the formation of nests for cortical cell bodies (Cajal). In successfully impregnated sections the origin of the axon forming the nest could be detected from the body of a short-axon stellate cell (Fig. 36). An axo-somatic contact of a branch climbing obliquely upward and the body of a small pyramidal cell of layer II of the visual cortex was also observed in a monkey (Fig. 95, A). The axon branch ascending up to layers I–II may be either an axon collateral of a pyramidal cell or the ending of an association afferent fiber. It terminates in a small bouton in contact with the cell body. Another type is the contact formed *"en*

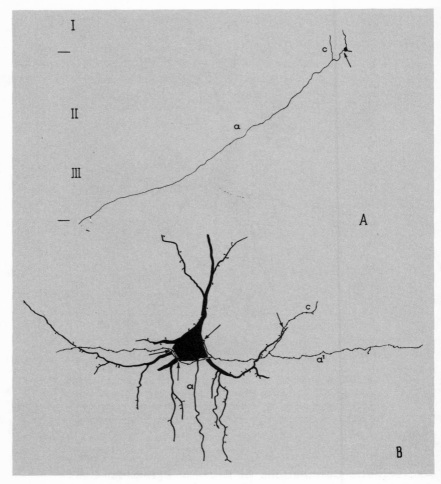

Fig. 95. A: Axo-somatic contact of an ascending axon collateral with the body of a small pyramidal cell in layer II of Area 17 of a monkey. B: Contact between the axon of a short-axon stellate cell and the body and basal dendrites of a pyramidal cell in layer IV of Area 17 of the dog. a, axon of pyramidal cell; a¹, axon of short-axon cell; c, axon collateral; arrows denote points of contacts.

passant" by the axon of a short-axon stellate cell (Fig. 95, B). One small collateral branch terminates in a bouton on the cell body, while other boutons along the course of the axon are in contact with the cell body near the place from which the basal dendrites emerge (shown by the arrows on the left). Another collateral of the same axon forms connections with the basal dendrite through a spine (arrow on the extreme right).

The third type of axo-somatic connections with bodies of pyramidal cells is represented by contacts *"en passant"* with axons of short-axon stellate cells. In this type of synapse (Fig. 96) several arrangements of contact are observed—either as coils with boutons at their end, or as one or several boutons along their course. The turns of the axon collaterals and their

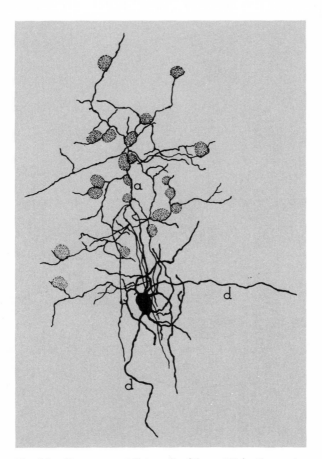

Fig. 96. Short-axon stellate cell of layer IV in the cortex of the green monkey (*Cercopithecus sabaeus*). The axon forms axo-somatic connections with surrounding bodies of neurons shown in the figure as stippled areas. (Shkol'nik-Yarros, 1963.)

terminal branches can be seen clearly to wind around the cell, matching its outlines. A typical axon of a stellate cell of layer IV of the visual cortex of the green monkey (*Cercopithecus sabaeus*) is illustrated in Fig. 96. Along the course of the axon, boutons contact surrounding cells, and frequently two or three boutons form synapses on the body of a single neuron. Sometimes the terminal branches of an axon form a cup-shaped hollow in which a cell body fits (the uppermost contact on the right). Some of the stippled structures illustrated in this figure are bodies of pyramidal cells, although the

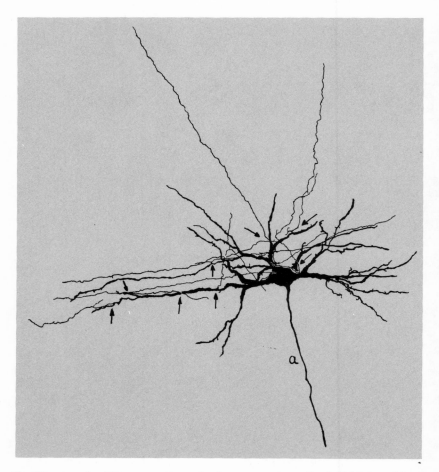

Fig. 97. Axo-dendritic connections of a long-axon star cell of Cajal in sublayer IVb of the visual cortex of a monkey. a, axon of Cajal's cell; arrows denote sites of contacts.

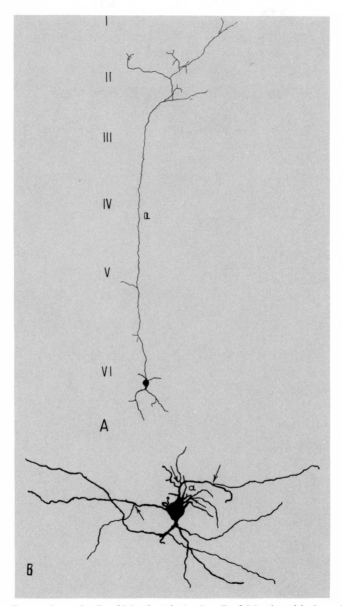

Fig. 98. Connections of cells of Martinotti. A: A cell of Martinotti in layer VI of the dog's cortex (Area 18). Ending of axon in layer I, of collateral in layer II. B: Axo-dendritic contacts of cells of Martinotti. Area 17 of adult man. Intracortical connections with association axons. a, axon; arrows indicate points of contacts between boutons of axons and dendrites of the cell depicted.

great majority of them are stellate cells of various types. It is interesting to note that contacts *"en passant"* with bodies of neighboring neurons are formed not only through thin preterminal branches of the axon, but also through its thicker, more proximal segments.

Axo-dendritic Contacts of Cortical Stellate Cells

Axo-dendritic connections with the star cells of Cajal are formed by means of long horizontal and smaller vertical axon collaterals (Fig. 97). Thin axon collaterals or endings, running in the direction of horizontal fibers of Gennari's band, form tangential contacts with spines or dendritic trunks. The predominant direction of the axons suggests that they are branches of afferent fibers which, as they arrive in the visual cortex from other parts of the brain, ascend vertically upward, and then ramify at right angles at the level of layer IV (Figs. 43 and 61).

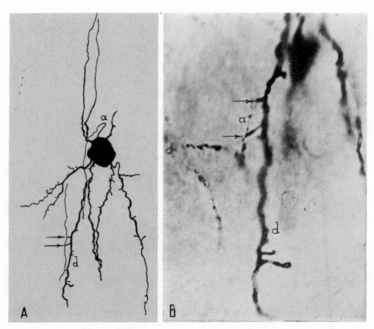

Fig. 99. Tangential contact of an axon collateral with the infrequent spines on dendrites of a short-axon stellate cell of the rabbit's cortex. Drawing (A) and photograph (B) of the zone of contact between the axon and spines. a, axon; d, dendrite; arrows show sites of contact. Immersion; 1500×. (Shkol'nik-Yarros, 1956.)

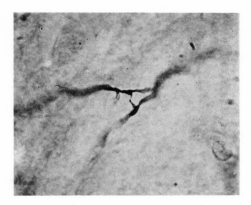

Fig. 100. Contact of an axon collateral with the spine on a dendrite of a short-axon stellate cell. Photomicrograph; immersion. Golgi preparation.

Connections are also observed with the large oblique afferent fibers, which are most widespread in the cortex of rodents and carnivores. These axons give off a branch running obliquely upward and forming contacts with spines on dendrites of stellate cells in layer IV.

Axo-dendritic connections with cells of Martinotti are formed by axonal endings running in different directions. Figure 98 shows that thin fibrils terminate in a small bouton almost on the dendrite itself. These thin fibrils are not the endings of afferent fibers, which have typical outlines; from their structure they can be regarded as intracortical connections. An intracortical connection in the form of axo-dendritic contacts is also observed on typical short-axon stellate cells. Long, thin spines on the dendrite of such a cell (Figs. 99 and 100) are connected by their heads with very thin axons running past them.

Axo-somatic Contacts of Cortical Stellate Cells

Axo-somatic connections with the bodies of stellate cells are formed most frequently, especially in layer IV of the visual cortex, by different types of afferent axons. A large afferent fiber from the stria of Gennari, running horizontally, gives off a thin branch, climbing upward, with numerous synaptic boutons, and two of its endings form connections with the body of a star cell of Cajal (Fig. 101) shown as a stippled area.

The completely impregnated ending of a specific afferent branch revealed the formation of numerous axo-somatic contacts along its course with bodies of small short-axon stellate cells in sublayer IVc in the visual

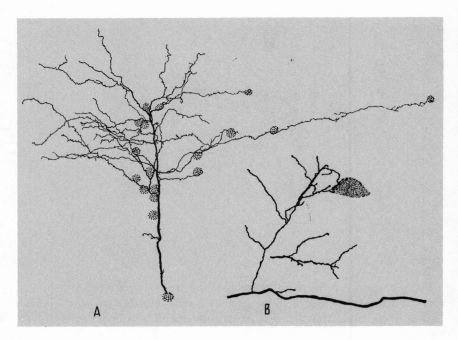

Fig. 101. A: Specific afferent in sublayer IVc of visual cortex of the green monkey (*Cercopithecus sabaeus*). Axo-somatic connection with bodies of surrounding small short-axon cells shown in the figure by stippling. B: Axo-somatic contact of specific afferent with the body of a star cell of Cajal. Sublayer IVb of Area 17 of man. The cell body is visible in the section and indicated by stippling (Shkol'nik-Yarros, 1961a).

cortex of the green monkey. The axon either keeps close to part of the cell body and then proceeds further or it forms a cup-shaped hollow at its end, in which the body of one of the neighboring cells fits.

In this way one afferent branch can bring many hundreds of neurons into a state of excitation at the same time (Fig. 101). Some afferent "brushes" run obliquely from above down, and the branches which they give off terminate as large boutons on the round bodies of short-axon cells concentrated in sublayer IVc (Fig. 102).

Besides this important connection between the cells described above and afferent axons entering the cortex, the short-axon cells are also connected with each other. The axon of each small cell forms a delicate and thin plexus for communication with neighboring round cells (Fig. 48). These connections are most numerous in sublayer IVc, where the cell density is highest. In other layers short-axon cells also form contacts with each other. A typical short-axon stellate cell of layer III with well-marked dendrites and axon is rep-

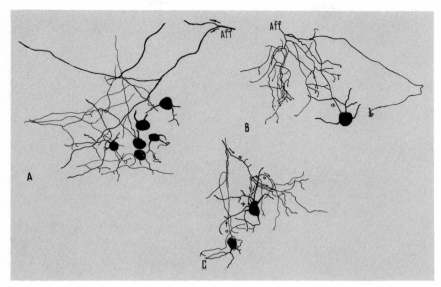

Fig. 102. Specific afferent ramifications in sublayer IVc of Area 17 of the green monkey. A: Large oblique fiber descending from sublayer IVb into sublayer IVc, thin axonal endings and the bodies of small, short-axon, stellate cells are also visible. B: Small short-axon cell of sublayer IVc; a, axon; Aff, afferent fiber whose endings have boutonlike thickenings and are of various shapes. C: Two short-axon cells in sublayer IVc; a, their axons; a[1], terminal ramification of axon whose collateral approaches the cell body; (+) synaptic boutons. Drawn under magnification of 600×. (Shkol'nik-Yarros, 1955a.)

resented in Fig. 103. It is clear that the axon is in contact with the body of neighboring cells either along its course (on the left) or at its end (on the right) by means of boutons, adapting its course to the shape of the cells. The shape of the shadowed area reveals that in this case (especially the uppermost contacts on the left) a synaptic connection exists with the bodies of stellate cells but not of pyramidal cells. The numerous ramifications of a particular axon, which cannot always be followed as far as its terminal branches, can influence very many neighboring neurons at the same time. Single terminal synaptic boutons or double or more complex endings are adapted for contact with the cell body. Bouton, loops, and coils along the course of the whole axon also form axo-somatic contacts *"en passant"* with the cell bodies. Figure 96 demonstrates the axon of a stellate cell forming numerous synapses with bodies of neurons, shown by stippling on the sections under high power.

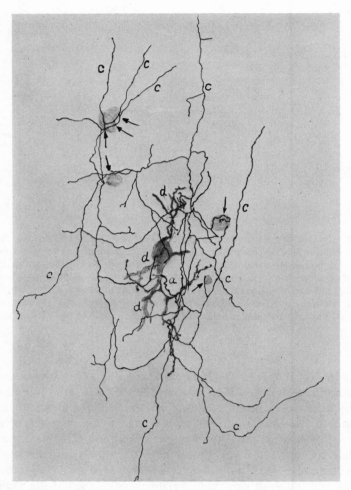

Fig. 103. Short-axon stellate cell of layer III in Area 18 of man. Ramifications of an axon are seen. The cell body, dendrites, and bodies of surrounding cells are shown by stippling. Drawn under magnification of 600×. a, axon; c, axon collateral; d, dendrite; arrows indicate sites of contacts.

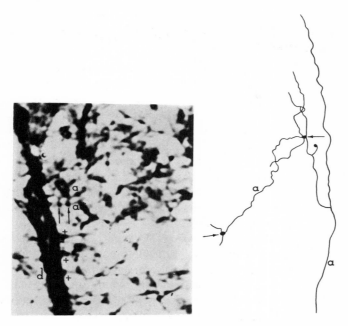

Fig. 104. Axo-axonal contacts. On the left: apical dendrite of a triangular cell in layer V of Area 17 of *Macaca mulatta*. Crosses (+) denote areas where axon boutons form synapses with a dendrite trunk. Arrows indicate axo-axonal contacts between two axons which terminate in axo-dendritic synapses. Photomicrograph; objective 150×, immersion. Golgi–Deineka method. On the right: axo-axonal connection between axon collateral and axon of two short-axon cells. Rabbit cortex. Drawing, Golgi's method.

Axo-axonal Connections in the Cortex

I also observed connections between axon and axon in the cortex. In some cases a small axon winds around a larger. This state of affairs was observed in layers VI and VII of the human visual cortex. The large axon is most probably the axon of a large pyramidal cell departing from the cortex. The small fiber winding around it is probably the axon collateral of a short-axon stellate cell. In other cases (Fig. 104), a typical synaptic bouton is in contact with an axon running vertically at right angles. By impregnation with Golgi's method and Glees' method, I demonstrated axo-axonal connections of a perpendicular character with axons running vertically.

Axo-axonal synapses are also observed on the axon hillock. Observations with the optical microscope thus demonstrate that such synapses may be found at the origin of the axon, along its course, and before its termination on the dendrite (see also Shkol'nik-Yarros, 1965).

Axo-dendritic and Axo-somatic Contacts of Cells of the Lateral Geniculate Body

The shape and distribution of synapses in the lateral geniculate body of the rabbit were studied by Glees (1942), and in the cat and monkey by Glees (1941, 1958), Le Gros Clark (1941), and Glees *et al.* (1958). In the rabbit Glees found terminal loops as large as the nucleolus, and sometimes they were joined into groups and formed clusters. Many endings were connected not only with the body, but also with the dendrites. In the cat, about 40 terminal loops of visual afferent fibers may be counted on the cell bodies and dendrites. Axo-dendritic synapses are more numerous than axo-somatic. One visual fiber covers with its terminal branches an area containing about 10 cells. Glees considers that the same area is supplied by other visual fibers as well, so that overlapping takes place.

Many textbooks (Glees and Le Gros Clark, 1941) give a scheme for the endings of visual fibers in the lateral geniculate body of the monkey. The workers cited used Glees's method. In alternate layers after division of the optic nerve they found degeneration of endings which are large, long, black in color, and clearly visible even under low power. Some endings showed less severe degeneration (mainly in the magnocellular layers), and sometimes a normal terminal loop was visible.

Glees and Le Gros Clark conclude that each visual fiber turns away from the fiber bundles and divides into five or six branches, with one large synapse at their ends in contact with the body of a single cell. The function of the lateral geniculate body is to transmit visual excitation to the cortex. They associated the unique structure of the synaptic apparatus with the precision of transmission of the visual image in primates.

I cannot accept the view that axo-dendritic contacts are absent, and I consider that this conclusion can be explained by the method which they used. If it were true, what would be the role of the dendrites? Other evidence against this conclusion is the number of branches of the visual fibers and the number of endings on each neuron (Shkol'nik-Yarros, 1961b) (Fig. 57). As was pointed out in Chapter 1, these fibers are highly variable.

Balmasova (1950) observed synapses of many different types on the bodies and dendrites of neurons in the lateral geniculate body of the rabbit, cat, and dog. Synapses consisting of terminal and *"en passant"* loops, rings, boutons, chains, networks, and very thin fibrils, and also more complex endings of brush type, are present on the large, medium-sized, and small neurons of the lateral geniculate body. More synapses are present on dendrites than on the body of the neuron.

Synapses on the proximal segments of dendrites form a continuous sleeve, but they are also visible on parts of the dendrite further from the cell body. Often synapses occur in groups. Balmasova postulates that a group of synapses belongs to the ending of one axon and suggests that grouping plays the role of summation of impulses and of their conduction in a particular direction. Endings are not so numerous on neurons of the lateral geniculate body of the rabbit as in the cat and dog, and complex synapses are absent.

Silva (1956) used the Nauta–Gygax method and obtained a picture of alternate degeneration of axons and terminal boutons in the lateral geniculate body of the cat, thus confirming Minkowski's results concerning representation of the eyes in layers. He accepts the possibility of ephaptic conduction of excitation, in an attempt to explain the discrepancy between strict separation of one layer from another and interaction between the layers (Bishop and Davis, 1953) and also the existence of cycles of spontaneous excitation (Bishop et al., 1953).

Degeneration of synapses on cells of the lateral geniculate body of the cat was also seen by Obukhova (1958, 1959). Normally between 2–3 and 40–50 synapses 0.5–2.5μ in diameter are seen on the cells (fewer of them on small cells). The synapses have the appearance of rings, loops, or are lanceolate; in some of them a network of neurofibrils is visible. Synapses are numerous in all parts of the dorsal nucleus, axo-somatic more so than axo-dendritic, and they are especially numerous on cells located between projection fibers and on cells (mainly on the dendrites) of the dorsal reticular formation.

Hayhow (1958, 1959) used the Nauta–Gygax method to study distribution of fibers in the lateral geniculate body of the cat. He considers that cells unilaterally supplied with synapses from one eye alternate with cells receiving preterminal branches from both crossed and uncrossed fibers. He accordingly counts as many as nine layers in the medial portion of the nucleus, postulating the existence of latent striation and fields of overlapping. Fibers of small caliber mainly end on medium-sized cells, larger fibers on large cells. The pars dorsalis B is supplied almost entirely with fibers of small caliber. Hayhow, Sefton, and Webb (1962) discovered latent striation also in the lateral geniculate body of the rabbit.

Synapses of the lateral geniculate body of the cat have been studied with the electron microscope. Szentágothai (1963b, 1965) and Szentágothai, Hamori, and Tömböl (1966) found complex synaptic glomeruli which included three types of axons forming contacts with the distal parts of dendrites of lateral geniculate body cells. Besides glomeruli, there are also axo-dendritic synapses along the course of the dendrites and occasional axo-somatic synapses. Guillery (1967a) found synapses richly supplied with nerve filaments (filamentous synapses), also forming a glomerular complex. According to Peters and Palay (1966), five types of axons form synapses with the principal neurons in layers A and A_1 of the lateral geniculate body in cats.

I shall now turn to the description of my own material.

Axo-dendritic connections in the lateral geniculate body differ depending on the type of neuron with which the synapse is formed. Contacts of this sort are particularly numerous on dendrites of cells resembling neurons with few branches in the reticular formation. Many terminal branches of axons approach the long dendrites from all sides and terminate in boutons. The axons are thinner than the dendrites which they approach, and sometimes possess boutons along their course. They frequently run perpendicular to the dendrite and sometimes have a distinct terminal bouton. Many axo-dendritic connections with the dendrites of cells with few branches in the human lateral geniculate body are demonstrated in Fig. 105.

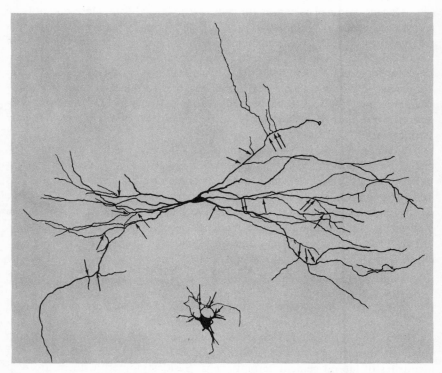

Fig. 105. Top: Cell with few branches in the human lateral geniculate body; arrows indicate formation of axo-dendritic contacts with axons approaching the dendrites. Below: Midget cell of the human lateral geniculate body with few dendrites spreading only a short distance. The endings of three single fibrils can be seen on the dendrites of this cell in larger synaptic boutons.

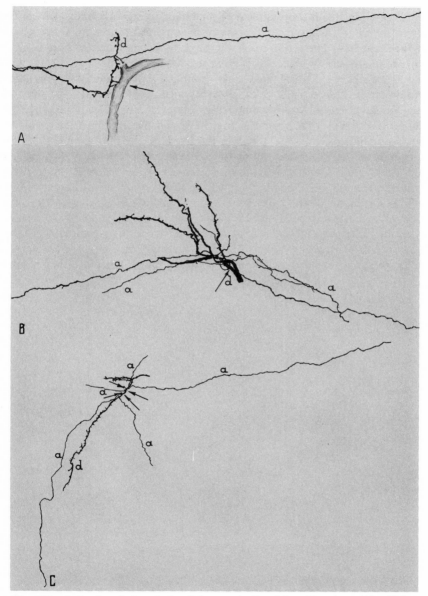

Fig. 106. Lateral geniculate body of the cat. A: Dendrite with spines with which an axon forms a contact "*en passant.*" The shadow of a capillary is shown, connected with the dendrite through its spines (arrow). B: Dendrite with spines. Axo-dendritic synapses with axons passing by them. C: Five terminal contacts on a dendrite; axon terminals approach the dendrite from different sides. a, axon; d, dendrite.

The midget cells more typical of the lateral geniculate body possess far fewer axo-dendritic contacts because of the small number and short length of the dendrites. Three thin axonal endings with large boutons in contact with dendrites of a midget cell may be seen in Fig. 105.

Drawings were also made of a number of successfully impregnated axo-dendritic connections in order to confirm the existence not only of tangential, collateral synapses on the dendrites, but also of terminal synapses. Tangential synapses are visible in Fig. 106B and five terminal axo-dendritic synapses can be seen in Fig. 106C. In the last case the thin axon collaterals, with boutons here and there along their course, are in contact with a thicker dendrite covered with spines. Axons run as single branches toward the dendrite from all sides, possibly indicating their completely different origin.

Axo-somatic connections in the lateral geniculate body also have the form of terminal and collateral synapses. The terminal synapses are formed by contact between a large terminal bouton or two or three terminal boutons, forming a cuplike hollow (Fig. 107), with the body of a neuron. Numerous collateral synapses can also be observed in this figure. They are very similar

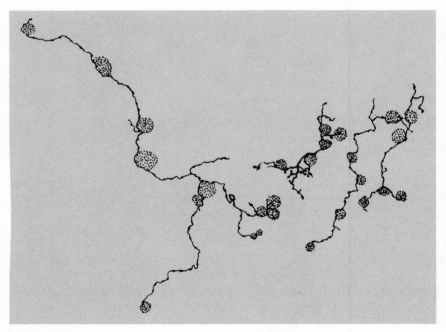

Fig. 107. Lateral geniculate body of the cat. Axo-somatic connections of afferent fibers from the retina with bodies of neurons indicated by stippling.

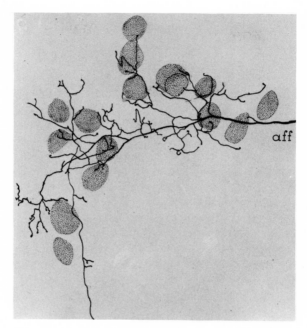

Fig. 108. Axo-somatic contacts of an axon branch in the pretectal nucleus of the dog's brain. Drawn under magnification of 600× with subsequent reduction. Cell bodies shown by stippling.

to the former, the only difference being that after the formation of the contact the axon does not terminate but runs on toward the next cell. Only the most distinct shadows of the bodies of neighboring cells are drawn, and in some cases the bodies hang like bunches of grapes from branches of large axons. A similar bunch of axo-somatic contacts was also seen in the pretectal nucleus of the dog (Fig. 108). Terminal branches from a large afferent fiber wind around the bodies of neurons, in contact with them through terminal boutons.

The drawing of one field in the lateral geniculate body of the cat shows the formation of pericellular structures from two or three axons. In some cases where complex interweaving of axons takes place (Fig. 109) the same axon can be seen to surround the cell body almost completely, while in other cases one afferent fiber is in contact with one side of the cell body and a second fiber with the other side. The presence of synaptic boutons from two different axons can be seen most clearly in Fig. 110. The largest afferent fibers give off thinner branches terminating in boutons or forming tangential

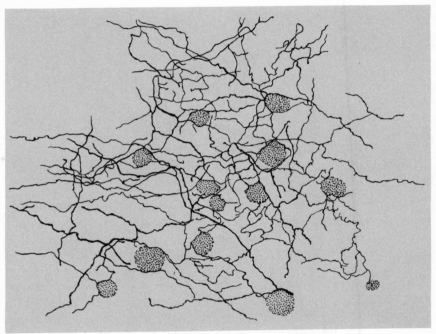

Fig. 109. Lateral geniculate body of the cat. One field of vision drawn under magnification of 600× with subsequent reduction. Complex interweaving of axons with the formation of tangential and terminal contacts on the bodies of neurons represented by stippling.

contacts with boutons on the body of a cell indicated by stippling. Terminal axo-dendritic contacts from more diffuse single fibers are also shown in the same illustration.

Hence, axo-somatic and axo-dendritic synapses can be seen in the lateral geniculate body. They may be either terminal or collateral. Their number depends on the type of neuron and the length of its dendrites.

Axo-dendritic contacts which have been found (Figs. 105, 106) are evidently not glomerular connections formed along the course of dendrites. Synapses with the bodies of cells are demonstrated in Figs. 107 and 109, a variety of synapse rarely detected by electron microscopic investigation. I observed axo-axonal connections in the human lateral geniculate body; small, thin axons formed contacts with large endings of visual fibers. Axo-axonal connections were discovered in the lateral geniculate body of the cat by Szentágothai (1963a,b), Peters and Palay (1966), and Guillery (1967a), and in that of the monkey by Colonnier and Guillery (1964).

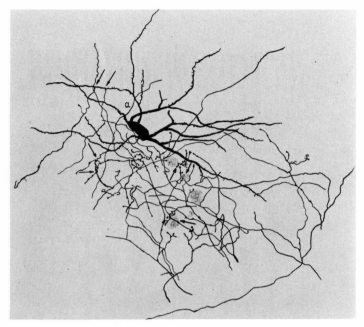

Fig. 110.   Lateral geniculate body of the cat. Long-axon cell surrounded by afferent fibers. Afferent branches form axo-dendritic and axo-somatic contacts (arrows). Axo-somatic contacts are formed mainly by clusters of endings with fairly large boutons. Usually single branches approach the dendrites. Bodies of neurons are shown by stippling. a, axon.

Connections in the Retina

A special description of the retina will be given later. At this stage I shall consider only the general scheme of the rod system of the retina (Fig. 111) based on my studies of the rabbit and dog retinas impregnated by the Golgi technique, and on published data.

The scheme shows the great variety of forms of synapses in the retina itself and their difference from synapses in the central part of the visual system. Dendrites and spines of bipolar cells vary in size and shape. The synaptic system may vary on the same bipolar cell. Differences in size and shape of synapses of the bipolar cells (Fig. 76A), amacrine cells, and horizontal cells (Fig. 76B) can be seen. Each type of neuron in the retina has its own distinctive morphology of its axonal and dendritic ending. This specificity is much more marked than in central parts of the visual system.

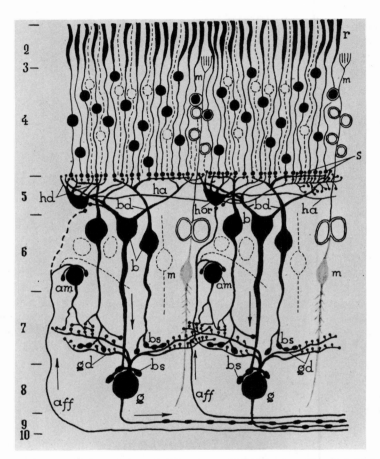

Fig. 111. Scheme of the rod system of the mammalian retina based on Golgi preparations of the dog's retina and also on published data. 2, layer of photoreceptors; 3, outer limiting membrane; 4, outer nuclear layer; 5, outer plexiform layer; 6, inner nuclear layer; 7, inner plexiform layer; 8, layer of ganglion cells; 9, layer of nerve fibers; 10, inner limiting membrane; r, rods; s, synaptic boutons of rods; b, bipolar cells; bd, dendrites of bipolar cells; bs, large terminal structures of axons of bipolar cells; am, amacrine cell; hor, horizontal cell; hd, dendrites of horizontal cell; ha, axon of horizontal cell; g, ganglion cell; gd, dendrites of ganglion cell; m, fiber Müller; aff, centrifugal fiber. The basic features of the rod system are illustrated in the scheme; cones and the cone system are not shown. Differences between the synapses of bipolar, horizontal, and amacrine cells are noteworthy.

The scheme also shows the centrifugal pathway starting from other parts of the nervous system and ending on the bodies of the amacrine cells (Cajal, 1909–1911; Dogel', 1895; Shkol'nik-Yarros, 1955b, 1961a, etc.) and also possibly on the bodies of the horizontal cells (Pilipenko, 1961).

Relationships between the photoreceptors (rods) and other retinal elements in a generalized form can be seen. However, I did not undertake any quantitative investigation.

Despite the many excellent electron microscopic studies of the retina (Sjöstrand, 1958; Kidd, 1962; Borovyagin, 1963, 1966; Dowling and Boycott, 1966; Dowling, 1968), I consider a preliminary investigation of the retina by bichromate-silver impregnation absolutely essential in order to obtain some idea of its general structure.

REALITY OF THE SYSTEMS OF SPINES ON DENDRITES; THEIR ORIGIN AND ROLE

The study of interneuronal connections was not conceived as a separate, special investigation, but from the numerous facts accumulated during the study of the visual cortex some generalizations can be deduced.

There would seem to be no doubt about the existence of spines on dendrites of neurons belonging to the central nervous system. However, many histologists are not convinced of the reality of these structures. Voronin and Kuparadze (1958) declared that structures found after experimentally induced swelling of axons and dendrites are very similar in the character of the changes and in their external appearance to the structures at present known as spines and synapses. This fact led them to express doubts about the existence of endings of the type regarded as axo-somatic and axo-dendritic connections. Similar doubts were also expressed by Cholokashvili (1958a). Vinnikov (1962) has repeatedly stated that he regards spines as an artifact or as part of the glial system. Other histologists and physiologists have repeatedly declared their scepticism concerning the existence of spines on dendrites.

Synapses consisting of terminal loops, rings and other forms, which are very clearly demonstrated in the spinal cord (Cajal, 1903; Hoff, 1932; Gibson, 1937; Zurabashvili, 1947; Lavrov, 1949; Pchelina, 1951; Plechkova, 1961; Zhukova, 1960) and in the subcortex (Glees, 1941; Glees and Le Gros Clark, 1941; Balmasova, 1950; Obukhova, 1958) are difficult to demonstrate in the cortex. The technical difficulties of demonstrating synapses in the cortex led to the view that pericellular structures in the cortex are mainly of the basket type, without special synaptic endings (Glees, 1946; Snesarev, 1950; Sholl, 1956) or alternatively, that only single synapses are present on cortical cells and that basket ramifications are completely absent (Yuv-

chenko, 1954). Smythies and Inman (1960) suggest that terminal axon structures can be stained only after degeneration, or that they are simply
breakdown products arising as a result of autolysis, and not synapses.
Boycott, Gray, and Guillery (1960), in a special study, put forward a theory
to explain the absence of end plates in the cortex in sections impregnated
with silver. According to this theory, synapses rarely contain filaments
corresponding to neurofibrils, and for this reason they cannot be revealed
by neurofibrillary stains.

However, as stated above, some workers succeeded in demonstrating
synapses quite clearly in the cortex by silver impregnation methods.

Details of interneuronal connections can now be determined by the
electron microscope, and relationships between processes and bodies of
neurons are gradually becoming known (Palay, 1958; Gray, 1959, 1961;
Hamlyn, 1963).

Living synapses were demonstrated originally in Lavrent'ev's laboratory and more recently again by Maiorov (1960).

The situation is different with respect to spines on the dendrites. In
reports of many electron microscopic investigations they are not mentioned,
and the reader may be left with the false impression that they are absent. It
seems necessary, therefore, to summarize the facts already given in the
survey of the literature (in pp. 124–127, 135–140) and in the description of
my own observations (pp. 127–134, 140–154), on the basis of which it can be
asserted that the spines are a component part of the dendrite, a contact
structure developing regularly in ontogenesis and phylogenesis:

1. Spines can be detected on dendrites not only by bichromate-silver
impregnation, but also by staining with methylene blue.

2. Spines are found with great constancy on the dendrites of many
neurons and with a definite localization.

3. Spines are regular in shape, they often appear as small branches in
continuation of the dendrite, and sometimes they have a head on their end.

4. Spines develop regularly in ontogenesis, appearing in a definite
order in areas and layers of the cortex.

5. Spines are present on dendrites of neurons not only in man, but also
in many different orders of mammals (insectivores, rodents, carnivores,
primates).

6. Lability of the spines relative to pathological agents has frequently
been demonstrated.

7. Contacts between spines and axon collaterals have been found.
Synapses of this type, confirmed by photomicrograph, have been described
by Polyakov (1955, 1961b), Shkol'nik-Yarros (1950a, 1955a, 1956, 1961b,
1963), Leontovich (1952, 1958), Zhukova (1950, 1960), Gray (1959, 1961),
and others.

Gray's work is particularly important in providing conclusive electron microscopic proof of the synaptic nature of the spine with a magnification of the order of $10,000 \times$.

8.   It has also been shown that during ontogenesis closure of temporary connections can only take place if spines are present on the terminal branches of dendrites, coinciding with the third stage of development of the neuron, i.e., with the appearance of definitive Nissl granules (containing ribonucleic acid) and a differentiated nucleolus (Ivanitskii, 1958).*

In the present study, several problems concerning spines are of interest: their variability, differences at different levels of the central visual system, varieties of contacts in which they take part, their resemblance to axon branches and, finally, their connection with particular structures of the neuron.

Variability of the spines is interesting from the point of view of the specialized structures of the visual system. Spines of the pyramidal cells are known to differ from spines of short-axon stellate cells in their length, the density of their distribution, and the character of their head (Polyakov, 1953). Spines on posterior horn cells of the spinal cord differ sharply from spines on the anterior horn cells (Geier, 1904; Zhukova, 1960). Definite differences are found between spines on dendrites of neurons of the reticular formation and of specific brain-stem nuclei (Zhukova, 1959), or between cells of the corpus striatum and the globus pallidus, or the specific and nonspecific nuclei of the thalamus (Leontovich, 1952, 1959b).

However, I consider that even on neurons of the same type there is considerable variability of the spines on their dendrites. The variability is expressed by differences in length, in the position and shape of the head, and in the number of boutonlike endings at the tip or along the course of the spine. Under high power, spines of many different shapes can be seen on the same dendrite (Figs. 78, 82, 84, 86), and sometimes all forms are represented from a short spine with the typical head to a long, narrow, rod-shaped process without a head. The direction and angle of inclination of the lateral appendage to the dendrite also varies widely. Spines were most varied on the cells of Martinotti in the rabbit cortex. Spines on pyramidal cells are more constant in shape but even they possess a wide range of variation.

The shape of the spine is mainly dependent on three factors (under normal conditions). The first factor is the type of neuron. Small, short-axon star cells of sublayer IVc of the monkey's cortex have spines on

---

* Changes are found in spines on dendrites of pyramidal cells in layer IV of the visual cortex of mice after loss of visual input; they decrease in number (Valverde, 1967) or change in shape (Globus and Scheibel, 1967). For a survey of some of the most recent research concerning dendritic spines, see Scheibel and Scheibel (1968).

their dendrites only very rarely, for varicosities are a more characteristic feature. Conversely, large, star cells of sublayer IVb have on their dendrites appendages similar to the spines on the dendrites of pyramidal cells. However, this is by no means a rigid law or general rule, for I have shown that several typical short-axon cells in layer IV of the visual cortex of the rabbit and dog possess dendrites covered with spines (Fig. 80). The second factor of importance is the direction of the axonal ending or collateral as it approaches the dendrite and spine. In some cases the spine appears to be the direct continuation of the axon branch, and a gap between them can be detected only with the electron microscope; in other cases the spine looks as if it is drawn toward the axon collateral as it runs close by.

Finally, the mobility of these tiny appendages may perhaps play a role. The normal mobility of small appendages of nerve tissue was described by the classical neurologists.

In neural tissue cultures Troitskaya (1954) also observed mobility of dendrites. Pomerat (1952) recorded mobility of the processes of neurons and neuroglia by microcinematography. Mobility on a very small scale, a property of all living tissues observable under normal conditions, is mentioned by Veize and Frank (1960). An inspection of all the illustrations (with magnifications of the order of $10,000\times$) given by Gray (1959, 1961) shows that all spines differ, within narrow limits, in their various characteristics such as length, thickness, direction, and so on. Consequently, differences reflected in my own drawings (made under high power), and photographed, can be regarded as fully objective, and they provide evidence to support the view that small processes and endings normally possess mobility (Figs. 78, 82, 84, 86, etc.).

Various opinions are held on the origin of spines. Besides the "artifact theory," already mentioned, two other principal theories exist. Cajal (1935), until the last years of his life, was doubtful of the existence of contacts on spines and he considered that they are a component part of the dendrite. This view has also been adopted by many other workers. Bodian (1940) was in no doubt whatever about the opposite view, i.e., spines are a part of axonal endings approaching a dendrite. Lorente de Nó (1934) was unable to state definitely whether spines are axonal endings or part of the dendrite. Fox and Barnard (1957) also vacillated, and did not rule out the possibility that spines may be axonal in origin.

My own studies of the structure of spines and axo-dendritic connections began in 1948. I frequently found pictures in the cortex of different mammals which created the impression of the axonal origin of a spine, especially if it has not one, but several heads along its course. In these cases the longer part of the axon was not impregnated, while the part of it close to the dendrite together with its characteristic boutons appears on the specimen. In Fig. 112,

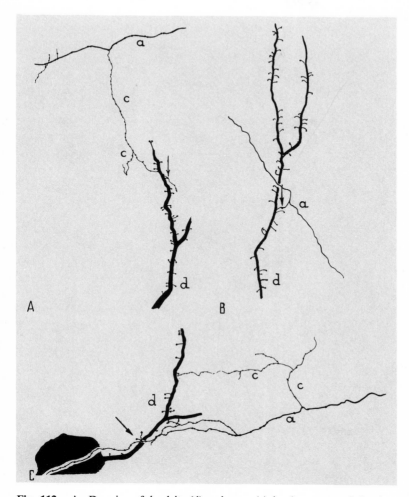

Fig. 112. A: Drawing of dendrite (d) and axon (a) in the cortex of the dog. Axon gives off branches with boutons which could be taken for spines of a dendrite (arrow). B: Drawing of a dendrite and axon in the rabbit cortex. Axon collateral (c) approaches dendritic spine (arrow). C: Drawing of dendrite in the dog cortex. Axon intersects dendrite (arrow). Oil immersion; 1450×.

axon collateral, dendrites, and spines merging both with the axon and dendrite can be distinctly observed in the cortex of rabbit and dog. In the most successfully impregnated cases, a gap can be observed between two heads, one connected with the dendrite, the other with the axon (Fig. 86).

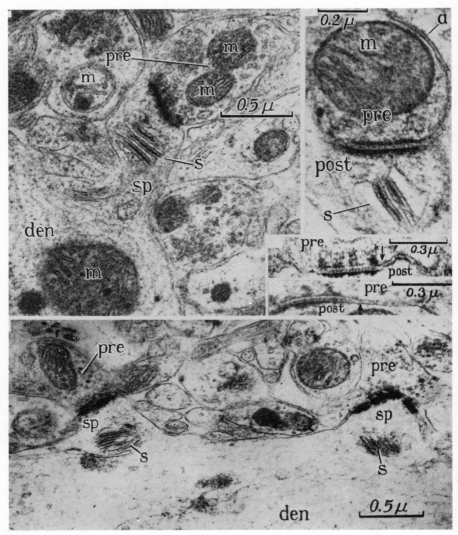

Fig. 113. Different types of synapses in the cortex. den, dendrite; m, mitochondria; sp, spine on dendrite; pre, axon ending; s, spine system; post, postsynaptic part of synapse. The photomicrograph on the left gives a clear idea of the ultrastructure of a synapse with participation of the spine of a dendrite. (After Gray, 1959.)

As Gray (1959, 1961) discovered, this type of contact corresponds to his type I synapse, in which an axonal ending runs up to a spine on a dendrite. The distance between the two processes is only 200 Å, and the oil immersion magnification in Fig. 112 was therefore too small to detect it; only with electron microscopic magnifications could the evidently narrow gap be seen between the axonal and dendritic part of the head. The type of contact which I discovered in 1948, in which heads of an axonal ending and spine lie close together coincides completely with Gray's observations (Fig. 113). There is thus strong evidence that the spine is the postsynaptic part of a synapse connected with the dendrite.

Very little is yet known about the manner of termination of dendrites of the cortical neurons and the functional significance of these endings. The retina has been studied more closely in this respect, and clublike thickenings on dendrites of the ganglion cells have been described and interpreted as baroreceptors (Shibkova, 1956). Can neurons be linked together into functionally united groups through connections of their dendrites? Such a possibility was regarded as probable in relation to dendrites of cortical neurons by Bekhterev (1898), and in the case of dendrites of retinal neurons by Dogel' (1892). Support for the view that cortical neurons are connected through their dendrites was recently given by Kaplan (1958) and van der Loos (1959, 1964). Dendro-dendritic connections are also accepted by Estable (1961).

By means of bichromate–silver impregnation, it can be seen under high power that dendritic endings of cortical pyramidal cells have a specific shape. They are usually tapering filaments, terminating in a single branch and sometimes having a bouton at or near their end. Sometimes the ending is shaped like the claws of a foot or like a bowl (Fig. 83), very similar to the shape of axonal endings adapted for contact with the cell body.

As regards the significance of these endings, two possibilities can be suggested:

1. Endings of this type are adapted to the shape of the neighboring cell body. Dendro-somatic connections of this nature were described by Estable in the reticular formation of the brain stem, the retina, spinal cord, and oculomotor nucleus. In the cortex, dendro-somatic connections have not yet been described, and the hypothesis that they exist has not yet been confirmed by facts.

2. The dendritic ending is part of a dendrite with a spine stretched out to meet the axon. Evidence of this is that in cortical sections a connection can be found between an axon collateral arriving from a distant part and the end of a dendrite (Fig. 90). A bouton is present at the point of contact, and bichromate–silver impregnation gives the impression that it is a single structure, although under very high power its structure can be seen to be

complex. The ending of the dendrite thus is indistinguishable from the remainder of its surface, and it terminates in a spine making contact with approaching axonal branches.

STRUCTURE OF INTERNEURONAL CONNECTIONS IN THE CORTEX

The first point of interest is the origin of synaptic endings in the cortex. At least nine possible origins of synapses can be distinguished: from axons of short-axon stellate cells, from stellate cells with an ascending axon, from axon collaterals of pyramidal cells, from axon collaterals of fusiform cells, from axon collaterals of the original cell, from specific afferents from sub-cortical structures, from nonspecific afferents, and from association and commissural fibers.

If the visual cortex is examined specifically, collaterals of some types of long-axon stellate cells must also be added to this list. Association fibers do not all end in the same layer and not all in the same manner. Finally, specific afferents may also differ, first, depending on the type of cell giving rise to them in the lateral geniculate body and second, because they also arrive from other sensory systems, as physiological data have shown (Jung, 1961; Skrebitskii and Voronin, 1965). Consequently, at the least possible estimate, from the point of view of origin there must be 15 different categories of synaptic termination. This least estimate likewise fails to take into account the sharp difference between concentrated and scattered types of cortical stellate cells.

The rich variety of synaptic structure thus makes classification very difficult. The term axo-dendritic synapse can be taken to mean a connection between a dendrite and the axon of a short-axon stellate cell, or with an association or nonspecific afferent ending. An axo-somatic synapse may take place not only with a specific afferent, but also with the axon of a short-axon stellate cell and with the collateral of a pyramidal cell axon.

The present investigation showed that one criterion alone is not enough for the study of interneuronal connections. The origin, shape, and mode of termination of each process must be taken into account, and the connection between structure and function judged from several different points of view.

The facts of the situation as they are known at the present time are described briefly below.

Specific afferent fibers usually terminate in a brushlike ramification. Thin endings equipped with synaptic boutons and also boutons along the course of the afferent fiber and its loops are adapted to the shape of the bodies of surrounding neurons (Fig. 101), against which they are evidently tightly pressed. No particularly large bulbs or glomerular endings are present in these cases. Consequently, axo-somatic contacts, principally on stellate cells of layer IV, are formed by bouton synapses from specific afferents. Connections between specific afferents and dendrites are much less common (Figs. 87 and 91). Collaterals from specific afferents branching from them in layers V and VI terminate on neurons of these layers. Some afferents branching in layers V and VI are similar in shape and thickness to specific afferents. They are almost certainly connected with dendrites of pyramidal cells.

Endings of specific afferent branches in the cortex are extremely varied in shape. Besides brushes climbing vertically upward, sometimes appearing like umbrellas, thick, ascending oblique fibers are observed (Fig. 26). The first type forms numerous (hundreds or more) synaptic endings on small neurons of sublayer IVc, which themselves form fewer contacts. Specific afferent branches in layers V and VI, however, form fewer still synaptic connections. Connections with large numbers of small axon cells in sublayer IVc were discovered in monkeys, but no such pattern was found in the cortex of rodents or even of carnivores.

Descriptions and drawings of specific afferents published previously (Cajal, 1900–1906, 1909–1911, 1935; Lorente de Nó, 1922, 1943; Polyakov and Sarkisov, 1949) made their identification in my own material easier. However, the descriptions give no information whatever about some varieties of specific afferents or about their differences in members of different orders of mammals. These differences must be connected with differentiation of neurons in the lateral geniculate body. In the rabbit, in which the neuronal composition of the dorsal part of the lateral geniculate body is fairly uniform (Fig. 7), branches of specific afferent fibers without any sharp differences are in fact found in layers III and IV of the cortex (Fig. 10,1). The situation is quite different in primates in which, in addition to complex brushes, long, single branches and numerous small, thin preterminals are found, branching from the main horizontal trunk (Figs. 42, 43, 61, 101).

Complex differentiation of neurons of the lateral geniculate body associated with the well-developed vision of primates accounts for this great variety of afferent structures.

Endings of nonspecific fibers in the cortex are less well known. They are represented somewhat differently in the existing drawings of Lorente de Nó (1943) and A. and M. Scheibel (1958a,b). I regard the single branches stretching from the white matter vertically upward and sometimes reaching the uppermost layers of the cortex as nonspecific. They give off small collaterals, mainly connected with dendrites.

Endings of the association fibers also are varied in character, and they terminate in layer III, very rarely in layer I, and sometimes in layer V also. Branches of association fibers also are single, they do not form brushes, and consequently they extend to far fewer neurons than specific afferents. These single endings resemble axo-dendritic synapses.

In my material, connections of short-axon neurons were revealed best. Their axons can form synapses with surrounding neurons by means of basket ramifications or nests (Figs. 36 and 73), i.e., typical axo-somatic contacts, by means of single synaptic boutons (also an axo-somatic contact; Figs. 73, 95, 96, etc.), by means of multiple collateral synapses with dendrites (Figs. 91 and 92), and by means of single terminal synapses on dendrites. Consequently, axons of stellate cells connect with bodies and dendrites of neighboring neurons both by terminal and by collateral synapses.

Some drawings show multiple connections of basal and other dendrites (not only bodies) of pyramidal cells with these axons (Figs. 91 and 92). The endings of these axons are small boutons and in sections treated by neurofibrillar stains loops and rings are obtained.

Bichromate-silver impregnation also sheds light on the fine details of the connections seen in sections under high power. Synapses may occur: (1) between axonal ending and dendritic spine (Fig. 86); (2) between axonal ending and dendritic trunk (Figs. 87, 97, etc.); (3) between axonal ending and neuron body (Figs. 95, 96, etc.). In these cases the contact may be formed by a single axon collateral, a complex ramification of the axon, or on the other hand, by bunches of synapses from endings of basket or nest type; (4) a synapse can be found simultaneously on the dendrite and body from the same axon (Fig. 95); (5) an axon may be connected with several dendrites from different cells (Fig. 88); (6) an axon may be connected with bodies of many neurons (Figs. 96, 101) at the same time (even hundreds); (7) an axon may wind many times around a dendrite (Fig. 85), and in these cases sliding contacts may be seen (Fig. 84); (8) an axon, by means of its collaterals, may form contacts with dendrites of its own neuron (Figs. 93 and 94).

I observed all these eight types of contacts between neurons in the cortex. Besides these connections described above, connections have also been found in the central nervous system between neuroglial processes and neurons; among dendrites, axons, and capillaries, between dendrites, and between axons. In some sections I found connections between a dendritic spine and capillary (1961b), between axonal endings and capillaries (Skrebitskii and Shkolnik-Yarros, 1964), and axo-axonal connections (1961b, 1965).

Each of these types of connection may vary because of differences in the shape and size of the synaptic ending. The second type, between axonal ending and dendritic trunk, varies sharply, depending on its location. In the cortex, association and nonspecific afferent fibers are connected in this way with dendrites of pyramidal cells. They have thin, single ramifications without forming large synapses. In the retina the axon of a bipolar cell forms contacts with dendrites of a ganglion cell by juxtaposition of very large, bulbous synapses. Clearly the microstructure (number of mitochondria) and cytochemistry of these two synapses are completely different, and this is related to their completely different functions. In the first case the axo-dendritic contact provides for complex associations involving dendrites of pyramidal cells or for raising the tone of cortical cells through nonspecific afferents. In the second case the specific peripheral transmission of visual excitation must take place in the area of contact between the bipolar and ganglion cells. It is evidently there that a different level of oxidative activity and energy expenditure is required, and this is reflected in the special size of the synapse.

Excellent modern investigations of synapses in the central nervous system (by neurofibrillar stains), carried out mainly in Leningrad and Moscow, have revealed with a previously unattainable level of perfection the number, shape, size, and localization of synaptic endings. However, it is still very difficult to judge from whence, from which neuron, these numerous loops and rings arise. Even the best electron microscopic sections of synapses containing mitochondria and vesicles with acetylcholine cannot help to elucidate the origin of the contact. These difficulties give rise to mistaken or biased conclusions. Consequently, before cytochemical study, before electron microscopic investigation, and even before the use of neurofibrillar stains, it is essential to study the ramification of neurons by a method revealing them in their entirety. Failure to use such a method has led, for example, to the erroneous idea firmly rooted in the literature that no axo-dendritic connections are present in the lateral geniculate body of primates. The role of the dendrites is thus oversimplified, convergence of excitation in the lateral geniculate body is completely ruled out and it is not then clear how the central sensory systems interact with each other or with the reticular formation at the subcortical level.

Éntin's conclusion that nearly all cortical synapses originate from subcortical afferents cannot be accepted. The view that basket ramifications of axons are not present in the cortex (Yuvchenko) must certainly be rejected, but the existence not only of basket ramifications in the cortex, as Cajal, Snesarev, and others were inclined to believe, but also of typical boutons and loops, must be equally affirmed. The view that basket ramifications around the bodies of cortical neurons modify their excitability, while the axo-dendritic connection is a pathway for the direct transmission of excitation (Sepp), cannot withstand a simple examination of the morphology of synapses. Often very similar loops are found on the dendrites and bodies of neurons (Éntin) and also on blood vessels (Dolgo-Saburov), and the same axon may terminate both on a dendrite and on a cell body (Fig. 95B); specific afferents carrying visual excitation most commonly terminate on the bodies of neurons (Fig. 101), while on dendrites connections of a winding type are observed, among others (Fig. 85), which are most probably concerned with the modification of excitability.

If an analog of the Renshaw cells of the spinal cord exists in the cortex, as some investigators believe, it must be sought among the short-axon neurons. The function of the Martinotti cells must be complex. They collect excitation, presumably intracortical, mainly in the lower layers, and transmit it upward into layer I (sometimes forming contacts with dendrites along their course). In layer I they form baskets for stellate neurons of this layer (Cajal), and these in turn form axo-dendritic connections with the apical dendrites of pyramidal neurons.

In my study I discovered several hitherto unknown types of interneuronal connections which shed light on the organization of vertical and horizontal connections. For instance, large afferents ascending to layer IV may terminate not only in brushes, but they may also give off horizontal branches stretching a considerable distance (Fig. 61). Consequently, in addition to the shortest association connections effected in the lower layers of the cortex, the long axon collaterals of pyramidal neurons running horizontally, and the horizontal arrangement of certain neurons forming nests (Fig. 36), the horizontal plexuses also include branches from large afferents, possibly specific in character.

Vertical relationships between neurons are especially interesting. Lorente de Nó (1938) first observed that the cerebral cortex is divided into vertical elementary units, consisting of a chain of neurons lying in all the layers of the cortex. Vertical "columns" were subsequently discovered electrophysiologically (Mountcastle, 1957; Hubel and Wiesel, 1963, 1965; Rabinovich, 1964).

Some details of the interneuronal connections described in this book supplement the existing concepts of vertical contacts. Axons descending from the upper layers of the cortex, for instance, form numerous connections along their course with the dendrites of neighboring neurons (Fig. 84a). Other types of axons form tangential contacts, not with dendrites, but with the bodies of neighboring neurons lying in the lower layers (Figs. 75, 96).

An interesting attempt to interpret the vertical relationships between cortical neurons has been made by Colonnier (1966).

The drawings of neurons of Areas 17, 18, and 19 and the scheme (Fig. 128) given in this book reveal that these vertical relationships undergo very substantial changes which depend on the general structure of the particular area. Every cytoarchitectonic area is characterized by its own arrangement of vertical chains.

Attempts to examine the morphology and classification of neurons and interneuronal connections of the neocortex in the light of inhibitory and excitatory functions have not yet produced definitive results. Different views are held on the fine morphological structure of the inhibitory system. Sepp (1949) thought that inhibition of neurons in the central nervous system is carried out by the baskets plaited around their bodies. Some have stated more specifically that inhibition in the cortex is associated with short-axon neurons (Szentágothai, 1965; Shkol'nik-Yarros, 1965; Skrebitskii and Shkol'nik-Yarros, 1967). The suggestion has been made that Gray's type I synapse is excitatory and his type II synapse is inhibitory (Eccles, 1964). Uchizono (1965) considers that synaptic vesicles of an oval shape and small size are characteristic of inhibitory synapses, while large, circular vesicles are characteristic of excitatory synapses

Despite progress in electron microscopy, it is quite obvious that the examination of a structure as a whole lays the foundation for the subsequent study of its parts. From this point of view the list of the principal varieties of synapses—axo-somatic and axo-dendritic (Cajal, 1935), terminal and collateral (Lorente de Nó, 1933; Polyakov, 1953), types I and II (Gray, 1959) might well be supplemented by yet another, based on the area of contact between two neurons and the number of synaptic endings. It is very important to remember that some of the connections described cannot be completely distinguished by ultrastructural electron microscopic investigation because of the thinness of the section used in this method. The first variety is characterized by considerable extent and number of its synaptic ending. This variety includes the baskets and nests described earlier in the human motor cortex by Cajal (1911), and subsequently confirmed by O'Leary (1941), Polyakov (1955, 1965), and Shkol'nik-Yarros (1959b, 1965) (see Figs. 17, 36, 37, 48, and 73).

Short-axon stellate cells forming nests or baskets can be subdivided into several varieties. The first consists of neurons in the lower layers with the main branch of the axon horizontal. It gives off secondary branches upward and downward, and these in turn give off fine collaterals, with boutons along their course and terminating in complex synaptic structures around the bodies of neighboring neurons. Nests of neurons of this type unite the large pyramidal cells of layer V into a functional unit.

The second variety consists of neurons in layers II, III, and IV forming nests which do not run horizontally but in the neighborhood of the body of the original cell. If a basket-type cell is located in layer II, the baskets are most often formed by descending branches of the axon, surrounding the bodies of cells in layer III (see, for example, cell 3 in Fig. 17A). If the original cell is in layer III, the baskets surround the bodies of neurons in the same layer, both close to the original cell or some distance from it (Fig. 73).

The third variety is characterized by the formation of nests or baskets in very close proximity to the body of the original cell. These neurons are most common in layer IV of the visual cortex (Fig. 48). Nests can also be formed by descending axons passing down from layer IV into layer VI (Fig. 50B, axon 1). In such cases, the original cell is probably a pyramidal cell with a short, descending axon, not departing into the white matter.

Other interneuronal connections of considerable extent are the several varieties of axo-dendritic contacts described above, especially contacts of winding type (Shkol'nik-Yarros, 1956; Figs. 85 and 85a). It was difficult to determine precisely from which cells the axons winding around ascending dendrites of pyramidal cells in the visual cortex are derived. These connections cover a large surface of the dendrite, providing the necessary conditions for synchronized effects at different levels of the dendrite. Contacts parallel to the apical dendrites of pyramidal cells (Figs. 84, 84a) are formed either by axons of double-tufted neurons or by descending axons of pyramidal cells, or again by ascending afferent branches (Fig. 85D).

The second type of connection is characterized by small area and few synapses. These connections are adapted for discrete transmission to particular parts of the soma or dendrite, and they are usually formed by axons from different sources.

Connections of the extensive variety cover a large part of the body or dendrite. They are formed by the axon of one neuron, and if this neuron is in an active state it can evidently act on a considerable part of a neighboring cell at once. From descriptions of inhibitory neurons in other parts of the nervous system (Andersen, Eccles, and Voorhoeve, 1964; Andersen, Eccles, and Løyning, 1964), and from interest which has been shown in the search for inhibitory systems in the cortex (Eccles, 1964; Szentágothai, 1965), there was a strong case for examining the data concerning neuronal structure of the cortex from this point of view. It can be envisaged that the neurons are in fact connected with the basket ramifications of axons with inhibitory function. Only a few such neurons are present in the cortex as is clear from the drawing of cortical neurons given by Cajal (1911), Lorente de Nó (1922, 1938), and Polyakov (1953, 1955, 1965).

The hypothesis of the presence of inhibitory interneurons in the cortex has been strengthened by the investigation of Holubar, Hanke, and Malik (1967), who were able to distinguish between pyramidal and short-axon cells by intracellular labeling. The labeled cells differed in size, shape, and character of activity when penicillin was applied to the surface of the cortex. These workers regard the small neurons as cortical inhibitory interneurons.

The latest results obtained by Colonnier (1968), who found few synapses on the bodies of pyramidal neurons in layer II of the cat visual cortex, cannot be regarded as an argument against the views expressed above. Ultrathin sections do not allow any estimate to be made of the total number of synapses on the soma of a given cell, or still less, of the origin of these synapses.

Chapter 3

DIFFERENCES IN STRUCTURE AND CONNECTIONS OF THE VISUAL SYSTEM AT CORTICAL AND SUBCORTICAL LEVELS

THE CORTICAL LEVEL

Connections of Pyramidal Cells and Their Significance

The fully developed pyramidal cell possesses a complex system of branching dendrites receiving excitation at various levels and, without doubt, from various sources. Figure 114 is a scheme of the connections of a pyramidal cell in layer III based on the study of a large number of sections. For the sake of convenience the pyramidal cell can be divided into five parts, each of which forms connections with surrounding and distant neurons. The material of the preceding chapter (Figs. 83–95) can be briefly summarized.

The apical dendritic bouquet forms contacts with horizontal and other axons in layer I. Axons of layer I arise from Martinotti cells which are present in all layers of the cortex but are largest and most conspicuous in the lower layers. The axons of layer I also arise from Cajal–Retzius cells. Numerous branches of axons from short-axon cells in the upper layers and layer I itself and endings of collaterals of the long axons can next be observed here. Consequently, in layer I alone, through their apical bouquet, the pyramidal cells receive impulses from a vast number of intracortical cells.

The trunk of the apical dendrite of the pyramidal cell receives excitation from afferent fibers coming from other parts of the brain and also from intracortical short-axon neurons.

Basal dendrites of the pyramidal cells possess different connections depending on the layer in which the cell body is situated. Descending basal dendrites of cells in layer III are adapted for reception of impulses from specific afferent endings. Basal dendrites of pyramidal cells of Meynert have their long axis in the horizontal direction and they evidently receive infor-

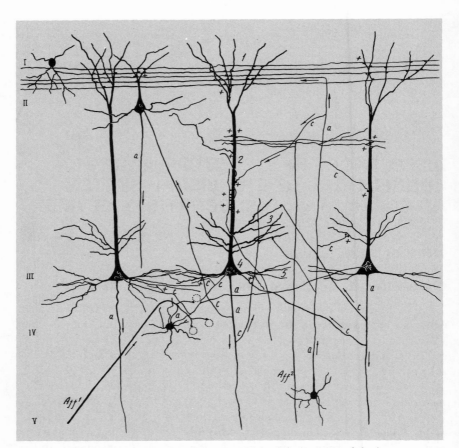

Fig. 114. Diagram of connections of a pyramidal cell in layer III of the human cortex based on studies of Golgi material. The pyramidal cell in the center of the scheme is divided into five parts. In layer I of the cortex horizontal axons of cells in layer I and axonal endings of Martinotti cells with ascending axon are in contact with its apical dendrite (1). In layers II and III afferent fibers arriving from other parts of the nervous system, axons of Martinotti cells, and numerous other axons presumably from cortical short-axon stellate cells are in contact with the apical dendrite (2). Axon collaterals of pyramidal cells, of Martinotti cells, and of the original pyramidal cell itself (self-contact) contact dendrites in the lower third of the trunk (3). Axons of stellate cells and axon collaterals of other pyramidal cells contact the body (4) of the pyramidal cell. Axons of stellate cells contact the basal dendrites (5). Each short-axon stellate cell contacts several pyramidal cells. Aff[1] represents afferent from subcortical structures reaching layer IV and forming contact with short-axon stellate cell. Aff[2] afferent fiber reaching upper levels of layer III and contacting dendrites of pyramidal cells. a, axon; c, axon collateral. Arrows show direction of transmission of excitation; + denotes site of contact.

mation *"en passant"* from long, horizontal collaterals of axons of other pyramidal cells coming from a distant region.

Pyramidal cells form an extremely large number of connections with surrounding short-axon neurons. Sometimes these connections are formed with the body of a pyramidal cell, sometimes with a dendrite at any level, and sometimes with both body and dendrite (i.e., axo-dendro-somatic connection). My observations also show conclusively that dendrites of pyramidal neurons may receive endings of collaterals of the axon belonging to their own cell.

It follows from this brief survey that the pyramidal cell is a complex integrating system on which impulses converge from many different sources, the role of intracortical connections being particularly important.

It also follows from the facts described in Chapters 1 and 2 that the structure and number of the pyramidal cells vary considerably in members of different orders of mammals. In the hedgehog and even in the rabbit there are no cells similar in the richness of ramification of their dendrites to the pyramidal cells of carnivores and primates. One pyramidal cell may have up to 60 or 80 dendritic branches, and several thousands of spines, i.e., post-synaptic portions of synapses, on its dendrites. On some particularly large and successfully impregnated pyramidal cells in the cortex of carnivores and primates, the whole bouquet of dendritic branches in the lower third of the ascending trunk is revealed, providing yet another thousand synapses.

Finally, the vast increase in number of pyramidal cells in the phylo-genetically new areas of the human cortex, connected with the increased development of association and commissural connections, is particularly important.

These observations here described can be compared with data in the literature. Sukhanov (1896) considered the pyramidal cells special psychic neurons. Pyramidal cells receive excitation from different sources and possess several zones of dendritic contacts (Lorente de Nó, 1938; Bodian, 1952; Shkol'nik-Yarros, 1950b, 1958c).

Polyakov (1956) obtained important new quantitative data: according to his calculations pyramidal cells account for between 71 and 79.3 % of all cortical cells.

The greatest number of synapses in the cortex is found on the pyramidal cell. Actual figures for these quantitative relationships are given by several authors. Éntin (1954a), for instance, demonstrated several hundreds of synaptic endings very clearly on the body of the pyramidal cell and initial segments of its dendrites. Polyak (1957) mentions 1000 synaptic endings on dendrites of a solitary pyramidal cell of Meynert. Polyakov (1953) counted 4000 spines on one pyramidal cell in the human cortex and also described a covering of synaptic endings. I counted 2600 spines on dendrites of a large pyramidal cell in layer III of the dog's cortex (Shkol'nik-Yarros, 1950b). The spine is part of a synapse, and it is therefore perfectly correct to count them along with the loops and rings. The largest number is given by Young (1958), who considers that there are 10,000 synapses on a cortical pyramidal cell. If the synaptic endings form palisades upon the neuron (Palay, 1958), it may be that Young's figure is close to the truth.

During ontogenesis of the cortical pyramidal cell, the body increases in size and becomes conical in shape, with the appearance of secondary and tertiary branches of the dendrites, axon collaterals, synapses, and spines and with changes in their chemical properties (Cajal, 1900–1906, 1909–1911; Polyakov, 1951, 1954; Conel, 1939–1959; Glezer, 1958; Tsinda, 1959, 1960; Ivanitskii, 1958). The same process can be seen in phylogenesis, as Cajal previously demonstrated schematically. The number of branches of the dendrites and the shape of the body of the pyramidal cell depend on the level of development of the mammal (Figs. 5, 11, 28, 63, 72).

Considerable change has been discovered, especially in pyramidal cells located in layer III of the cortex, in disease (schizophrenia, Pick's disease, Alzheimer's disease). Death of nerve cells, with their disappearance and fragmentation of the processes mainly in the upper layers of the cortex were observed by Snesarev in schizophrenia.

Growth of phylogenetically new areas in primates, so well demonstrated in work carried out at the Brain Institute (Filimonov, 1932, 1933; Shevchenko, 1938; Kononova, 1940; Blinkov, 1955) leads to a very large increase in the number of pyramidal cells. The greatest accumulation of pyramidal cells takes place in layer III in these phylogenetically new areas, in which they are arranged in three sublayers. Growth of this layer is particularly conspicuous during phylogenesis of the cortex.

Another characteristic feature of phylogenetically new areas is an increase in the degree of radial striation, i.e., the appearance of clearly defined vertical stripes. As was fully described above, this morphological sign is dependent, in turn, on the increase in number of pyramidal cells whose axons are gathered into bundles. In the hedgehog, radial striation in the cortex is absent altogether, in the rodent and carnivore it is ill defined, and in primates it is well developed. Consequently, radial striation is a specific reflection of the process of progressive development of the cortex and of the increase in number of pyramidal cells connecting near and remote portions of the brain.

My own results and those reported in the literature concerning structure, connections, development, and pathology of pyramidal cells suggest their extreme importance for basic cortical function.

If the great enlargement of Areas 18 and 19 in the series of primates is recalled, and it is assumed that on the average pyramidal cells account for

70–80 % of the total number of cells in each area, and each of these cells can form several thousands of contacts with other neurons, it will be clear that these neurons, along with others, must play a decisive role in the activity of higher levels of the central nervous system.

Only the Purkinje cells of the cerebellum and certain neurons of the optic lobes in birds can be compared with the cortical pyramidal cells in their receipt of impulses from many different sources.

Recent electrophysiological investigations of convergence of impulses on neurons of the reticular formation (Scheibel *et al.*, 1955) and on neurons of the visual cortex (Jung, 1958, 1961; Akimoto and Creutzfeldt, 1958; Skrebitskii and Voronin, 1965), and the theory of convergence put forward by Fessard (1958), in which the cortical pyramidal cell is regarded as a highly complex modulating and integrating apparatus, attach definite interest to these data for the multiple connections of pyramidal cells. Unquestionably the morphology of the pyramidal neuron and the great variety of its connections indicate that this neuron forms the anatomical substrate for the most complex connections and the most highly developed convergence of impulses in the cortex. The pyramidal cell may be responsible for interaction between processes taking place in other parts of the cortex with local processes and, in addition, with the activity of the original cell itself. Most probably these combinations and interactions may be manifested as the most complex forms of activity of the human brain.

The importance of pyramidal cells for basic cortical functions has recently been assessed in the latest work by Beritashvili (1968). In his opinion, activity of neurons of this type is connected with memory. Beritashvili describes the very small number of short-axon stellate cells in the gyrus proreus of the dog. According to counts made by Polyakov (1959), only a very small percentage of short-axon neurons is present in the cytoarchitectonic areas of the human frontal cortex. The frontal lobes, of course, are most intimately related to the programming of action (Luria, Pribram, and Khomskaya, 1966). If the frontal region is ablated, there is no integration of various excitations (Shumilina, 1949; Anokhin, 1965, 1968).

In primates the area of the frontal lobes rises sharply from the marmoset to man (Kononova, 1962). In the bear, the structure of the frontal region is much more complex than in other carnivores (Svetukhina, 1959).

Hence, psychological, physiological, morphological, and comparative-anatomical methods confirm the importance of pyramidal neurons in highly complex cortical functions.

Connections of the Long-Axon Star Cells of Cajal

Dendrites of Cajal cells are found in sublayer IVb, sometimes spreading far and wide in a horizontal direction as well-developed branches (Fig. 46,

21, 23), sometimes spreading radially from the cell body (Fig. 46, 27). Star cells of Cajal are particularly richly supplied with synapses (Éntin, 1954a), found both on their body and dendrites. In sections in which the fibers of Gennari's band are successfully impregnated, it can be seen that thick, horizontal afferent fibers give off thinner branches, ending on the body of a stellate cell visible as a shadow (Fig. 101). My material also revealed connections of dendrites of star cells of Cajal with thin axon collaterals and endings running in the direction of Gennari's band and also from above downward, from the higher layers (Fig. 97). Synapses on these neurons are thus principally endings of visual afferent fibers from the lateral geniculate body. These connections, clearly specific in character, are mainly axo-somatic. The axo-dendritic connections are evidently mainly intra-cortical. The arrangement of these cells among a mass of endings of fibers belonging to the optic radiation and their failure to develop in the case of developmental defects of the eyes (Leonova, 1896) demonstrate their important role in visual function.

In von Bonin's (1942) opinion, a quantitative relationship exists between cones, rods, and stellate cells in sublayer IVb. He considers that the cones present in the macula lutea bear a 1:1 ratio to the large star cells, and that for each of the remaining stellate cells there are 125 receptors. The study of the structure of layer IV in different animals does not allow von Bonin's views to be accepted fully, because the star cells of Cajal are a very constant element, presumably relatively independent of the cone system. In the visual cortex of cats and dogs, for instance, with a predominantly rod type of retina, they may also be observed. However, these cells are most varied in character and very numerous in the cortex of animals with highly developed vision (squirrels, primates).

The study of the course of the axons shows that they run into the white matter (Fig. 33); in this respect my material confirms Cajal's (1900) opinion but does not agree with Polyak's diagram (1957). As was stated above, there is indirect evidence of degeneration of the bodies of Cajal cells after division of the cortical white matter, from which it may be concluded that their axons run to subcortical structures. Large size, abundant synaptic connections, and a thick axon are evidence of an effector function, so that my morphological data suggest that these cells play a role in reflex move-ments of the eyes. Endings of visual afferent fibers simultaneously on Cajal cells and stellate cells of sublayer IVc suggest the simultaneous formation of the visual image (IVc) and eye movements (IVb) (Shkol'nik-Yarros, 1958b). On the basis of morphological observations, Beritov (1960, 1961) put forward a theory of the cortical genesis of the orienting reaction. Many cortical and subcortical structures can be assumed to take part in the complex process of the orienting reflex, including autonomic components (Sokolov, 1958).

Axons descending from the cortex and running toward the superior colliculi may be a link in such chains as: cortex–tectum–spinal cord (tectospinal tract), cortex–tectum–reticular formation (tectoreticular tract), or cortex–tectum–oculomotor nucleus (tecto-oculomotor tract).

Connections of Short-Axon Stellate Cells and Their Significance

Bekhterev (1896–1898) described the stellate cells as "unifying." Richness of the cortex in short-axon cells reflects the complexity of function of the human cortex (Cajal, 1909–1911; Lorente de Nó, 1938). Sarkisov (1948, 1960) and Polyakov (1949, 1953, 1955, 1959) consider these cells very important. According to Sarkisov (1960), they play a special role in formation of an impression of external stimuli and in the retention of this impression. Polyakov emphasizes that it is the stellate short-axon cells which redistribute and relay impulses in the cortex. He demonstrated neurons of complex shape possessing axonal systems with selectivity of direction as characteristic features of the human brain.

Beritov (1960) linked the psychogenic function of the human brain directly with the activity of these neurons. In later papers (1961, 1963a) he suggested calling the short-axon stellate cells "sensory," in view of their role in the reception of impulses, and he assigned a special role to them in the recreation of shape.

Turning now to the visual cortex, where these cells are particularly numerous, the statements of Cajal (1900, 1911), Henschen (1930), and Polyak (1957) must be considered. Cajal suggested that small short-axon cells amplify visual excitation while transmitting it to other neurons. Henschen, who judged cells not by their shape as a whole, together with their processes, but merely from the appearance of their bodies and nuclei (Nissl preparations), divided all neurons in layer IV of Area 17 into two types: photosensitive and color-sensitive, thus accepting their role in the perception

Table II. Percentage of Neurons with Long Axons and of Neurons with Short Axons in a Cross Section of the Cortex[a]

Cells	Area						
	3	1a	1b	1c	2	40	39
Pyramidal	71.0	79.3	79.2	71.1	77.4	72.9	73.9
Fusiform	5.1	5.4	6.5	9.2	8.2	9.5	7.1
Stellate	23.9	15.3	14.3	19.7	14.4	17.6	19.0

[a] From Polyakov (1956).

of visual stimuli. According to Polyak, the very great number of small, short-axon cells in layer IV is a barrier to the spread of visual excitation, which is thus kept within definite limits.

According to Polyakov (1956), there is one stellate cell to every 4–5 pyramidal cells in the upper layers of the cortex and to every 10–11 pyramidal and fusiform cells in the lower layers (Table II).

The number of these neurons varies in different areas of the cortex from 14 to 24%. In the cat's cortex Cajal (1900, 1911) and Sholl (1956) found an accumulation of short-axon neurons in layer IV of the visual cortex, as well as in other layers but in smaller numbers. Zhukova (1953) found no appreciable accumulation of short-axon cells in particular layers in the motor cortex of the hedgehog, rabbit, dog, or monkey.

Popova (1960a,b), after comparing her data for short-axon cells in areas of the dog's auditory cortex and my observations (Shkol'nik-Yarros, 1954, 1959b), considers that axon collaterals are more concentrated in the visual cortex. These differences in the stellate cells, in conjunction with differences in the subcortical structure of the auditory and visual systems (Zvorykin, 1960), enabled Popova to explain the differences which she observed in the dynamics of neural activity during the production of reflexes from the auditory and visual systems. A more rapid response was observed during auditory conditioning, the reflexes were stabilized faster, and their latent period was shorter, while visual conditioned reflexes were more slowly stabilized and their aftereffect was longer.

No accurate estimates have yet been made of the number of the principal types of neurons in the cortex of different animals. However, the following conclusion can be drawn from the results of my qualitative investigations: the visual cortex of the hedgehog contains few short-axon stellate cells; the visual cortex of the rabbit has very many of them in all its layers, but mostly in layer IV, and they vary considerably in shape, size, and direction of their axons. In layer I the direction of their axons is mainly horizontal, while in layers II, III, and IV the axons are predominantly of the narrow-branching type, with the formation of baskets and nests; in layers V and VI the axons mainly run upward and horizontally. Short-axon cells are of the following types: diffusing, with narrowly and widely branching axonal systems, and concentrating, with single contacts. Consequently, the types and distribution of short-axon cells in the rabbit's visual cortex indicates, first, that complex and varied types of these cells are present in the rodent cortex, as Lorente de Nó had clearly shown previously in mice, and second, that certain principles govern the transmission of excitation within the visual cortex.

Two types of axons are also present in the visual cortex of the dog: widely and narrowly branching. Wide ramifications of axons communicating with neurons over wide areas of the cortex are most characteristic of the dog's cortex. However, in layer IV itself, more narrowly concentrated axons with a small area of distribution of their collaterals are frequently found.

In Area 17 in monkeys the greatest concentration of short-axon cells is observed in layer IV, the density and stratification of which vary depending on the properties of vision in each monkey and the structure of its lateral geniculate body and retina. In other layers (Fig. 46), numerous short-axon cells of different types can also be seen (Shkol'nik-Yarros, 1954, 1955a, 1961b; Polyak, 1957). Areas 18 and 19 contain somewhat fewer short-axon cells than Area 17. This is explained by the particularly high cell density of layer IV in Area 17.

The distribution is different in Areas 18 and 19; for they are more uniformly arranged in layers II, III, and IV, although their concentration is greater in layer IV, as is clearly demonstrated by the compactness of their cell bodies on cytoarchitectonic photographs.

Very many different types of neurons are seen in the monkey's cortex. Neurons of shrub type are more characteristic of the upper layers. In sublayer IVc cells with helical dendrites and a descending, arcuate axon can be distinguished. Ramification of the dendrites of these neurons is mainly of the narrowly branching type, and they form numerous connections with similar cells lying alongside. In the lower portion of sublayer IVb some neurons, similar in their general appearance to long-axon cells of Cajal, in fact have a short axon which is distributed there and then in the cortex.

I made more or less the same observations when studying areas of the human occipital cortex. The main difference between the human and monkey cortex, in my opinion, is not the qualitative differences between short-axon stellate cells, but their relative numerical proportions. Typical double-tufted neurons are evidently absent in rodents. In carnivores, the axons form fewer vertical branches. The double-tufted cells are adapted for the formation of vertical contacts with pyramidal cells. Consequently, the fact that they reach their highest level of development in man can also be connected with their pyramidization. They are most numerous in the phylogenetically newest areas. Because of the much smaller areas of the cortical surface occupied by phylogenetically new areas in monkeys, there will also be far fewer double-tufted cells in those areas.

The visual cortex, which is extremely rich in all the types of short-axon neurons described above, provides a convenient example for studying their importance. The main collections of stellate cells in the visual cortex are found in layers receiving afferent fibers from the subcortex, and it therefore seems correct to regard them as playing an important role in the reception of external stimuli. This fact is illustrated particularly clearly in the visual cortex of the macaque. In this monkey the unusual complexity and fineness of structure of the retina are reflected in the high cell density and sharply defined lamination of the lateral geniculate body (Fig. 38), and also in the particularly high concentration of cells in sublayer IVc of Area 17 (Fig. 41), higher even than their concentration in man.

Consequently, with the visual cortex as an example, a relationship can be clearly seen among the number of short-axon cells in layer IV of the cortex, the degree of differentiation of this layer, and the height of development of visual function. The number of double-tufted cells depends on the pyramidization and size of the cortex bordering Area 17. According to my observations, the main distinguishing feature of the human cortex is its abundance of pyramidal cells filling the wide layer III in the phylogenetically new areas. A high concentration of short-axon stellate cells is characteristic of layers receiving external stimuli (what von Economo calls the koniocortex). It is certain that visual perception unconnected with higher functions (reading, writing, etc.) is extremely well developed in the macaque, and this is undoubtedly reflected in the high development of layer IV of the visual cortex with its abundance of short-axon cells.

Pyramidal cells with arcuate axons are also of the short-axon type. The dendrites of these neurons are short and medium-sized. Consequently, they lie in the zone of spread of visual excitation through specific afferent fibers and their collaterals (layers VI and V; Figs. 46, 62, and 128). The dendritic bouquet of these neurons is not extensive and is adapted for the formation of individualized contacts. Axons emerging from the lower surface of the body run for a short distance downward, then turn upward in an arch and ascend vertically to sublayer IVb (Fig. 62). According to Cajal they reach layer III. The terminal branches of the axons do not form dense baskets, but simply two or three individual endings incorporated into Gennari's bands.

Two hypotheses can be put forward to explain the function of cells with an arcuate axon. First, on account of their position and their special arrangement (the ending of the axon is often in the same layer as the apical dendrite) it seems that these neurons may participate in the formation of closed cycles of propagation of excitation in the cortex. They may help to retain visual images. Second, the small size of these cells, their round shape, and their individualized contacts suggest that they may be a part of the cone-midget system. Only further research can shed light on this important problem.

Very different opinions are thus held on the functions of short-axon stellate cells. They are unifying (Bekhterev), they create the impression of external stimuli reaching the cortex (Sarkisov), they are the principal mechanism for redistribution and relaying of impulses in the cortex (Polyakov), they act as specialized amplifiers of excitation (Rusinov), they are sensory in nature (Beritov, 1961; Beritashvili, 1963a), and they reflect the precision and complexity of activity in the human brain (Cajal, Lorente de Nó).

The study of the visual cortex, which is exceptionally rich in short-axon stellate cells, provides additional evidence for judging the importance of these cells. The short-axon neurons are the first link in the chain of various cortical neurons concerned 'in the complex process of reflection of the external environment and reception of external stimuli.

These differing opinions on the role of short-axon stellate cells enumerated above are not mistaken. It must be realized that these cells exist in several different types, and a concentrating cell can hardly act as amplifier whereas a diffusing cell can amplify, relay, and unify simultaneously. A special variety of short-axon cell, with basketlike ramification of its axon, possibly plays the role of an inhibitory interneuron. (See also the section "Structure of Interneuronal Connections in the Cerebral Cortex," p. 182). The most complex types of brain activity, speech and intellectual activity, are in my opinion connected with the activity of all cortical neurons, which are (both literally and metaphorically) interwoven. Neurons of layer IV and the lower level of layer III are more directly concerned with the reception of external stimuli, while the double-tufted neurons of layers II and III may participate in complex, indirect circuits converging on pyramidal neurons.

The stellate cells of layer IV are frequently interconnected by numerous contacts, so that what Zavarzin describes as a screen is created. The double-tufted cells play a more important role in associative activity.

THE SUBCORTICAL LEVEL

Neurons of the Lateral Geniculate Body

In the lateral geniculate body I found (Shkol'nik-Yarros, 1958b) five main types of neurons: (1) long-axon cells with radial dendrites (Fig. 115A, 1, 3); (2) long-axon shrub cells (Fig. 115A, 4); (3) long-axon cells with few branches and widely spreading dendrites (Fig. 115A, 2); (4) long-axon cells with a few, short dendrites (midget) (Fig. 115B, 5); (5) short-axon cells (Fig. 115A, 6, 8; Fig. 115B, 6).

The composition of the neurons varies with the order of mammals and the state of visual function. In dogs, for instance, there are very few midget cells which are typical of the upper four parvocellular layers of the human lateral geniculate body (Fig. 115B; Figs. 59, 60). Of the typically human neurons there are many shrub cells with a dendritic bouquet running in one direction (Fig. 115B; Figs. 59, 60).

Four of the five cell varieties give off long axons into the cortex. Differences in the structure of the long-axon neurons can be attributed to differ-

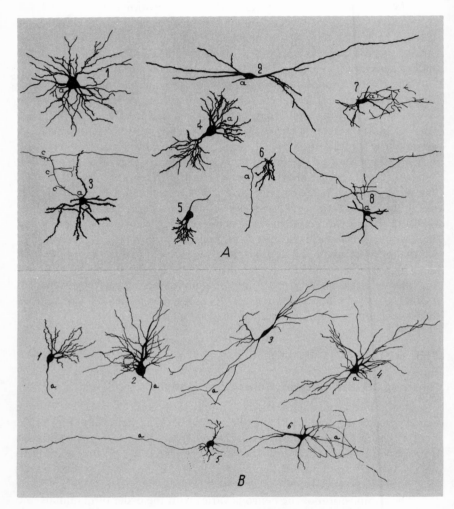

Fig. 115. A: Types of neurons in the lateral geniculate body of carnivores. 1, 3, long-axon radial cells; 4, 6, long-axon shrub cells; 2, long-axon cell with few branches (marginal); 6, 7, 8, short-axon cells. B: Types of neurons in the human lateral geniculate body. 1, 2, shrub (fan-shaped) long-axon cells; 3, long-axon cell with few branches; 4, long-axon radial cell; 5, small long-axon cell with a few short dendrites (midget); 6, short-axon cell; a, axon.

ences in the type of ramification of their dendrites which, in turn, is connected with the afferent fibers reaching these cells.

A comparative study of the lateral geniculate body in the hedgehog, rabbit, dog, cat, monkey, and man shows that most neurons are of the long-axon type. A very small percentage of short-axon cells is present in this nucleus in all animals and man. In the hedgehog there are no short-axon cells whatever and only a few in the dog. They are more numerous in the cat than the dog. In man, despite the large number of cells with long axons which I have drawn, only a few are of the short-axon type (Fig. 115B, 6). Polyak (1957), 14 years after his work demonstrating the absence of short-axon cells in the lateral geniculate body, gave a drawing of a short-axon cell which he found in Golgi material and which he called an association cell, thereby overthrowing the hypothesis which he himself created and defended. In explaining his earlier statement that all cells of the lateral geniculate body without exception degenerate after removal of the cortex, he felt that short-axon (association, in his terminology) cells as well as long-axon cells must disappear. It was this total degeneration which had previously led him to conclude that short-axon cells were absent.

Because of the small number of short-axon cells in the lateral geniculate body they cannot be considered to play a fundamental role in the reception and transmission of visual excitation. The whole nucleus is permeated by visual afferent fibers forming numerous contacts with surrounding long-axon cells (Figs. 24, 57, 107).

Thus results accumulated over many years demonstrate that von Monakow was in error in believing that transmission of visual excitation must take place through internuncial cells. Afferent fibers reaching the lateral geniculate body from the retina terminate mainly on long-axon cells giving off axons directly to the cortex. This is shown, first, by the diffuse arrangement both of the long-axon cells and of afferent fibers from the retina throughout the nucleus; second, by the presence of long axons on the smallest neurons, which some workers have evidently included among the short-axon type because of their small size; third, by Obukhova's findings (1958, 1959) showing that after division of the optic nerve, synapses disintegrate not only on small but also on large cells of the lateral geniculate body. This does not mean, however, that the possibility of more complex interconnections between the neurons of this nucleus can be ruled out. Collaterals of long-axon cells have repeatedly been observed in dogs, where they evidently do not leave the lateral geniculate body (Figs. 22, 23). These collaterals and axons of the short-axon cells provide interconnections between the neurons, about which very little is yet known. They may possibly be responsible for cyclic connections discovered electrophysiologically (Bishop *et al.*, 1953) or for inhibition of surrounding cells.

Collaterals have also been observed leaving for the optic tract (Cajal, 1911; O'Leary, 1940) and also for nuclei of the reticular formation and other subcortical structures.

The neurons of the lateral geniculate body with few branches have long and straight dendrites, also with few branches. I found similar cells in the lateral geniculate body of the dog in 1952, and later in the ventral part of this nucleus in the rabbit (Fig. 8) and in its dorsal part in man (Fig. 105). They are very similar to the cells with few branches described by Leontovich (1952, 1959b) and Zhukova (1959). Cells of the lateral geniculate body with few branches exhibit bifurcation of their axon (Fig. 115). This very important structural detail explains how interconnection with other structures can take place at the subcortical level.

Midget cells (Fig. 115B, 5; Fig. 105) are very rare in the lateral geniculate body of the dog, absent in that nucleus in the hedgehog, and are the principal cells completely occupying the upper four parvocellular layers in the subcortical division of the human visual system (Fig. 59).

Electron microscopic discoveries in recent years have enabled an integrative structural unit to be distinguished in the lateral geniculate body of the cat (Szentágothai, 1963b, 1967), consisting of a specific visual afferent fiber, axons of Golgi type II cells, axons descending from the cortex, and spines on dendrites of the principal cells of the lateral geniculate body. Future investigations will reveal the relationship between these structural units and the various types of neurons and the changes taking place in them, depending on the character of vision and level of development of the central nervous system in mammals of different orders.

The Main Differences Between Neurons of the Visual Cortex and Lateral Geniculate Body

The principal criteria used for comparison of neuronal structures are: first and foremost, the architectonics and grouping of neurons; varieties and types of neurons; characteristics of the receptor part—the dendrites and their lateral appendages; characteristics of the efferent part—the axon, its collaterals and endings; the number and type of synapses in which the cell participates.

Architectonic differences between the cortex and subcortex are very important. According to Zavarzin there are two types of centers: screened centers in which synapses are formed in several layers, and nuclear centers in which neurons are concentrated in groups with the character of a nucleus; synaptic connections are limited to these groups of cells. If the auditory cortex and medial geniculate body of primates are examined, as an example, in this case the cortex has all the features of a screened center and the medial geniculate body those of a nuclear center, because the subcortical center of hearing has no stratification. The situation is quite different with the visual centers. In primates and in man the visual cortex and lateral geniculate body are sharply stratified structures and it is virtually impossible by architectonic methods alone to establish the principal differences between these two parts.

My observations, which are summarized in composite drawings of neurons in the cortex (Figs. 31, 67) and lateral geniculate body (Figs. 24, 63), reveal these differences sufficiently clearly. In the second case there is a laminated nuclear center, i.e., concentrations of neurons form several layers —three in the cat, four in the dog, six in man, and a variable number of layers in different monkeys. Visual afferent fibers entering each layer of this nucleus form contacts mainly with the cells of that particular layer. Dendrites of the cells of each layer of the lateral geniculate body do not extend into neighboring layers, and consequently they do not form connections with afferents of the other layers.

The situation is quite different in the cortex. Its most important cells are pyramidal cells whose synaptic surfaces occupy several layers. For example, besides the large dendritic receptor synaptic surface, consisting of the basal dendrites in layer V itself (Fig. 63), the pyramidal cell in layer V has an ascending trunk forming axo-dendritic connections in layers IV, III, and II and an apical bouquet in layer I, receiving impulses arising in this layer. Pyramidal cells of the other layers are connected in the same way with all other layers. Lorente de Nó was certainly correct when he considered that architectonic division of the cortex into areas purely on the basis of the arrangement of bodies of the neurons is inadequate.

The first and foremost difference between the cortex and subcortex is thus the presence of cells with plurisynaptic connections formed at several different levels of their structure. The second distinguishing feature is the variety of neuron types, which is large even in rodents.

In this short section I shall attempt, on the basis of my own observations, to distinguish the main type of neurons in the visual cortex and lateral geniculate body from the whole range of varieties, in order subsequently to compare them. These principal types differ in different orders of mammals depending on the state of visual function. In the narrow meaning of the term, the visual cortex is Area 17, present in both higher and lower mammals and, accordingly, the most stable and phylogenetically oldest portion of the cortex.

The most important types of neurons in Area 17, the central part of the visual cortex, are (Fig. 116): (1) the pyramidal cell with a long axon, (2) the fusiform cell with a long axon, (3) the star cell with a long axon, (4) the Martinotti cell with an ascending axon, (5) the pyramidal cell with an arcuate

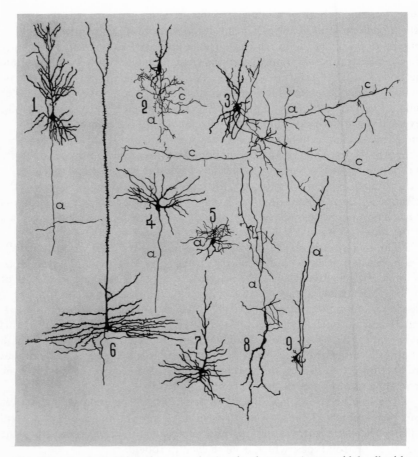

Fig. 116. Some varieties of neurons in the visual cortex. 1, pyramidal cell with long axon from layer III; 2, short-axon stellate cell with narrowly branching system from layer II; 3, short-axon stellate cell with widely branching axon system in layer IV; 4, star cell with long axon (star cell of Cajal); 5, short-axon stellate cell with narrowly branching axon system from layer IV; 6, solitary pyramidal cell of Meynert from layer V; 7, fusiform cell with long axon from lower layers; 8, cell with ascending axon; 9, pyramidal cell with ascending arcuate axon.

axon, (6) the short-axon stellate cell with widely branching axonal system, and (7) the short-axon cell with a narrowly branching axonal system (Shkol'-nik-Yarros, 1955a, 1958b).

Three of the principal varieties of neurons in the cortex thus have long axons extending into other parts of the nervous system, while the four varieties with short axons are responsible for complex interaction between neurons within the cortical layers themselves.

The four principal varieties of neurons in the lateral geniculate body have long axons extending into other parts of the nervous system; only a few short-axon cells are present for communication within the nucleus itself.

In the cortex the most characteristic and typical feature is that of the dendrites of pyramidal cells which may have as many as 80 dendritic branches. Several thousands of presynaptic terminals contact the body and dendrites of the cortical pyramidal cell, and several thousand spines can be counted on its dendrites. Dendrites of the fusiform cells have fewer branches but they are extensive and may spread through all the layers; dendrites of all the other cells in the cortex (stellate cells) are similar to dendrites of cells in the lateral geniculate body and other subcortical structures.

Just as in other subcortical nuclei, in the lateral geniculate body there are no cells resembling pyramidal cells in their receptive parts, nor as stated above, are any found in the brain stem, striopallidum, thalamus, or spinal cord. The pyramidal cell is typically cortical.

Dendrites of neurons in the lateral geniculate body may have up to 45 branches, but in the overwhelming majority of cases the number is much smaller, sometimes 10–15 (cells with few branches and midget cells). The number of spines is small. According to Glees (1941) and Obukhova (1958, 1959), up to 40 synaptic endings can be found on cells and dendrites of the cat's lateral geniculate body.

The length and degree of ramification of the dendrites increase in phylogenesis and ontogenesis. This process accompanies growth and development of the rest of the neuron—its body, axon, and axon collaterals. With growth and appearance of secondary and tertiary branches of the dendrites in ontogenesis, the number of spines, and synaptic endings approaching the dendrites, increases (Polyakov, 1951; Éntin, 1956). Growth of branches of axons and dendrites is different for different types of neurons. The length and pattern of the dendrites and the number of axon terminals approaching them are mutually related. The longer the dendrite and the more extensive its ramification, the greater its contact surface for communication with other neurons.

In the human lateral geniculate body I distinguished five main types of neuron (Fig. 162). Midget cells and cells with few branches differ most clearly in the arrangement of their dendrites. The midget cell (Fig. 115 B,5) as I have pictured it, is a component of the cone midget system conducting color stimuli as well as other visual sensations. Only a few visual fibers reach this cell. Besides these cells, other specific neurons—densely branching, double-tufted and radial—also are present in the lateral geniculate body, but the total number of their dendrites does not exceed 20 to 30 and the number of spines on their dendrites does not exceed 200. Their dendrites do not cover a wide area and they are only a little longer than dendrites of the midget cell.

The cells with few branches differ considerably in the arrangement of their dendrites. Whereas only a few axon terminals approach the short dendrites of the midget cells, a much greater number touch synapses with the long dendrites of these cells with few branches (Fig. 105). Only those axon terminals approaching dendrites which were successfully impregnated are shown in the figure, but even with this partial impregnation it is possible to visualize the vast quantitative differences observed simply on account of the length of the corresponding dendrites.

Enough has been said about the importance of spines as synapses. The morphological material demonstrates the intense development of the pyramidal cells in phylogenesis, their particular development in the upper layers, and the many and varied connections (Fig. 117). Compared with other cortical and subcortical cells, the pyramidal cell forms the greatest number of connections. It is beyond question that the conditioning function of the cortex, the complex chains of conditioned-reflex connections must be effected through the pyramidal cells, which have the leading role in this process. The association between qualitative and quantitative changes in the dendritic system of the pyramidal cells and increasing complexity of higher nervous activity is equally indisputable.

The subcortical neurons selected for comparison differ sharply in this respect from cortical cells. The subcortical midget cell of the visual system, concerned with the transmission of specific stimuli, has few connections with strictly definite systems of neurons. The cells with few branches have many connections whose nature can be conjectured. Work by Kravkov's school, together with modern electrophysiological research, has demonstrated interaction between analyzer systems, and especially between the visual and auditory systems at the subcortical level. It may be postulated that in the visual system it is the cells with few branches that are responsible for interaction with other sensory systems and also with the reticular formation at the subcortical level.

Consequently, the length and degree of ramification of the dendrites are important criteria determining the number of possible connections with other neurons. Some consider that the density of synaptic endings is maximal on neuron bodies. However, the surface area of the dendrites and the number of spines must indicate a larger number of axo-dendritic connections on pyramidal cells. In this respect my observations confirm Sarkisov's (1948) view that axo-dendritic contacts are more numerous in the cortex than in the subcortex.

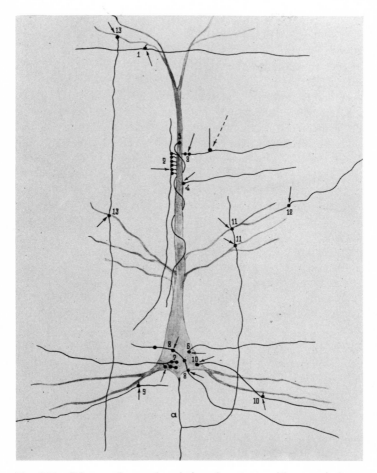

Fig. 117. Scheme of several varieties of contacts with a cortical pyramidal cell. 1, collateral contact between axon and apical dendrite through spine; 2, collateral contact between axon and trunk of apical dendrite through several spines; 3, terminal contact between axon and head of spine; 4, terminal contact between axon and dendrite trunk; 5, winding contact; 6, single terminal contact on body; 7, terminal contact on body with a cluster of synapses; 8, collateral contact on body; 9, collateral contact with spine of basal dendrite; 10, contact of axon simultaneously with dendrite and body; 11, contacts of axon collateral of original cell with dendrites, self-contact; 12, terminal contact of axon on end of dendritic branch; 13, contacts of ascending axon with dendritic branches. Golgi preparations. (Shkol'nik-Yarros, 1963.)

According to my observations, many neurons of the lateral geniculate body have no axon collaterals (Fig. 115B, 5); a small proportion of neurons have few collaterals (Fig. 115A, 6, 7, 8) and bifurcations (Fig. 115B, 3). The number of axon collaterals of the short-axon cells (Fig. 115A, 7, 8) is much smaller than the number of axon collaterals of cortical stellate cells (Figs. 36 and 73).

These facts all indicate that neurons of the lateral geniculate body have much less extensive connections both within the nucleus and with other parts of the nervous system than cortical neurons. However, as already mentioned, the presence of a few bifurcations and collaterals cannot be ignored because they may serve to connect different sensory systems at the subcortical level. This seems the more possible because numerous axo-dendritic contacts have been demonstrated with cells of the lateral geniculate body with few branches, i.e., a morphological basis for the convergence of excitation has been found even in such a highly specific nucleus as the lateral geniculate body.

Careful examination of lateral geniculate body neurons of different mammals led to the suggestion that interaction at the subcortical level is greater in carnivores than in primates. In the lateral geniculate body of the dog, which I have studied, axon collaterals and bifurcations were found more frequently than in primates. These unusual facts agree fully with Zvorykin's (1954, 1960) view regarding the importance of subcortical structures and also with the existence of greater structural and functional specialization and differentiation existing in primates.

Highly complex connections are characteristic of axons of cortical cells. Besides the principal axon, extending into other areas or into the subcortex, the long-axon pyramidal cells have numerous ascending or horizontal collaterals connecting one neuron with cells or dendrites in other layers of the cortex and sometimes with dendrites of the original neuron. Axons of fusiform cells and some axons of star cells of Cajal also have collaterals. Consequently, the highly complex system of interaction between cortical layers provided by all types of short-axon cells is also supplemented by a rich system of connections from long axons. All layers of the cortex are intercon-nected most intimately.

The four types of short-axon cells forming interneuronal connections in the immediate cortex also differ very considerably. Stellate cells with an ascending axon join all the layers (III, IV, V, VI, VII) with the upper layers as far as layer I. These neurons contact dendrites of pyramidal cells as their axon climbs upward, but their principal connections are formed with the cells of layer I.

The pyramidal cell with arcuate axon (Figs. 46, 62, 116) is a special type of short-axon cell. This intracortical mechanism of communication, according to Lorente de Nó (1922) is observed in all cortical areas but, as the result of my study of the visual areas has shown, it is seen much more frequently in Area 17 than in Areas 18 and 19. The axons evidently constitute an important part of Gennari's band and form intracortical connections.

Small short-axon cells with a narrowly looped axonal system are found in all layers of the cortex, but they are mainly concentrated in sublayer IVc of Area 17 and layer IV of Areas 18 and 19. Dendrites of these neurons are often coiled around the body and possess few spines; along the course of the dendrites fusiform thickenings are observed (Fig. 51). In sublayer IVc of Area 17 (a typical cell is shown in Fig. 116, 5) of the primate cortex the number of these small neurons, corresponding to "granules" in the cytoarchitectonic picture, is very great.

Stellate short-axon cells with widely branching axons contact many pyramidal and stellate neurons far from the original cell. They are particularly numerous in layers III and V (Fig. 116, 3).

The following conclusion can be drawn from this short survey. Excitation is carried from the visual cortex by neurons of three types: pyramidal cells, fusiform cells, and star cells of Cajal. Within the cortex itself, interneuronal connections are provided by at least four types of neurons (pyramidal cells with an arcuate axon; cells of Martinotti with an ascending axon, short-axon stellate cells with widely or narrowly branching axonal systems), and also by numerous axon collaterals of Golgi type I cells. Finally, these countless mechanisms of interconnections are strengthened by a special type of synapse—contacts of the cell on itself (Polyakov, 1955; Shkol'nik-Yarros, 1956, 1961b).

According to Beritov, activity of axo-dendritic synapses is important for neuron inhibition. I consider that changes in excitability of the neuron brought about through dendritic activity make an important contribution to the understanding of the structural differences between the cortex and subcortex. The great length of the dendrites and the variety of connections of the pyramidal neurons (Shkol'nik-Yarros, 1956, 1961b, 1963; Hamlyn, 1963) are among the many factors lying at the basis of the mosaic of inhibition and excitation so clearly revealed by electroencephalographic studies of the cortex (Livanov and Anan'ev, 1955, 1960). Because of the structural properties of cortical neurons, they can be involved either simultaneously or successively in excitation and inhibition, thus providing the material basis for complex cortical function, including the higher forms of cortical activity.

Structural properties in the lateral geniculate body—ramification of dendrites and axon collaterals, connections between neurons—are much less complex.

Chapter 4

STRUCTURE OF THE CENTRAL VISUAL SYSTEM AND PATHWAYS

CORTICAL ANALYZER AND DIFFUSE ELEMENTS

Pavlov advanced the idea that the general nature of the activity in all parts of the cortex was similar, although he, of course, accepted the existence of special cortical analyzers. He considered that for each sensory modality there is a corresponding region of the cortex which represents its precise projection. Morphologically he defined the cortical analyzer as the largest concentration of cells, with the most compact arrangement. This structural concept "explained the existence of special analyzers, where the exceptionally dense concentration of elements makes the synthetic and analytical activity of the analyzer possible."*

Pavlov's concepts of the visual analyzer are based on the following arguments: (1) projection of the retina on the cortex of the visual analyzer has been proved; (2) the visual analyzer, the organ of higher synthesis and analysis of photic stimuli, is located in the occipital lobes. Pavlov supports this statement by the existence of hemianopia associated with damage to the occipital lobe; (3) Pavlov regarded constriction of the visual fields as a disturbance of higher analysis and synthesis of visual stimuli; (4) besides the central part of the visual analyzer, located in the occipital lobes, there are other elements scattered diffusely throughout the cortex and performing more elementary visual functions. However, the work of Pavlov's school so far has not fully explained the structure and organization of the visual analyzer.

---

* I. P. Pavlov. *Lectures on the Operation of the Cerebral Hemispheres* [in Russian], 2nd ed. Moscow-Leningrad (1927), p. 294.

Many facts have been accumulated indicating that three occipital areas—17, 18, and 19—are united in their structure and activity. According to the results of neuronographic studies in monkeys, Area 17 is closely connected by short association fibers with Area 18, which in turn sends fibers into Area 19. If Areas 17, 18 and 19 are stimulated electrically eye movements are obtained. Cytoarchitectonic studies (Preobrazhenskaya and Filimonov, 1949) reveal that the structure of these areas have much in common—the small size and dense arrangement of their cells, their narrow cortex and well-marked striation. However, their morphological differences are also very apparent.

Areas 17, 18, and 19 develop differently in ontogenesis. Area 17 is basically mature by the fourth year of life. Areas 18 and 19 develop more slowly and mature later (Preobrazhenskaya, 1948). As was pointed out above, Areas 18 and 19 attain a very large size in man, whereas in monkeys Area 17 occupies the whole outer surface and Areas 18 and 19 are merely narrow bands surrounding area striata (Filimonov, 1933).

Consequently, both the ontogenetic and phylogenetic data demonstrate the later development of Areas 18 and 19, a result which is certainly related to the different relationships of these areas with the brain as a whole and with the external environment.

Considerable differences are observed between patients with lesions of Area 17 on the one hand, and Areas 18 and 19 on the other. Bekhterev (1890, 1911) demonstrated that separate areas exist for physiological and psychological blindness; pathological foci in the lateral cortex (i.e., in Areas 18 and 19) give rise to psychological blindness. Henschen, starting in 1890, conducted spirited arguments with other neurologists (Munk, Monakow, and others), defending his views on the role and significance of the visual areas. According to Henschen's clinical and pathomorphological data, the outside world is reflected in the area striata, because it is the fixed projection of the retina. When pathological foci develop in the region of the calcarine fissure, blindness is present, its extent corresponding to the size of the focus, but optical ideas and recollections are intact. They become changed if the lateral visual cortex, i.e., Areas 18 and 19, is destroyed. Filimonov (1957) considers that the function of Area 17 is less complex, while Area 19 is the most complex part of the occipital cortex. Hartridge (1952), when speaking of Areas 18 and 19, describes them as the "visuopsychic" area, repeating Campbell's (1905) terminology. Bailey and von Bonin (1951), in their latest map of cytoarchitectonic areas, unite Area 17 with the other receptor areas, and clearly distinguish Areas 18 and 19 as associative in character.

According to Luria (1966), the visual agnosia found in patients with lesions of the "general visual sphere" is a complex disturbance of synthesis of the elements of visual perception, a disturbance of the unification of these elements into simultaneously perceived groups. Lesions of Area 17 do not give rise to visual agnosia, but only to hemianopia.

By electrical stimulation of the human cortex, Penfield and Jasper (1954) obtained various visual responses, most frequently accompanied by movement. Whereas in stimulation of Area 17 objects move in the opposite visual field, in stimulation of Areas 18 and 19 the object frequently is visible ipsilaterally. Penfield suggests that Area 17 is simply a relay station on the path to higher levels, while Areas 18 and 19 are connected with the integrative system where vision is represented as a whole and bilaterally (visual integration).

Preobrazhenskaya (1952) studied patients with lesions of the occipital region after penetrating wounds of the skull, and identified three syndromes resulting from such a lesion. In the first the lesion affects mainly the "first signal system," while in the second and, in particular, the third syndromes, complex manifestations of activity of the "second signal system" (disturbances of praxis and gnosis) are present to a varying degree.

Modern workers have approached the question of the place of Areas 17, 18, and 19 in the visual analyzer from the standpoint of Pavlov's theories. Their views on this matter conflict. Filimonov (1951), for instance, recognizes the presence of nuclei of analyzers of the "first signal system" in the cortex, among which he includes Area 17. Preobrazhenskaya (1954) considers that the nucleus of the visual analyzer includes all three areas of the occipital cortex: 17, 18, and 19. Interesting views have been expressed by Davydenkov and Dotsenko (1956), who divide the visual analyzer into two parts: that of the first signal system (calcarine fissure) and that of the second signal system (the left gyrus angularis). Polyakov (1956) distinguishes between the central area of the analyzer (Area 17) and peripheral areas (Areas 18 and 19). The central area has its highest concentration of stellate neurons in layer IV, the peripheral area in upper layers of the cortex.

Many interesting data concerning the function of these areas have been obtained in experiments on animals. Khananashvili (1960b, 1962), in an extensive investigation on dogs, removed Areas 17, 18, and 19 separately. His results show that removal of Area 17 always disturbs direct perception of objects, while Areas 18 and 19 are concerned with the normal course of internal inhibition and participate in the fine analysis of visual stimuli.

Sikharulidze (1962), working in Beritov's laboratory, likewise clearly demonstrated the different functions of these areas in dogs. After bilateral extirpation of Area 17, a disturbance of visual perception of objects was observed; after removal of Areas 18 and 19, spatial orientation and the normal course of delayed responses to conditioned stimuli were disturbed. Some authorities find no justification for differentiation between Areas 18 and 19 and consider that the minor cytoarchitectonic differences are of no importance. From my study I consider that every architectonic characteristic, however trivial, corresponds to a different pattern of interneuronal connections, and from this point of view I regard architectonics (connections) as being of prime importance. The differences are especially significant when neurons of Areas 17, 18, and 19 are compared. This has been very clearly demonstrated by microelectrode electrophysiological investigations carried out on cats (Hubel and Wiesel, 1963, 1965). The functional boundaries of Areas 17, 18, and 19, defined in accordance with the degree of complexity of single unit responses, coincide precisely with their cytoarchitectonic boundaries.

However, a study of the neurons in the human occipital cortex suggests a more specific role for Area 17 in the act of vision and a less specific role, more mixed with other functions, for Areas 18 and 19.

This conclusion in no way contradicts the great increase in the surface of the phylogenetically newer Areas 18 and, in particular, 19, together with Areas 39, 40, and others, in man.

Morphological analysis shows that these facts are not antithetical. The extreme structural complexity of Area 17 and its high concentration of visual afferent fibers are conclusive evidence of its decisive role in the analysis and integration of visual stimuli. The lamination which characterizes all visual centers—the retina, lateral geniculate body, and cortex of Area 17, which Zavarzin (1950) emphasized, may be recalled. Projection of visual fibers on the cortex is confirmed by Polyak's (1933) experiments, where portions of Area 17 of different shapes were removed and the degeneration produced in the lateral geniculate bodies corresponded to these shapes.

The latest experimental evidence has completely confirmed the precise projection of the retina on the lateral geniculate body, and then on the cortex of Area 17 in monkeys. An important mathematical analysis of this matter has recently been made by Daniel and Whitteridge (1962), who demonstrated the linear dimension of the cortex of Area 17 relative to each degree of the visual field. In this way fresh evidence has been obtained that the visual analyzer is located in Area 17.

By virtue of its structure and connections, the area striata is thus best adapted for analysis and integration of specific visual stimuli. This is supported by considerable experimental evidence (Minkowski, 1913, 1920b; Lashley, 1934a,b; Polyak, 1933, 1957) and also by many pathological and clinical investigations.

Surrounding areas, differing in structure and, consequently, in function, are connected differently with the periphery and surrounding parts of the brain. These areas (18 and 19), which have grown to a particularly large size in man, I regard as a further addition to the analyzer, adapted for association connections as well as for specific, visual function. These areas play a greater part in complex and specifically human functions connected with visual gnosis.

I should emphasize once more that the organization of the visual system is substantially different in primates and other mammals. This is apparent not only from a comparison of neurons in the occipital cortex, but also from examination of electrophysiological data and results of the study of nerve pathways.

In monkeys, for instance, according to the latest experimental data, fibers of the optic radiation terminate precisely at the border of Gennari's band, while in cats these fibers can be traced into neighboring areas: Area 18 and part of the suprasylvian gyrus (Wilson and Cragg, 1967). Termination of fibers from the lateral geniculate body outside visual areas 17, 18, and 19 in the cat have also been described by Sprague (1966); projections in the rabbit are observed not only to Area 17, but also to Area 18 (Rose and Malis, 1965). This agrees with earlier electrophysiological data indicating higher amplitudes of evoked potentials in the cortex bordering on Area 17 in cats (Doty, 1958), recently confirmed by Berkley, Wolf, and Glickstein (1967) and by Krol' (1968), and also showing that in cats the visual perception of objects may require integrity of more than the area striata (Doty, 1961).

The problem of the diffuse elements of the visual analyzer is much less clear. It is often claimed that they do not exist (Belenkov and Kalinina, 1963). Supporters of this view regard their acceptance as scientific dogmatism. Other neuroscientists remain undecided, not finally rejecting the possibility of diffuse elements, yet at the same time not finding concrete methods for studying them. Finally, there are those investigators who continue to work in this direction and who accept diffuse elements in the cortex. Kukuev (1955), for instance, considers that motor neurons scattered among other cortical systems are diffuse elements of the motor analyzer. This view is unquestionably the right one and it is confirmed by many morphological investigations.

So far as the visual system is concerned, I accept the presence of diffuse elements in both its centrifugal and its centripetal parts (Shkol'nik-Yarros, 1958a, 1961b; Skrebitskii and Shkol'nik-Yarros, 1964).

It would be wrong to regard the centrifugal pathways of the visual system in isolation purely as bundles of fibers descending from the visual cortex. The relationship of the anterior oculomotor areas of the cortex, temporal areas, and, finally, occipital areas to movements of the eyes is well known from clinical observations and experiments on animals (Bekhterev, 1896–1898; Gerver, 1899, 1937; Foerster, 1936; C. Vogt and O. Vogt, 1919; Szentágothai, 1943; Adrianov, 1951, 1953; and many others). Since the visual act cannot be separated from movement of the eyes, the visual system in the broad meaning of the term must include all parts of the cortex giving rise to movements of the eyes when stimulated electrically. If the visual system is considered from this point of view, Pavlov's diffuse elements immediately come into the picture. Obviously these motor pathways of the visual system do not arise from zones where the principal neurons receiving visual excitation are concentrated. They lie outside the visual analyzer.

Some of my own observations made on diffuse elements of the centripetal part of the visual system are interesting in this respect. After removal of the eye or division of the optic nerve, degeneration appears not only in the usual brain stem and subcortical structures, but also in various regions of the cortex. I discovered this originally by the use of Marchi's method (starting in 1952), and later by Nauta's method (1960, 1961), and the results are described in my doctoral dissertation (1961b). Later, also using Nauta's

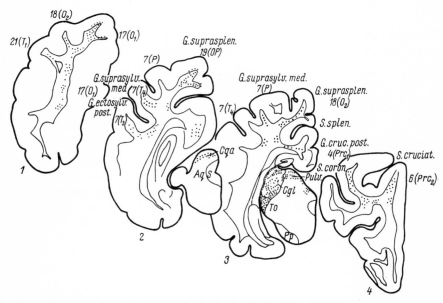

Fig. 118. Frontal sections through the brain of dog No. 195. Topography of direct centripetal fibers connecting retina with cortex shown semischematically by dots. 1: Section at level of occipital pole. 2: Section through mesencephalon. 3: Section through lateral geniculate body. 4: Section through cruciate sulcus: Cqa, superior colliculus; AqS, aqueduct of Sylvius; Cgl, lateral geniculate body; To, optic tract; Pp, cerebral peduncle; Pulv., pulvinar. Marchi's method. Identification of areas after Gurevich and Bykhovskaya; in parentheses, after Adrianov and Mering. (Skrebitskii and Shkol'nik-Yarros, 1964.)

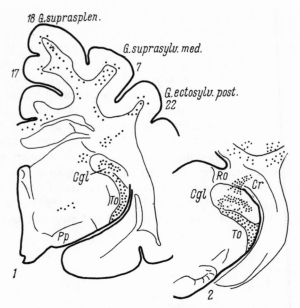

Fig. 119. Frontal sections through cat's brain after enucleation. 1: Section through lateral geniculate body, Marchi.
2: Section at same level, Nauta; Ro, optic radiation; Cr,
corona radiata. Remainder of abbreviations as in Fig. 118.
Identification of cytoarchitectonic areas after Gurevich and
Khachaturyan. (Skrebitskii and Shkol'nik-Yarros, 1964.)

method, Biryuchkov (1963) obtained similar results in extensive experiments on rodents, carnivores, and primates. Recently, Svanidze (1964)
confirmed the direct pathway from the eye to the occipital and other regions
of the cortex in rats.

I removed the eye or divided the optic nerve surgically in rats, rabbits,
cats, and dogs; operations were performed on 11 animals altogether.

No special investigation was made of connections of the optic nerve
with the brain stem and subcortex. Recent work, using new methods, has
filled in many important details in our knowledge (Silva, 1956; Obukhova,
1959; Hayhow, 1958, 1959; Novokhatskii, 1957; Biryuchkov, 1963; Laties
and Sprague, 1966; Garey and Powell, 1968). In brief, my observations
confirm those of others on the termination of visual fibers in the lateral
geniculate body (dorsal and ventral parts), superior colliculi, pulvinar,
and pretectal nucleus. A few fibers can be traced into the medial geniculate
body, the reticular formation of the brain stem, and possibly also into the
nucleus of the oculomotor nerve, and the hypothalamus.

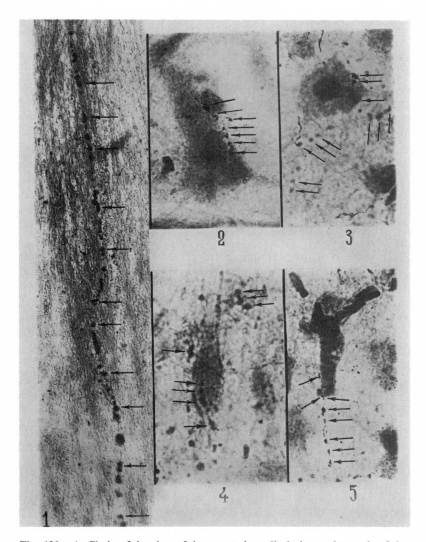

Fig. 120.   1: Chain of droplets of degenerated myelin in internal capsule of dog No. 195. Droplets located along course of bundle of fibers. Marchi's method, 140×. 2: Cortex of cat. Large pyramidal cell of layer III in Area 17. Degenerated preterminal axon endings are shown by arrows. Nauta; immersion; 750×. 3: Cat cortex. Stellate cell of layer IV in Area 17. Degenerated preterminal axon endings on body of a neuron and in other parts of cortex are shown by arrows. Nauta; immersion; 750×. 4: Cat cortex. Fusiform cell of layer VI in Area 22. Degenerated preterminal axon endings on body of a neuron and in other parts of cortex shown by arrows. Nauta. 5: Cat cortex. Capillary in layer IV in Area 17. Degeneration of axon connected by preterminal endings with capillary shown by arrows. Nauta; immersion; 750× (Skrebitskii and Shkol'nik-Yarros, 1964).

In all 11 cases I found degeneration in the cortex. With Marchi's method this degeneration was less marked than by Nauta's method.*

The most conspicuous degenerated fibers in the dog's cortex, demonstrable in all the histological sections, are found in the suprasplenial marginal gyrus, especially in its posterior parts corresponding to Areas 17 and 18 (Fig. 118, O_1 and O_2). Scattered fibers are definitely present in the middle part of the marginal gyrus and the middle and posterior suprasylvian and middle and posterior ectosylvian gyri, while fewer signs of degeneration are present in the posterior and anterior cruciate gyri. These changes are thus observed in Areas 21, 22, 7, 4, and 6 (T_1, T_2, T_4, P, Pc_1, and Pc_2). Degeneration was clearly marked both contralaterally and ipsilaterally relative to the side of operation. Degeneration was also found in the corona radiata and internal capsule (Fig. 120). The presence of chains of droplets located precisely along the course of bundles of fibers was the criterion used to assess degeneration in these cases.

Distribution of the degenerated fibers was also studied after removal of the eye or division of the optic nerve in cats, rabbits, and rats. The topography of distribution of degeneration in the cat's cortex is similar to that in the dog (Skrebitskii and Shkol'nik-Yarros, 1964). Its localization corresponds to Areas 17, 18, 21, 22, and 30 (Fig. 119, 1). Definite chains were visible in the internal capsule. By means of Nauta's method, which I used in the cat, the course of the diffuse fibers and their endings in the cortex could be demonstrated precisely. Fibers passing through the lateral geniculate body without interruption into the optic radiation and corona radiata are shown in Fig. 119, 2; degenerated axons thereafter can be seen as scattered fibers throughout the gyri. In the cortex itself, chains of degenerated axons are observed (Fig. 120, 5), and in some places preterminal fibrils and degenerated synaptic endings are visible as irregularly shaped deposits. Degenerated axo-somatic connections of this type were observed in the visual cortex (Areas 17 and 18), on pyramidal neurons of layer III (Fig. 120, 2), on stellate cells of layer IV (Fig. 120, 3), and in Area 22 on the fusiform cells of layer VI. In some sections degenerated preterminal fibrils could be seen on capillaries and glial cells.

In rabbits, degenerated fibers were most numerous in the area striata (Area 17) and Areas Par_3 and Par_4 (5–7) (Fig. 121), and more diffuse fibers in Areas Occ (18), T_1 (21), and Par_4 and Par_5 (7). Single granules were found in the area precentralis agranularis (4) and area postcentralis (3). Degeneration was also clearly visible in rabbits in the internal capsule (Fig. 121). Just as in the cat's cortex, degenerated synaptic endings were found by Nauta's method on the bodies of neurons, notably the pyramidal cells of layer V.

---

* Some of the morphological data given in this section were described at a meeting to discuss the physiology of analyzers (organs of the senses) in Leningrad in May, 1961.

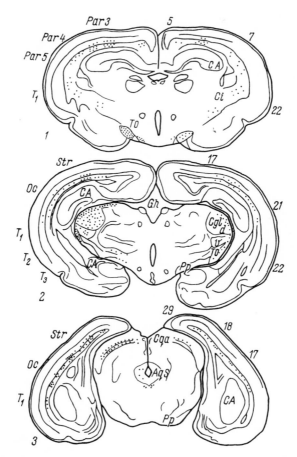

Fig. 121. Frontal sections through brain of rabbit No. 1230 (right eye removed). 1: Sections at level of optic tract. 2: Section at level of lateral geniculate body. 3: Section at mesencephalic level. Nomenclature of cytoarchitectonic areas after Rose on the left; Par, parietal; T, temporal; Oc, occipital; Str, striata. On the right, after Brodmann. Marchi's method. CA, hippocampus; Cgld, dorsal part of lateral geniculate body; Cglv, ventral part; Ci, internal capsule; Gh, habenula. Remainder of legend as in Figs. 118 and 119. (Skrebitskii and Shkol'nik-Yarros, 1964.)

The few fibers which can be seen after staining by Marchi's method could have been overlooked by investigators studying the brain after removal of the eyes. Their presence and distribution in the cortex provide a morphological explanation of the observations made previously by electrophysiologists who described changes in potentials in the parietal, temporal, and motor areas after enucleation of the eye (Sarkisov, 1939), and also of the many later findings of direct changes in the EEG in different parts of the cortex during excitation of the visual system (Leushina, 1961, 1963; Skrebitskii, 1960; Skrebitskii and Shkol'nik-Yarros, 1964). Biochemical changes in the rabbit cortex observed by Pigareva (1958, 1960) after enucleation are also interesting in this respect.

These results also suggest that short-latency potentials obtained in recordings from different points of the lateral suprasylvian and posterior sigmoid gyri (Areas 17, 18, T_1, T_4, P, Prc_1 respectively) are explained by a direct connection between the retina and cortex. Although some eminent authorities in the past have denied that such connections exist, and although no mention of them is made by Polyak (1957), I still feel that such connections are possible.

Direct connections between retina and cortex could explain the phenomenon, observed by Livanov, of the spread of excitation over the whole cortex in rabbits before its concentration in the analyzer.

The question of the increase in "tone" of cortical cells under the influence of visual stimuli must be considered afresh. Whereas previously the view was accepted that the only possible pathway is that through the reticular formation, with its projection to the brain as a whole, it now seems that a direct influence on extensive cortical territories can be effected in a second way. In each of these cases the pathway and point of termination of the corresponding fibers will differ. In the first case termination on dendrites of the cortical cells is more probable; in the second case termination is on the bodies of these neurons.

It is interesting that a pathway of visual impulses to areas of the cortex outside the analyzer, via the lateral geniculate body, has also been demonstrated electrophysiologically by Vastola (1961).

Pavlov's theory of diffuse elements of analyzers in the cortex and the fact that such elements have been discovered in the form of diffuse fibers in the central visual system explain new data on the convergence of different types of excitation in the cortical projection areas (the polysensory neurons of Jung and others). Interesting results from this point of view were obtained by Babayan (1955), confirming Bekhterev's (1906) earlier descriptions of visual and motor disturbances following removal of the parietal region in dogs. Babayan concluded that diffuse elements of the visual and motor analyzers are present in the dog's parietal cortex.

My method of examination showed that direct pathways running from the retina to the cortex are not concentrated in bundles and can be detected only histologically. The suggestion is that in man, where a direct pathway in the form of a bundle was demonstrated by Dzugaeva (1958), connections of a more diffuse character also exist with other parts of the cortex. The results of my investigation also indirectly confirm my hypothesis put forward in 1958 suggesting that the centrifugal fibers of the retina arise from diffuse elements in various cortical areas.

Filimonov's theory of plurality of functions of the cytoarchitectonic structures of the brain is thus confirmed. A concrete reflection of this theoretical situation is the diffuse elements demonstrated in the visual system in my investigations. These pathways running directly from receptor to cortex provide the latter with its necessary tone.

Naturally, the foregoing data on direct retino-cortical pathways require further confirmation, and the existence of such paths is thus indicated only tentatively by dashed lines in Fig. 128.

EFFERENT CONNECTIONS OF THE VISUAL CORTEX

Despite many investigations, significant gaps and uncertainties remain in knowledge of the visual pathways and centers. As stated above, the phylogenesis and ontogenesis of the visual cortex and the projection of the retina on the lateral geniculate body and of the latter on the cortex have been studied in detail. Considerable attention has been paid to centrifugal pathways from the visual cortex, although they have not yet found a place in many textbooks. Most frequently only the centripetal parts are shown in schemes of the central visual system.

The need for clarification of the course of efferent fibers from the visual cortex has been stressed by Klosovskii (1939) and Le Gros Clark (1942), among others.

Other aspects of the structure of central visual connections likewise remain undecided.

The theory that Area 17 is isolated from other areas, based on the work of Le Gros Clark (1942) and Dusser de Barenne and McCulloch (1938), is still widely held in the West. In their opinion, the association connections of Area 17 do not go beyond its boundaries, for they were traced for only 5 mm from a lesion or point of stimulation. On the basis of these studies, Hartridge (1952) considers that a special feature of the visual pathways and cortex connected with them is their isolation. However, this view was not confirmed by the work of Nauta and Bucher (1954) who demonstrated a large number of association fibers in the rat's brain in the presence of very small lesions in Area 17.

The existence of commissural pathways from Area 17 is denied by some although others have observed them. Van Valkenburg (1913), for example, using the methods of Nissl and Weigert, showed that the area striata has no commissural connections; Krieg (1947), in experiments on rats, confirmed the absence of commissural fibers from Area 17. Kononova (1926), Polyak (1927), Mettler (1935) and others described degeneration of commissural fibers after lesions of the visual areas.

Many investigators are doubtful of the existence of projection fibers from Area 17 to structures of the diencephalon and mesencephalon, and the data which are available are highly contradictory. The marked discrepancy between the results and between the conclusions deduced from them may evidently be explained by differences in the species and methods used.

Monakow (1889) considered that the large pyramidal cells of layer III of the visual cortex, which he regarded as solitary cells, connect the cortex with primary visual centers, and he observed degeneration of these pyramids after division of the posterior limb of the internal capsule. Monakow declared most emphatically that the cortex has centrifugal connections with the superior colliculi, and these are reflected in his scheme of the visual pathways.

In his doctoral dissertation, Gerver (1899) discussed the centers for eye movements. He removed the occipital cortex from dogs and, using Marchi's method, traced degenerated fibers into the corona radiata, the posterior portion of the internal capsule, the posterior portions of the thalamus, the optic tract, lateral geniculate body, posterior commissure, superior colliculi, posterior longitudinal fasciculus, and the medial parts of the ipsilateral reticular formation. On the side opposite to the lesion degenerated fibers were observed in the thalamus, optic tract, and superior colliculi, although in smaller numbers. On the opposite side degeneration was considerable in the posterior longitudinal fasciculus.

For cats and dogs Probst (1902) gave a detailed account of the changes taking place after removal of part of the occipital cortex. Degenerated fibers were found in the white matter of the three lateral gyri of the occipital cortex, in the sagittal layers, the fasciculus subcallosus, symmetrical areas of the opposite hemisphere, the ipsilateral superior colliculus, the posterosuperior part of the opposite superior colliculus, the lateral part of the cerebral peduncle and pons, the pulvinar and lateral thalamic nuclei, and the stratum zonale of the thalamus.

Minkowski (1911) reached similar conclusions. He considers that more marked degeneration of projection pathways of the visual cortex is observed after destruction of the ectosylvian gyrus in dogs than in the presence of foci in Area 17. Degeneration is clearest in the superior colliculi.

Kononova (1926) removed gyri from the medial surface of the occipital lobe in dogs corresponding in Klempin's scheme to Areas 17a, b, c and 18. She traced the course of the degenerated fibers by Marchi's method into neighboring gyri, into symmetrical and asymmetrical gyri of the opposite side, and into the subcortex: lateral geniculate body, more marked in its dorsal and anterior portions, the lateral nucleus of the thalamus, and deep layers of the superior colliculus of the same side, and much less marked in the superior colliculus on the opposite side. After removal of gyri on the lateral surface of the occipital lobe in dogs, followed by the use of the Weigert–Pal method, Kononova obtained considerable changes in the pulvinar and lateral thalamic nucleus, which were reduced in size; a decrease in volume of the superior colliculi and pallor of its fibers also were observed. After this operation the lateral geniculate body was not reduced in size, and only a few degenerated fibers penetrated into it.

Centrifugal pathways of the visual system were also studied by Cords (1926) in connection with the problem of oculomotor nystagmus. As a result of a thorough study of the literature dealing with the pathology of visual centers and tracts in man, Cords drew up a scheme of pathways to explain the loss of optical reflex movements of the eyes after destruction of the oculomotor areas. He considers that the corticifugal pathways run through the posterior portion of the internal capsule and lateral part of the cerebral peduncle to the center for rotation of the eyes close to the nucleus of the sixth pair of cranial nerves.

Polyak (1927) describes centrifugal pathways from the visual cortex of Area 17 in cats (Marchi's method) to the superior colliculi (superior and middle layers). He calls this projection the dorsal cortico-mesencephalic fasciculus of the occipital region. Very thin fibers run through the fasciculus subcallosus to the head of the caudate nucleus. He traced paths from Areas 18 and 19 to the superior colliculi and nuclei of the pons.

Mettler (1935), also using Marchi's method, studied corticifugal connections of the occipital region in monkeys (*Macaca mulatta*). Besides numerous association and commissural connections, he describes pathways from the superior lip of the calcarine fissure to the lateral geniculate body, mesencephalon, pulvinar and lateral nucleus of the thalamus, tectum, the central gray matter around the aqueduct of Sylvius, the nuclei of the third and fourth pairs of cranial nerves on both sides, the red nucleus, the medial longitudinal fasciculus into the tectum, and (problematically) to the sub-thalamic region and globus pallidus.

On the basis of the results of removal of parts of the visual cortex in cats, Barris, Ingram, and Ranson (1935) completely reject any direct centrifugal connection between the cortex and lateral geniculate body.

Brouwer (1936) sums up the results obtained by others for centrifugal pathways of Area 17. He believed that these fibers arise from the solitary cells of Meynert and, possibly, the large pyramidal cells of layer III. A large bundle runs into the stratum medullare superficiale of the superior colliculus; this pathway is probably concerned with inborn reflexes and carries visual impulses to the motor centers. Türck's bundle begins not only from the temporal and parietal regions, but also from the occipital. It may transmit visual excitation through the pons to the cerebellum. Brouwer considers that the pathway from the cortex of Area 17 to the lateral geniculate body is responsible for changes in excitability of the neurons of this nucleus.

In his doctoral dissertation on the mechanism of vestibular nystagmus and its participation in cortically controlled eye movements, Klosovskii (1939) concludes that the visual cortex is connected with the triangular (medial) nucleus of the vestibular system, where the whole mechanism of coordinated combinations of eye movements involving the nuclei of the sixth and third pairs of cranial nerves and the whole vestibulo-oculomotor system is triggered. Klosovskii stresses that much remains unexplained and debatable in the problem of centrifugal cortico-bulbar pathways, and considers that further clarification of their course is essential.

Le Gros Clark (1941), in a paper on association connections of the visual cortex in monkeys (three monkeys, Marchi's method), categorically supports the presence of corticotectal, corticopontine, and, perhaps, corticogeniculate pathways. He also (1942) observed retrograde degeneration of Meynert's cells in Area 17 of macaques one week after destruction of the superior colliculi, demonstrating that their axons participate in forming corticomesencephalic pathways.

Krieg (1947) used the Marchi technique on albino rats after removal of parts of Area 17 and Area 18. He observed considerable degeneration of pathways running from Area 17 to the cerebral peduncle but saw no degenerated fibers to the lateral geniculate body. Krieg also denies that Area 17 has commissural connections; in his opinion pathways run from Area 18 to layers IV and II of the superior colliculus, the tectum, the lateral geniculate body, the lateral nucleus of the thalamus, and through the corpus callosum to the opposite hemisphere, to Area 17, and to the auditory and sensory areas of the ipsilateral cortex.

Brazovskaya (1951, 1953) detected an occipitopontine pathway by fine anatomical dissection in dogs and man. She found that in man there are three bundles in the occipital region: anterior occipitopontine, posterior occipitopontine (from Area 18), and superior occipitopontine (from Area 19). She suggests that corticopontine fibers from the occipital as well as from the temporal and parietal regions originate from large cells of layer III[3].

Corticifugal projections of the occipital areas (mainly Area 18) to the intralaminar nuclei of the thalamus, pulvinar, mesencephalic reticular formation, substantia nigra, and subthalamic region have been observed electrophysiologically (Jasper, Ajmone-Marsan, and Stoll, 1952).

Crosby and Henderson (1953) consider that besides the medial corti-cotectal tract which Crosby described in conjunction with Huber, there is also a corticotegmental tract, running directly from the occipital lobe to the opposite nucleus of the abducens nerve and to the medial and lateral vestibular nuclei.

Walberg and Brodal (1953), using Glees's method in cats after extirpation of the temporal and occipital cortex, traced corticospinal fibers running through the cerebral peduncle as far as the lumbar region of the spinal cord. In their opinion some fibers pass through the corpus callosum to the opposite internal capsule, peduncle, and pyramid, being components of the pyramidal tract. Many of these fibers are of medium or small caliber.

Nathan and Smith (1955), in a detailed survey of long pathways arising from the cortex, later cast doubt on the presence of occipital and temporal components of the pyramidal tract.

Nauta and Bucher (1954) destroyed Area 17 in albino rats. They used a new method introduced by Nauta and Ryan, and showed that Area 17 is connected with the lateral geniculate body (with its dorsal and, more especially, its ventral nucleus), with the posterolateral nucleus of the thalamus, the pretectal region, the superior colliculi, the zona incerta, and the pons. Association fibers connect various parts of Area 17, and also connect Area 17 with Area 18 and with the medial part of Area 18a, while commissural fibers connect with Area 17 and Area 18a of the opposite hemisphere.

Electrophysiological experiments on monkeys demonstrated the connection between the paraoccipital region and the bulbar reticular formation (French, Hernández-Peón, and Livingston, 1955). These workers showed by application of strychnine that the pathway they describe terminates at a place to which fibers run from the sensorimotor cortex, the frontal oculomotor areas, the anterior limbic gyrus, and other parts of the cortex.

Polyak (1932 and 1957), describing the results of an experiment on a monkey (Marchi's method), found that besides numerous short association connections within Area 17 and a longer pathway to the angular gyrus, there are other pathways running through the pulvinar toward the ipsilateral superior colliculus. However, he is very guarded, or even skeptical, in his remarks about this bundle. As regards the very thin fibers running to the superior portion of the lateral geniculate body, Polyak was also doubtful whether these descending fibers were corticogeniculate or the result of very limited retrograde degeneration of some cells of the lateral geniculate body.

Rossi and Brodal (1956) described fibers from Areas 18 and 19 descending to the bulbar reticular formation.

I also used Marchi's method (Shkol'nik-Yarros, 1958a). Small parts of the visual cortex in Area 17 were removed in rabbits, cats, and dogs. In rabbits, degenerated fibers were traced to the lateral geniculate body (dorsal and ventral parts), the stratum opticum of the ipsilateral superior colliculus (some fibers cross to the other side), the pretectal zone, zona incerta, and lateral part of the cerebral peduncle. In cats and dogs degeneration was seen in the dorsal part of the lateral geniculate body, the pulvinar and posterior nucleus of the thalamus, the pretectal zone, superior colliculus (the largest number of fibers), and the lateral portion of the cerebral peduncle. If large foci of destruction were present, degenerated fibers were found in the optic tract and nerve.

Dzugaeva used fine anatomical dissection. In a special article (1958) on the optic pathways she concludes that in man a few direct connections exist between the cortex and optic tract. She suggests that they may include both centripetal and centrifugal fibers.

Beritov (1960, 1961) believes that the star cells of Cajal give rise to pathways serving the purpose of directing and fixing the eyes on an external object. The pyramidal cells of Meynert, in his opinion, are concerned with activation of the coordinating apparatus for head movement. The cortex thus contains a trigger mechanism for the orienting reflex: movements of the eyes and head.

Obukhova (1960) removed parts of Areas 17, 18, and 19 in dogs and used Marchi's method to trace pathways running to structures in the subcortex. Degenerated descending fibers were traced from Area 17 to the pretectal region, the posterior nucleus and pulvinar of the thalamus, the superior colliculi, and in very small numbers to the lateral geniculate body. Degenerated fibers from Area 18 were traced to the pretectal region, pulvinar and posterior nucleus of the thalamus; and from Area 19 to the posterior nucleus of the thalamus.

Obukhova also studied descending connections of various parts of Area 17 in dogs. After removing the inferior part of Area 17 on the lateral surface, she found degenerated fibers only in the pretectal region, but after removal of the superior part she found them in the posterior nucleus and pulvinar of the thalamus and in the pretectal region.

Kusama, Otani, and Kawana (1966) described special topographical features of the descending pathways in cats. For instance, fibers from the occipital pole run to the middle third of the superior colliculi, and fibers from the anterior parts of the visual areas run to its lateral third. Fibers were traced to the posterior part of the lateral geniculate body from the postero-lateral gyrus, and to the anterior part of the lateral geniculate body from the posterior third of the anterior marginal gyrus. Descending pathways are distributed uniformly to the pretectal zone regardless of the topography of the areas removed.

Consequently, different methods (fine anatomical dissection, Marchi degeneration, silver impregnation by the methods of Glees and Nauta, study of brain pathology, used on different species such as rats, rabbits, cats, dogs, monkeys, and man led to many conflicting conclusions. Sometimes the same method, used on the same species but by different investigators, led to contrary conclusions. As was mentioned above, Polyak found no descending connections from Area 17 to almost all the subcortical structures in monkeys and was even doubtful about the corticotectal tract which, in his opinion, arises from Area 18. Mettler, on the other hand, found connections between Area 17 and 11 different subcortical structures.

Polyak's opinion was reflected in his scheme of the structure of connections of Area 17, where only short-axon neurons are found. It is not clear from an examination of Polyak's scheme how movements of the eyes are obtained in response to electrical stimulation of the visual cortex.

What are the actual pathways along which impulses for conscious and unconscious eye movements are transmitted from the occipital cortex? Does the cortex participate in regulation of the flow of afferent impulses, regulation of the abundant visual information arriving from the external environment? If regulation is carried out by cortical structures, through what specific structures do they act? Finally, many investigations during recent years, both electrophysiological and studies of conditioned-reflex activity, have demonstrated the great importance of cortical connections in closing not only intracortical, but also cortico-subcortical pathways. Consequently, the conclusion is reached once again that the study of centrifugal cortical pathways is of great importance.

In my own investigations I therefore concentrated on the study of efferent pathways of the visual cortex and centrifugal system as a whole. This was justified by the need for clarification of the morphological mechanism of visual regulatory systems. Some of the most instructive observations made in the course of an investigation in 1958 are given below.

Case 1.

At operation on an adult rabbit (KO El) Area 17 of the right hemisphere was removed. The rabbit was sacrificed 15 days later. A large piece of the superior part of the area striata in the right hemisphere had been removed, together with the area peristriata and part of the retrosplenial cortex (Rsgβ according to Rose's classification). The integrity of the white matter was considerably disturbed.

Marchi staining was used to study the pathways which run through the stratum sagittale internum et externum, and then turn downward and pass

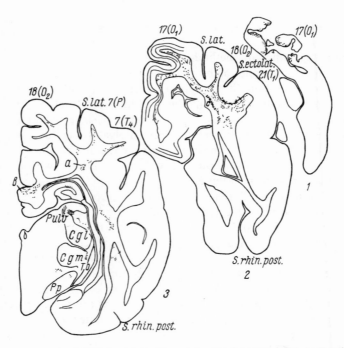

Fig. 122. Frontal sections through brain of dog No. 206. 1: Surgical focus at occipital pole, Area 17. Degenerated fibers can be seen as droplets (black dots in projections). 2: Course of degenerated association bundles to neighboring gyri. A projection bundle (c) can be seen. 3: Section at diencephalic level. Degeneration of association, commissural, and projection connections can be seen. Droplets in lateral geniculate body, pulvinar, and cerebral peduncle. a, long association bundle; Pulv, pulvinar; Cgl, lateral geniculate body; Cgm, medial geniculate body; To, optic tract; Pp, cerebral peduncle; b, chain of droplets in corpus callosum; c, degenerated projection fibers. Cytoarchitectonic areas according to Gurevich and Bykhovskaya denoted by numbers. Cortical areas according to Adrianov and Mering given in parentheses. (Shkol'nik-Yarros, 1958a.)

through Wernicke's area to structures of the diencephalon and mesencephalon, where many degenerated droplets could be seen. The fibers terminated in the dorsal and ventral nuclei of the lateral geniculate body, layers III and II of the superior colliculus, and the pulvinar. In the upper layers of the superior colliculus the fibers are divided transversely; larger in layer III and smaller in layer II. In layers IV and V (after Winkler and Potter, 1911), the fibers are divided longitudinally, and have a necklacelike appearance.

Some fibers run to the pons, some along the dorsal tegmental decussation; individual fibers run into the central gray matter and toward the midline.
Case 3. Dog No. 206

In this case (Fig. 122) the cortex of Area 17 at the right occipital pole was removed. The dog was sacrificed 12 days later. Examination showed the entire focus lay within Area 17, except, perhaps, for slight damage to the white matter of Area 18 at its most posterior part, in the lateral portion of the pole. There was no hemorrhage in the region of the focus. Degenerated fibers run from the focus of extirpation in three principal directions.

1. *Association Pathways.* Degenerated fibers run as short association bundles to all neighboring gyri and to others not bordering on the focus: the splenial, suprasplenial, suprasylvian, and marginal gyri. Droplets of degenerated myelin can be traced in the white matter of other parts of Area 17 and also in Areas 18 (O_2),* 21 (T_1), 7 (T_4), 7 (P), and 5 (Pc_1) (very few droplets in the last two). In Area 2 a more concentrated bundle is present, while in other areas there are only a few fibers. The chain of droplets runs from the white matter into the cortex not only at the apices of the gyri, but also at the lip and floor of the fissure. On the apex of the middle suprasylvian gyrus droplets can be seen radiating fanwise into the cortex along the course of the radial bundles. In the corona radiata above the level of the corpus callosum fibers running from the occipital lobe to the parietal region are divided transversely. These fibers can be regarded as a long association bundle connecting Area 17 of the occipital cortex with areas of the anterior parts of the cortex. In my specimens it can be traced in the direction of Area 5 (Pc_1).

2. *Commissural Fibers.* These run into the left hemisphere through the splenium of the corpus callosum. Fibers crossing to the left are divided longitudinally and can be seen as distinct necklacelike chains of larger caliber than those of the association fibers. A few droplets cross to the other hemisphere in the middle third of the corpus callosum. Degenerated droplets in the left hemisphere initially run anteriorly, then come together into a more concentrated bundle which runs both posteriorly and anteriorly in a sagittal direction. These transversely divided fibers are distributed in precisely the same part of the corona radiata as the long association bundle of the right hemisphere. The termination of the commissural fibers can be seen in gyri of the occipital lobe; isolated scattered droplets can be traced into other gyri.

3. *Projection Pathways.* These pathways in the stratum sagittale internum et externum run downward and anteriorly and give off two branches: one main branch running through Wernicke's area into the

---

* Designations of the cytoarchitectonic areas in accordance with the terminology of Adrianov and Mering (1959) are given in parentheses.

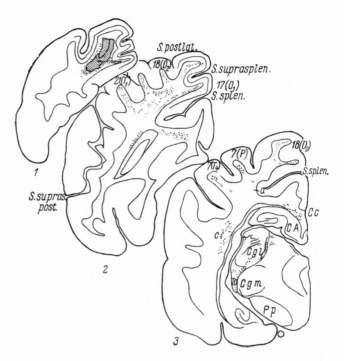

Fig. 123. Frontal sections through the brain of dog No. 259. 1: Hematoma in white matter of Area 17 and part of Area 18. 2: Degenerated bundles divided into three parts—commissural, projection, and association. 3: Section at diencephalic level. Droplets of degenerated fibers visible in lateral geniculate body, optic tract, and pulvinar. Cc, corpus callosum; remainder of legend as in Figs. 121 and 122. (Shkol'nik-Yarros, 1958a.)

diencephalon, and another descending to the internal capsule. In the diencephalon and mesencephalon endings of fibers can be traced in the superior portions of the lateral geniculate body, the pulvinar, the pretectal zone, the posterior nucleus of the thalamus, and the stratum opticum of the superior colliculi. A very small proportion of the fibers from the internal capsule runs into the cerebral peduncle, into its lateral portions. A much larger proportion of the droplets in the posterior portions of the internal capsule breaks up and disappears at the level of the posterosuperior part of the reticular nucleus of the thalamus. Some droplets are spread out over the internal capsule near the cells scattered within it. A few droplets can be traced running toward the ventral nuclei of the thalamus. Some fibers run into the external capsule.

Case 5. Dog No. 259

Part of Area 17 at the left occipital pole was removed and the dog sacrificed 12 days later (Fig. 123). Examination showed the focus lay at the occipital pole; beneath the focus, in the white matter of Area 17 was a hematoma, partly affecting also the white matter of Area 18. Division of degenerated pathways from the focus of extirpation into three parts can be seen.

1. *Association Pathways.* Degenerated fibers run in short association bundles into the splenial, suprasplenial, middle suprasylvian, and

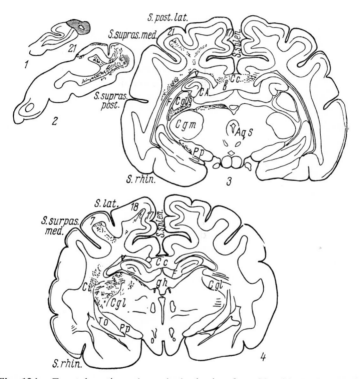

Fig. 124. Frontal sections through the brain of cat No. 31. 1: Focus of extirpation at occipital pole, Area 17. 2: Degenerated fibers in gyri next to focus. 3: Section at mesencephalic level. Degenerated association fibers run into auditory cortical areas. Degenerated commissural fibers run into opposite hemisphere (b). Projection fibers in lateral geniculate body, superior colliculus, cerebral peduncle. 4: Section at diencephalic level. Projection fibers in lateral geniculate body, pulvinar, and pretectal zone; Ci, internal capsule; V, ventricle; gh, habenula; f, fimbria. Remainder of legend as in Figs. 121–123. (Shkol'nik-Yarros, 1958a.)

marginal gyri. Droplets can be traced in the white matter of the following areas respectively: 17 (O_1), 18 (O_2), 21 (T_1), 7 (T_4), 7 (P), and 5 (Pc_1) (only a few droplets in the last mentioned). Long association fibers have the same distribution as in the previous case.

2. *Commissural Pathways.* Fibers run from the left hemisphere into the right through the splenium of the corpus callosum. They collect into a bundle in the corona radiata on the floor of the splenial fissure, from which they spread out along the gyri of the occipital region; a few droplets are also present in other gyri.

3. *Projection Pathways.* These run through the corona radiata, stratum sagittale internum et externum, and Wernicke's area into: (a) the lateral geniculate body, (b) the pulvinar, (c) the superior colliculi, (d) the pretectal nucleus, (e) the posterior nucleus of the thalamus, and (f) the optic tract. Another very small bundle runs downward through the internal capsule to the lateral portion of the cerebral peduncle.

Case 6. Cat No. 31

Part of Area 17 at the left occipital pole was extirpated in a fully grown cat which was sacrificed 14 days later (Fig. 124). Examination showed the focus of extirpation lies at the occipital pole entirely in Area 17. The white matter beneath Area 17 is only slightly affected. No hematoma was present. Division of degenerated pathways into three main parts begins from the focus of extirpation.

1. *Association Pathways.* Degenerated fibers run as short association bundles into the marginal, splenial, suprasplenial, and suprasylvian gyri. Droplets can be traced in the white matter of Areas 17, 18, and 21, and in smaller numbers in Areas 7 and 5. The line of droplets runs from the white matter into the gray not only at the apex of the gyri, but also at the floor of the fissure. At the apex of the gyri association fibers enter the radial bundles running fanwise into the cortex. No long association fibers can be found.

2. *Commissural Fibers.* Degenerated fibers can be seen running from the injured to the intact hemisphere through the corpus callosum in a section at the level of the mesencephalon and posterior part of the diencephalon. In the right hemisphere droplets run toward the occipital pole and reach the marginal and suprasylvian gyri (in small numbers), Areas 17 and 21 respectively, i.e., they are found not only in symmetrical (relative to the focus), but also asymmetrical parts of the cortex.

3. *Projection Pathways.* Droplets of degenerated myelin can be traced through the corona radiata, stratum sagittale internum et externum, and Wernicke's area in the following structures: (1) lateral geniculate body, (2) pulvinar, (3) pretectal zone, (4) superior colliculus, (5) optic tract (a small number), (6) posterior nucleus of the thalamus. Through the internal capsule

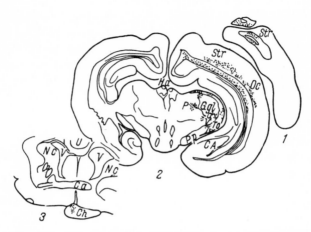

Fig. 125. Frontal sections through the brain of rabbit E4. 1: Part of focus of extirpation in area striata. 2: Section at diencephalic level. Degenerated association and projection fibers. Droplets in lateral geniculate body (dorsal and ventral portion), in pedicle of superior colliculus, in posterior nucleus of thalamus, optic tract, and lateral portion of cerebral peduncle. 3: Section at the chiasma level. Degenerated myelin droplets can be seen running to the left part of the chiasma; Nc, caudate nucleus; Ca, anterior commissure; Ch, chiasma; Cgld and Cglv, dorsal and ventral portion of lateral geniculate body; P, pulvinar; Ha, habenula; Pp, cerebral peduncle; To, optic tract; Str, area striata; Oc, occipital cortex. (Shkol'nik-Yarros, 1958a.)

fibers run into the cerebral peduncle, in its lateral and middle parts, and the corresponding occipitopontine and, perhaps, corticospinal tracts.

Case 7. Rabbit KO E4

Extirpation of Area 17 of the right hemisphere was carried out on an adult rabbit which was sacrificed 11 days later (Fig. 125). Examination showed the extirpation affects a large part of the area striata (only the superior layers of the cortex in the most posterior part), and a small part of the area peristriata and the retrosplenial cortex (Rsgβ according to Rose). The lesion thus certainly affected not merely a large part of the visual cortex, but other parts of the cortex as well.

1. *Association Pathways.* Droplets in degenerated fibers are present in other parts of the visual cortex Str and Oc, and in Areas Par_1, Par_2, Par_3, T_1, Praec. agr., and Postcentr. (few in the last mentioned).

2. *Commissural Fibers.* These are thin and run into Areas Str and Par of the opposite hemisphere.

3. *Projection Pathways*. Degenerated fibers can be traced through the corona radiata, stratum sagittale internum et externum, and Wernicke's area in the following structures: (1) lateral geniculate body, especially its ventral and dorsal parts, (2) stratum opticum of the superior colliculus; some fibers run further and cross to the left side, (3) pretectal zone, (4) zona incerta, (5) optic tract, (6) chiasma, optic nerve, and retina. Fibers run through the internal capsule into the lateral part of the cerebral peduncle and external capsule. Fibers of a large, longitudinally divided pathway are clearly visible in the optic tract. Degenerated fibers can be seen to cross through the chiasma. Droplets are located in the temporal portion of the left optic nerve.

Efferent fibers from the visual areas originate from long-axon cortical cells. The distribution of neurons in the visual cortex was shown above; obviously a very large number of axons from pyramidal and fusiform neurons in different layers and large star cells in layer IV leave the cortex.

Association connections of Area 17 in the animals which I studied are very extensive. After extirpation of small parts of the cortex (Case 3, dog No. 206, for example) numerous connections could be seen as degenerated fibers not only within the visual system, but also with the auditory system and the system for cutaneous sensation. So far as the extent of the association connections is concerned, my results agree with those described by Kononova (1926), Polyak (1927), Mettler (1935), Nauta and Bucher (1954), and others. The connections of Area 17 with the parietal region which I found were confirmed by the work of Iontov and Ermolaeva (1961). Using the Golgi–Deineka method they demonstrated bilateral connections between Areas 17 and 7 of the cat's cortex. Degeneration of synapses was observed along the course of the radial fibers and in horizontal bundles in the upper layers of the cortex.

How should the existing view concerning the isolation of Area 17 now be interpreted? This view was based on results obtained on monkeys, in which the specialization of Areas 17, 18, and 19 has reached a higher level than in the carnivores. Nevertheless, the total number of association connections in primates must be greater than in carnivores for the following reasons: (1) the quantity of white matter beneath the cortex is greater; (2) the surface of Area 17 itself is greater and, consequently, so also is the number of cells giving axons into distant parts of the brain; (3) vision is improved and more intimate functional links are established between the sensory systems.

On theoretical grounds it can thus be assumed that the number of association pathways in phylogenesis must increase and not decrease. Dzugaeva (1949) particularly stresses the qualitative differences between tracts in man and animals. In primates, evidently, most association connections originate in Areas 18 and 19, which also follows from the neuronal structure of these areas (Shkol'nik-Yarros, 1954), while Area 17 is connected principally with subcortical structures and the periphery. This conclusion is also supported by the narrowness of layer III of Area 17 in primates. Electrophysiological investigations have also demonstrated numerous connections between Areas 18 and 19 and other parts of the brain.

It should be emphasized that many association fibers, differing considerably in the animals investigated, together with powerfully developed projection pathways, originate in Area 17 in carnivores and rodents (cats, dogs, rabbits). In the rabbit, for instance, neither fissures nor gyri are present, the cortex is undifferentiated, there are few association connections and no typical U-fibers, and a very small quantity of white matter in general. In cats, where numerous short and medium association fibers are present, there are no long association bundles; in dogs the association connections are more numerous still, including some long association fibers, corresponding to the much greater development of the frontal areas and the appearance of variability of fissures and gyri.

Many recent investigations of conditioned-reflex activity after operative dissociation of the visual and somatosensory systems have led to the view that long association connections either are completely absent (Klosovskii, 1958) or play a minor role in conditioned-reflex activity. Sperry *et al.* (1955) categorically rejected the role of association connections, even the shortest, in the act of vision.

The data of evolutionary morphology have established the unique development of association connections in the human brain. Clear evidence of this is given by comparing the area of the peripheral organ of vision with the area of the brain as a whole in a series of vertebrates and mammals (Zvorykin and Shkol'nik-Yarros, 1953) (Fig. 1). The existence of abundant association connections between the areas and regions and the anterior and posterior parts of the hemisphere is an essential feature distinguishing the human brain.

In the frontal region only a small percentage of cells are of the short-axon stellate type (Polyakov, 1959). This phylogenetically new cortical region, the cytoarchitectonics of which was studied by Kononova (1935, 1938, 1940), is characterized by an enormous number of pyramidal cells. It is the pyramidal cells, of course, which give rise to association connections.

Morphological data concerning the structure and development of the frontal lobes are in agreement with clinical observations. As Luria (1966) and his collaborators showed, different parts of the frontal cortex and Areas 4 and 6 participate differently in the complex activity of the human brain, but there is no doubt whatever about the special importance of the frontal areas (together with the inferior parietal) for specifically human, goal-directed activity. In animals, without a second signal system, with feeble development of their frontal lobes and the other phylogenetically new areas, the association connections must obviously be less important.

In my material I was able to observe the caliber and mode of ending of the degenerated association fibers, the size of which is very small compared with that of the projection fibers. The results showed that association bundles are not uniform either in their direction or in their mode of ending in the cortex. They include groups of vertical fibers running directly upward from the white matter as far as layer III.

They also include fibers where terminals running slightly obliquely can be seen to depart from the vertical trunk. Horizontal fibers are also present in layer V. Finally, a few droplets can be detected in layer I (these fibers are the least numerous, occurring singly, so that less definite conclusions can be drawn about them). These observations were made on dogs using Marchi and Nauta techniques, the latter being superior. Short association fibers terminate mainly at the apices of the gyri and they run in the radial bundles, but droplets are also present in the gray matter of the lip and floor of the fissure. The small diameter of the association fibers suggests that they originate from medium-sized and small long-axon cells in Area 17.

The descending pathways from the visual cortex have until now been the greatest source of disagreement between investigators. According to my observations, in carnivores (cats and dogs) degenerated fibers can be traced along the course of projection pathways to structures in the diencephalon and mesencephalon: lateral geniculate body, pulvinar, posterior nucleus of the thalamus, pretectal area, and superior colliculi [where they are most numerous (Figs. 122 and 123)]. A few projection fibers also run into the internal capsule, the lateral part of the cerebral peduncle, the subcallosal bundle, and the external capsule.

I cannot accept the view of those who deny the existence of a centrifugal connection between the cortex and lateral geniculate body (Polyak, 1927; Barris, Ingram, and Ranson, 1935). In my material droplets of a few degenerated fibers of small caliber could be traced through Wernicke's area into the lateral geniculate body, where they were scattered as tiny dustlike dots over the myelin interlayers of the nucleus. In the most typical case they were observed in the superior part of the dorsal portion, but it is possible that had the cortical lesion been situated elsewhere, the distribution of axons in the subcortex would have been different. It is interesting to note that Polyak (1957), in a later study of the lateral geniculate body in monkeys, described (possible) cortical axons in it, marking a change from his original opinion. A few fibers descending from Area 17 into the lateral geniculate body were also found by Obukhova (1960). Beresford (1962) and Guillery

(1967b) found a reciprocal connection between the visual cortex and lateral geniculate body.

Extremely convincing evidence of the existence of corticifugal connections of Area 17 with the lateral geniculate body was obtained by Meshcherskii (1963) electrophysiologically. He applied a weak concentration of strychnine (0.1–0.25%) to the cortex and observed facilitation of responses of the lateral geniculate body to flashes, while a higher concentration of strychnine resulted in the appearance of a late positive wave in the geniculate response attributable to synchronized discharge of corticifugal neurons by photic stimulation. He did not obtain these responses by stimulating Area 18. He thus maintains that it is the primary projection area of the visual cortex which modulates transmission of the afferent volley. Narikashvili and Kadzhaya (1963), in experiments on cats, observed an inhibitory effect of the visual cortex on the lateral geniculate body. In a more recent investigation the number of efferent neurons in the cat visual cortex has been counted (Fomin, 1967). The mean number of fibers of the optic radiation is 58,500, and the number of efferent fibers entering the dorsal nucleus of the lateral geniculate body is 3000, compared with 2300 entering the ventral nucleus.

My observations revealed a definite link between the cortex and pulvinar, although even in carnivores the pulvinar is very poorly developed by comparison with primates. The number of fibers running from the cortex into the pulvinar is small. Endings of cortical axons are also definitely seen in the pretectal area in carnivores. A large fascicle runs into the stratum opticum of the superior colliculus.

According to Brazovskaya (1951, 1953), occipitopontine fibers are present in the cerebral peduncle and can be traced from cells of the limes parastriati gigantopyramidalis. According to Walberg and Brodal (1953), axons in this region also enter the pyramidal tract. In my material droplets could be traced in the lateral parts of the cerebral peduncle, but only in one case were they found close to its middle third.

In rabbits the course of the projection fibers differs from that in carnivores as follows: a very few droplets of degenerated fibers can be traced in the dorsal part of the lateral geniculate body, and rather more in the very well-developed ventral part. Very many axons terminate in the superior colliculi. Endings of fibers in the zona incerta, pretectal area, and posterior nucleus of the thalamus were also clearly visible.

What is the function of the descending cortical pathways? Some of them play the role of intermediate link in motor acts. For example, stimulation of the occipital areas in monkeys and dogs (Gerver, Foerster, Vogt, Crosby, and many others) produces movement of the eyes. Crosby and Henderson (1948) carefully worked out a scheme of cortical automatisms of eye movements superimposed on a purely subcortical mechanism. The path which they described (for eye movement upward) runs from the inferior portions of Area 17 to neighboring parts of Area 18, the superior part of Area 19, and then through the corticotectal tract to the anteromedial part of the superior colliculus and the anterior division of the oculomotor nucleus. According to Foerster and Vogt, Area 19 is a specialized oculomotor zone of the cortex. However, the work of Crosby and Henderson shows that movements of the eyes are also obtained by stimulation of Area 18 and Area 17 (judging from their diagram, the focus of stimulation was in the anterior part of Area 17 on its lateral surface). The work of Crosby and Henderson was recently confirmed by Jampel (1960). In response to electrical stimulation of the brain in macaques he observed movements of the eyes, convergence, and constriction of the pupils not only from areas of the frontal cortex, but also from the occipital cortex (Areas 19, 18, and, evidently, the anterior part of Area 17).

How are the other pathways descending from the cortex into subcortical nuclei unconnected with motor functions, such as the pulvinar, lateral geniculate body, and pretectal nucleus, to be regarded?

Cases of division of the optic nerve or enucleation of the eyes (in cats and dogs) which I investigated showed that the majority of degenerated axons can be traced into the lateral geniculate body, and from thence into the superior colliculus, pulvinar, and pretectal area.

Solitary fibers run into the cerebellum, hypothalamus, and medial geniculate body, while scattered fibers run directly into the cortex. It may be concluded that the principal relay stations of the centripetal visual fibers in the subcortical nuclei and the points of ending of the descending cortico-subcortical pathways coincide. However, centripetal fibers are much more numerous than centrifugal, for example, in the lateral geniculate body. It may be supposed that it is in this way that the cortex regulates the process of transmission of visual information. The cortex may thus exert its influence on all stages of the visual process, starting with motor acts and ending with the transmission of visual excitation to the cortex. Its influence on motor acts is exerted through the superior colliculi and pretectal area, and its influence on the transmission of visual excitation to the cortex through the lateral geniculate body and pulvinar.

The well-marked differences in structure of the long-axon neurons in the visual cortex are evidence that centrifugal pathways differing in their function originate directly from Area 17. For example, the long-axon large star cells of Cajal have no apical dendrite, so that acts carried out with their aid can take place more rapidly, without special delay of excitation in the slowly conducting long apical dendrite. Examples of such unconscious and rapid acts are the pupillary reactions.

The cells of Meynert, with a large apical dendrite, are perhaps mainly connected with voluntary movements of the eyes through the superior colliculi.

It is easy to see that with the increase in area of the cortex, descending pathways attain a higher development, so that an increase in the role of centrifugal, motor, regulatory and other efferent (association) systems has taken place in the higher mammals and man (Shkol'nik-Yarros, 1961c).

That part of the centrifugal pathways not directly connected with motor adaptations may be responsible for regulation of the inflow of sensory information. Adaptive and regulatory systems have developed in the course of evolution in connection with adaptation of the organism to the external environment. This device can be regarded as one type of feedback in the living organism. Whereas the best-known type of feedback is that running from the muscle (the effector) back to the center, to control performance of the action, another type of feedback runs from the center to the transmitter organ to control the inflow of impulses. At the present time physiologists are paying particular attention to feedbacks in the visual system, and their regulatory role in the act of vision has been emphasized (Sokolov, 1958; Snyakin *et al.*, 1961; Demirchoglyan, 1961).

CENTRIFUGAL CONNECTIONS OF THE RETINA

The problem of centrifugal fibers of the retina is particularly interesting. According to Engelman (1885), the optic nerve contains centrifugal fibers, stimulation of which causes contraction of the inner segments of the cones. By impregnation with silver and staining with methylene blue, endings of fibers of an obviously centrifugal character have been detected in the retina, and their relationship to the amacrine cells demonstrated. A full account of these fibers in birds was given by Dogel' (1895) and Cajal (1889–1911). An interesting study of them was made by Elinson (1896), who considered that they were vasomotor fibers of the retina, running through the root of the oculomotor nerve. Monakow believed that these fibers originate in the superior colliculi. In some of Cajal's diagrams long axons reaching the retina from cells of the lateral geniculate body can be seen. Recently the view has been expressed that centrifugal fibers of the retina arise from cells of the hypothalamus (Weber, 1945; Rubino and Scoppa, 1955; Novokhatskii, 1964). Their origin from the cortex is described by Sepp (1949), who considers that this connection is firmly established and a characteristic feature of mammals.

Polyak (1957) has little to say about the centrifugal fibers of the retina. Possibly it is through these structures that the brain exerts its influence on the retina. They are described predominantly in birds and are less definite in other vertebrates, especially mammals. However, Polyak found endings of this type in the chimpanzee retina. Notwithstanding this, he emphasizes that in man, in cases of prolonged absence of the eye, the optic nerve degenerates completely and no myelinated fibers can be found in it, i.e., no descending fibers are present.

A different conclusion was reached by Wolter and Liss (1956), who studied two cases of prolonged blindness in man. One of their patients lived for 11 years after surgical removal of both eyes, while the other patient lived for 16 years after enucleation of the right eye. In both cases atrophy of the optic nerve was found, but thin nerve fibers running in a longitudinal direction and possessing swellings like a string of pearls were also discovered. They consider the efferent fibers in the human optic nerve centrifugal. In two-dimensional sections of the human retina fibers have been discovered, running from the optic disc and terminating at the level of layer VII, or occasionally layer V (Honrubia and Elliot, 1968).

Szentágothai categorically states that they are connected with the mesencephalic reticular formation. In a special investigation, Pilipenko (1961) observed retrograde degeneration of some neurons of the lateral geniculate body and superior colliculi, in cats and rats after division of the optic nerve.

Brindley and Hamasaki (1961) using Nauta's method, found only very late degeneration of optic nerve fibers after intracranial division of the nerve. They concluded that there are no centrifugal fibers connecting the brain with the retina, or that if there are, they differ fundamentally from all other fibers in the central nervous system.

Cragg (1962) concluded from his investigation that centrifugal connections are present in the rabbit's retina and he suggests that they are collaterals of thin fibers running in the supraoptic commissures.

These pathways have recently been fully confirmed and carefully studied in birds (Dowling and Cowan, 1966). Their existence in mammals, as before, has been rejected by several investigators (Brindley and Hamasaki, 1966; Ogden, 1968).

A completely opposite conclusion was drawn by Novokhatskii (1964), who describes precise quantitative results of an investigation of the centrifugal fibers. They vary in diameter from thick, medium thick, to thin; some are medullated, others nonmedullated. The approximate number of centrifugal fibers in the human optic nerve is 800–1000, of which 300–400 are medullated and 500–600 nonmedullated.

Physiologists consider that before the nature of the influence of centrifugal connections on the retina is discussed, their existence must first be proved. The cautious statement of Polyak also adds to doubts about the existence of these fibers. Some positive facts in this direction have recently been obtained by Granit and Dodt.

Electrophysiological results obtained by Dodt (1956) concerning centrifugal impulses in the rabbit's retina are very convincing. An electric pulse applied stereotaxically to the contralateral optic tract produced spikes in the retina 7–25 msec after the antidromic spike. Dodt interpreted the delayed response as evidence of a true centrifugal effect on the retina, its pathway including one or more synapses.

Granit (1956) observed either inhibition or facilitation of the retinal response to flashes during stimulation of the mesencephalic reticular formation. In his opinion the increase in sensitivity of the retina during stimulation of the reticular formation can be explained by posttetanic poten-

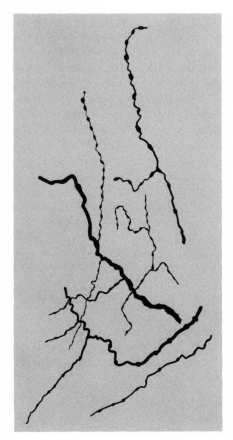

Fig. 126. Centrifugal fibers in the rabbit's retina. Axons of different caliber can be seen.

tiation. In a few experiments the facilitation was very obvious. Granit therefore considers that it is neuronal in origin. However, further investigations are necessary to rule out the possibility of vascular changes which may arise through activation of the centrifugal pathways.

The effect of central mechanisms on retinal neurons has also been demonstrated by Bogoslovskii and Semenovskaya (1959), Ostrovskii (1962), and others.

The importance of centrifugal influences for retinal activity can be seen particularly clearly in the work of Snyakin (1948), who always emphasized the role of central regulation. Similar problems affecting the auditory system have been discussed by Gershuni (1960) and Galambos (1956).

Although centrifugal fibers in the retina have been well studied in birds and some monkeys, very little is known about them in the rabbit and dog.

Using a technique of bichromate-silver impregnation (Shkol'nik-Yarros, 1955b, 1961a, b, c), I was able to demonstrate centrifugal fibers in the retina of rabbits and dogs and to observe differences in their structure.

Dichotomous division of centrifugal fibers in the rabbit's retina is demonstrated in Fig. 126. Some fibers are of considerable thickness; they differ in caliber, indirectly showing their origin from different structures. Besides these definitely centrifugal fibers, other thinner fibers of unknown origin with brushlike ramifications can also be seen in the rabbit's retina (Shkol'nik-Yarros, 1961b). What is the evidence that these fibers are ex-

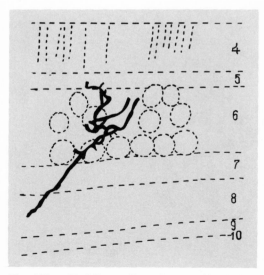

Fig. 126a. Forklike ending of a centrifugal fiber in layer 6 of the dog's retina.

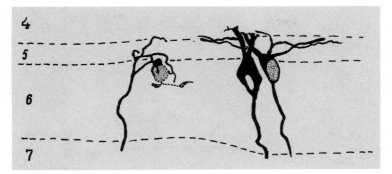

Fig. 127. Ending of a centrifugal fiber in the dog's retina. Axonal ending forms large cap-shaped axo-somatic contact on body of an amacrine cell shown stippled in the illustration. Two bipolar cells are visible on the right. (Shkol'nik-Yarros, 1961a.)

ogenous? (1) They run from the ganglion cell layer to outer layers. (2) They become thinner as they run outward. (3) They resemble axonal ramifications rather than dendritic (they have varicose thickenings at equal distances, a characteristic feature of many axons in the central portions of the nervous system). (4) The endings of these afferent fibers running from the brain form brushes typical of the endings of afferent fibers in other parts of the brain.

Two different types of afferent termination were observed in the dog's retina: in one case axons ascending obliquely from the layer of nerve fibers through the inner plexiform layer terminate by a fork-shaped ramification in the inner nuclear layer (Fig. 126a); in another case a fiber ascending less obliquely terminates as a cap-shaped axo-somatic synapse on the body of an amacrine cell (Fig. 127). The ending of the fiber forms a cap covering the body of the neuron and making contact with it by means of large, boutonlike thickenings (Fig. 127). In the dog's retina, just as in that of the rabbit, fibers with a less clearly defined pattern, running more vertically and spreading out fanwise in layer 7, could also be seen.*

Using a bichromate-silver impregnation technique I obtained indirect evidence of the origin of centrifugal fibers from the lateral geniculate body. In the human lateral geniculate body, for instance, neurons of the lower layers frequently give off axons running toward the optic tract. However, the possibility that they may subsequently turn and join the optic radiation cannot be ruled out.

In the lateral geniculate body of dogs, cells are found with an axon

---

* Pericellular plexuses and synapses on amacrine cells are clearly revealed by Campos's method (Shibkova and Koroleva, 1964).

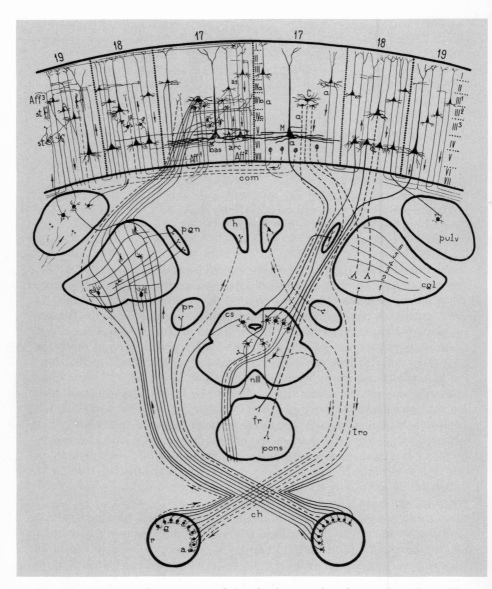

Fig. 128. Diagram of components of the visual system in primates. Top: Areas 17, 18, and 19. Layers of the cortex denoted by Roman numerals. Borders between areas shown by broken lines. On the left, centripetal connections; on the right, centrifugal. Subcortical structures are shown in the middle of the scheme and the retina below. The diagram emphasizes the principal quantitative and qualitative differences between neurons and connections of layers III and IV of Areas 17, 18, and 19, mutual connec-

giving off two principal branches. Although one of these has been shown to run into the cortex, it can be presumed that the other runs into the optic tract or into the reticular formation.

In some of my experiments described above, degeneration following removal of the visual cortex was traced in the optic tract and optic nerve. Similar results have been obtained by Mering (1962), Biryuchkov (1963), Haschke (1963), and Shibkova and Koroleva (1964). Biryuchkov, using Nauta's method, saw degeneration in the optic nerve of cats and rabbits after removal of the cortex.

I thus conclude that: (1) centrifugal fibers are present in the retina; (2) they differ in caliber and terminate in different places; (3) they differ in their cortical and subcortical origin (see also Shkol'nik-Yarros, 1958a).

Central tuning or regulation during the reception of visual information is thus found not only in birds but also in mammals. The small number of centrifugal fibers can readily be explained by the structure of the feedback circuits.

A SCHEME OF THE STRUCTURE OF THE VISUAL SYSTEM

By studying neurons and their connections some idea can be obtained, although in a very schematic form, of the manner in which excitation spreads in the central visual system. Leonova (1896) maintained that visual excitation is certainly relayed through interneurons of the lateral geniculate body to its principal cells and to the beginning of projection pathways from the pyramidal neurons of layer III of the cortex. In most modern schemes, consideration is paid either to neurons (for example, in Area 17, by Polyak) or only to pathways, without regard to connections with particular neurons (for example, by Kappers and Minkowski). The topography of corresponding

---

tions of the cortex and subcortical structures, and centripetal and centrifugal connections of the retina. All pathways for which insufficiently complete or conflicting data are available are shown as broken lines; more definite pathways are shown as continuous lines. C, star cell of Cajal with long descending axon; st, short-axon stellate cells; bas, cell with basketlike axon; Aff[1], oblique afferent fibers from lateral geniculate body; Aff[2], vertical afferent fibers of unknown origin, but probably also from lateral geniculate body; Aff[3], afferent fiber from other cortical areas; M, solitary pyramidal cell of Meynert; arc, pyramidal cell with arcuate axon; as, cell with ascending axon; pulv, pulvinar; cgl, lateral geniculate body; pgn, pregeniculate nucleus; h, hypothalamus; pr, pretectal nucleus; cs, superior colliculus; fr, reticular formation; com, commissural connections; III, oculomotor nerve; ch, chiasma; r, retina; g, ganglion cells of retina; a, amacrine cells of retina; tro, optic tract. Arabic numbers denote layers of lateral geniculate body: 1, 2, magnocellular; 3, 4, 5, 6, parvocellular; a, axon; c, axon collateral. Arrows show direction of transmission of excitation. Compiled from personal and other published data. Not all layers of cortex are shown. Retinotegmental tracts not shown.

parts of the retina, lateral geniculate body, and visual cortex has been most thoroughly analyzed. However, previous topographic schemes have been drawn up without regard to neuronal structure. I have tried to work out a scheme of interneuronal connections with centripetal and centrifugal pathways (Fig. 128).

My scheme shows the main difference between Areas 17 and 19 of the cortex and also, to a certain extent, the complexity of interrelationships within the visual system. The main distinguishing features of Areas 17 and 18–19 are concerned with neuronal composition and connections in layers III and IV. In Area 17, layer IV sublayers b and c are rich in various types of stellate cells—with both short and long axons. They are connected with afferent fibers of several different types: oblique and vertical, coming from the lateral geniculate body and giving off terminal branches simultaneously in sublayers IVc and IVb. This arrangement can be regarded as the morphological basis both for the visual image (IVc) and for reflex movements of the eyes (through the solitary pyramids of Meynert and long-axon cells of layer IVb). The most complex organization of these sublayers in primates corresponds to their highly developed visual function.

An important feature of Area 17 is the small pyramidal cell with an arcuate axon, evidently participating in the formation of the intracortical spread and preservation of visual excitation. In man the areas surrounding Area 17 are particularly well developed. They have the highest concentration of typical pyramidal cells and the most distinct (compared with Area 17) radial arrangement of cells, connected with the preferential development of association connections. Each long-axon pyramidal cell, which is much larger in the wide layer III of Area 19, subdivided into three sublayers, than in Area 17, is capable of forming thousands of connections with surrounding and distant neurons. This is the morphological basis for association of visual images with others, and it is still more marked in the cortex in the zone intermediate between occipital, the parietal, and temporal regions. The cell density of layer IV in Area 19 is not so great, and this layer does not include the special accessory descending pathway because of the absence of star cells of Cajal.

The chief centripetal pathways are found at relay stations with centrifugal pathways from the cortex. The former are very numerous; the latter only few in number. Centripetal pathways carry visual excitation through concentrated bundles to the many structures illustrated in the diagram. Diffuse fibers run to different parts of the cortex, the medial geniculate body, and the bulbar reticular formation. Fibers running to the hypothalamus are doubtful; in a special investigation, Novokhatskii (1956) demonstrated a direct connection between the optic nerve and hypothalamic nuclei in animals and man. Similar results were reported by Shapiro (1957). Despite the positive data in this direction, many authorities deny any connection between the hypothalamus and the eye. Szentágothai *et al.* (1962), in particular, attribute reports of such connections to incorrect interpretation of the morphological data. Hayhow (1966) and Kiernan (1967) likewise deny completely the existence of retino-hypothalamic connections.

Many other subcortical connections and also a few of the centrifugal pathways of the visual system are also open to question. Pathways to the retina are diagrammed not from a single structure but from many structures, as reported by different workers. This reflects my own view also; the optic nerve is essentially a projection bundle, containing both centripetal and centrifugal fibers from the cortex and many structures of the brain stem.

No interconnections between different sensory systems at cortical and subcortical level could be incorporated into the diagram; only one pathway is shown from other analyzers to the pulvinar. Data obtained by Lyubimov (1963, 1964), indicating the conduction of primary specific visual information to Area 17 not only along the classical pathway, but also via the corpus callosum and through a relay at the superior colliculi, likewise are not shown.

Hence, although my scheme of the visual system of primates has the advantage that in it the neurons are joined together by connections and a number of little-known pathways are included, it is still far from complete.

However, it does show how participation of long association connections with the motor cortex is not essential for the formation of motor reflexes directly from the visual cortex. Reception of the input and its transmission to many different neurons connected with reflex movements, with associative activity, and with memory can take place in the same area of the cortex. The pyramidal neurons, forming part of a system of distant connections, show the greatest degree of adaptation for integration and reflect the perfection of the human brain.

If this scheme is accepted as a model of the human visual system, what are the principal characteristics which distinguish it from that system in other mammals? The results of my investigations show that the main progressive features are as follows.

1. Growth of the rows of pyramidal cells in layer III of the cortex adjacent to the primary visual cortex (Areas 18 and 19). These rows of pyramidal cells have essentially unlimited capacity for the formation of new connections. No such areas of the cortex are present in the hedgehog, they are very small in the rabbit, and much larger in carnivores. In primates their growth is striking if monkeys and man are compared. It could be postulated that the artist or sculptor may perhaps be distinguished by the size of Area 19 and also by the cells of layer III in this area.

2. The presence of a mechanism providing a foundation for color and

stereoscopic vision in Area 17 itself. It is embodied in the structures of sublayers IVb and IVc, the differentiation of these structures to this degree is absent in other mammals not possessing complex and, in particular, color vision.

3.   Considerable phylogenetic changes are found in the size and density of distribution of the neurons. In primates the contrast between sizes of the neurons is much greater, reflecting the adaptation and specialization of the cells to differentiated function and, possibly, to a very rapid response of the extraocular muscles and to the more perfect visual perception of objects.

A well-defined lamination and specialization of its neuronal structure are characteristic of the lateral geniculate body.

SPECIFICITY OF STRUCTURE OF THE CENTRAL VISUAL SYSTEM

STRUCTURE OF NEURONS OF THE VISUAL SYSTEM AND THEIR COMPARISON WITH OTHER NEURONS

Comparative analysis of the neurons of various parts of the visual system is essential before it can be decided whether specialization and generalization are present, not only in peripheral parts of sensory systems so carefully studied histologically during recent years by Vinnikov (1947, 1963), but also of their central portion. I shall here compare my findings with other studies of neurons. Neurons of the motor cortex have been studied by Zhukova (1950, 1953), and of the limbic cortex by Tsinda (1959, 1960). Important work was also carried out by Polyakov (1949), Cajal (1900–1906, 1911), Lorente de Nó (1922, 1938), and de Crinis (1933).

If the study of neurons is made with constant comparison of the cyto-architectonic picture, it is found that for every mammal, as well as common characteristics of all areas of the cortex, there are special structural features of each particular cortical area. The specific features for Area 17 have been considerably modified during the long process of specialization.

Comparison of the motor cortex of the hedgehog (Fig. 129) with the visual area (Fig. 5) clearly shows how very similar in structure are these two functionally different areas. Common features of the whole cortex are: uniformity of neuronal structure, absence of cells differing sharply in shape and size, the small number of dendritic branches, feeble development of neurons in the upper layers of the cortex and dominance of the lower layers. Specific features of the visual cortex are ill defined in the hedgehog. In the rabbit the difference is much more marked, and consists mainly of the presence of more numerous and more varied stellate cells throughout the cross section of the visual cortex but especially at the level of layer IV, where the main branches of the specific afferent fibers terminate. Specific

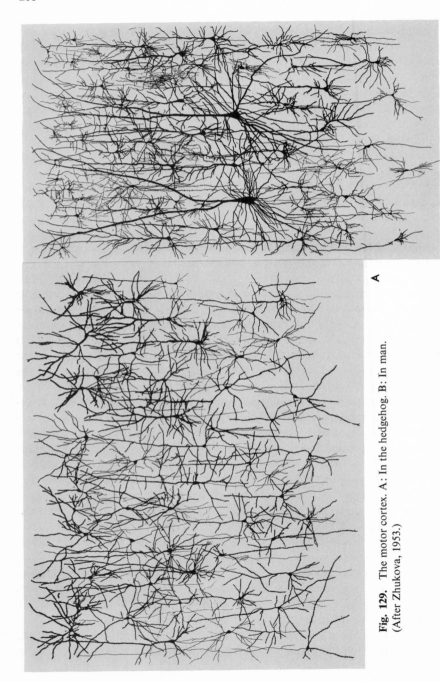

Fig. 129. The motor cortex. A: In the hedgehog. B: In man.
(After Zhukova, 1953.)

features of the visual cortex, in the form of striation and high cell density of individual layers, are seen much more clearly than in the hedgehog and distinguish this area from the motor cortex. Common features for the rabbit cortex as a whole are slight differences between structure of the pyramidal cells in different areas, considerable development of the lower layers of the cortex, and more numerous dendritic branches of pyramidal and stellate cells than in the hedgehog.

A much higher level of differentiation is found with the dog's cortex. True giant cells of Betz, which are absent in the hedgehog and rabbit, can be seen in the motor area. Pyramidal cells bearing some resemblance to the solitary pyramidal cells of Meynert are found in the visual cortex; no such neurons can be found in the cortex of either hedgehog or rabbit. The motor and visual areas of the dog's cortex differ considerably from the auditory cortex, as studied by Popova (1960a,b), which has neither Betz cells nor Meynert cells (nor cells similar to them).

A considerable difference is also found in the distribution and character of the stellate cells. In the motor cortex they are scattered fairly uniformly throughout its cross section. In the visual cortex they are concentrated mainly in layer IV, although they are also numerous in other layers; in the auditory cortex the largest concentrations are found in layer III. However, comparison of different parts of the cortex, including the limbic area (data obtained by Zambrzhitskii, 1954), reveals common features also in the dog for the cortex as a whole. These include, first, richness of dendritic branches of the pyramidal cells, the large size of the neurons, especially the pyramidal cells, great contrast in size of the cells, and well-developed upper layers (admittedly, layer III is not yet subdivided into sublayers as in the cortex of the anthropoid apes and man). The dog's cortex is also distinguished by its richness in short-axon stellate cells of different shapes and sizes, some types giving axons which ramify over a very wide area.

The structure of the motor and visual areas of the cortex is completely different in primates. In the motor cortex (Fig. 129), against a background of very wide upper layers and a gradually increasing caliber of the pyramidal cells from above downward, giant cells of Betz appear. These are extra-large pyramidal cells with a very large body (up to 130 μ) and with widely spread, large dendrites. Short-axon stellate cells are scattered throughout the cross section of the motor cortex.

As stated above, the visual cortex is characterized by concentration of small neurons in some layers, while other layers, containing numerous myelinated fibers, also possess large neurons. Of the varieties of neurons distinguishable in the visual cortex, the following are not present in the motor cortex: the pyramidal cells of Meynert, large and small star cells with a long, descending axon, pyramidal cells with an arcuate, ascending axon, and large concentrations of short-axon cells. Zones with large long-axon neurons and numerous horizontal myelinated fibers (layers IVb and V) particularly distinguish the visual cortex from all other parts of the cortex because of its well-marked striation.

Characteristic features of the whole cortex in primates are: marked specialization, as shown by precise differentiation of areas, layers, sublayers, and individual neurons.

If the motor and visual cortex are compared with the limbic cortex in man (studied by Tsinda), completely different neurons are seen in layer V of the limbic cortex. These are very large, fusiform cells with a corkscrew-like apical dendrite and very long, widely spreading dendritic branches, emerging from the body of the neuron. Giant cells such as those in layer V are never found in the human visual and motor cortex. A type of neuron was described in the temporal cortex (Cajal, 1911) which is not found in the visual, motor, or limbic cortex. This is the giant stellate cell of layer IV with a long axon and differing completely from the star cells of Cajal in the visual cortex by the character of ramification of its dendrite and axon. These stellate cells have a spread-out appearance, and whereas in the visual cortex, as I have described above, dendrites of the large stellate cells are similar to the wings of flying birds, in this case the dendrites have a completely different appearance.*

For my comparison of subcortical neurons I shall make use of a study of neurons of the striopallidum (Leontovich, 1952, 1954, 1959a), neurons of sensory structures—the trigeminal, vestibular, and visceral complexes of nuclei, and also neurons of the reticular formation of the brain stem (Zhukova, 1959, 1964, 1965, 1966), types of neurons from the specific nuclei of the dog's thalamus (Leontovich, 1959b), and neurons of the medial geniculate body of the dog (Popova, 1961).

Just as the visual and motor areas are the most different in primates, comparison of the subcortical visual and motor structures showed the greatest differences in primates. According to Leontovich, the variety of types of neurons in the corpus striatum of the monkey (Fig. 130) is exceptionally great. Long-axon neurons with dense ramifications or with only a few branches, divided into radial and fan-shaped types, can be distinguished. The very numerous short-axon cells of the monkey's corpus striatum are particularly rich in different forms. They include helical forms with repeatedly crossing dendrites forming a type of thick felt, and arachnoid

---

* I shall not describe the sharp architectonic differences between cortical areas because they are well known. For a detailed comparison of Areas 17 and 41 of the adult human cortex, see Blinkov (1941), and in ontogenesis, see Polyakov (1937).

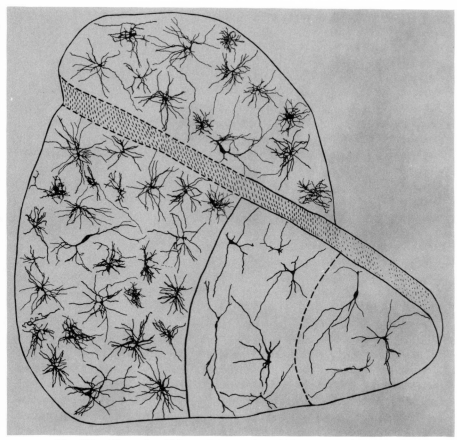

Fig. 130. The striopallidum of the monkey. (After Leontovich, 1959a.)

cells with a halo of many thin, twisted dendrites. The cells vary in size from very small to very large.

The lateral geniculate body of primates (Figs. 55, 59) shows a striking difference from the striopallidum, being distinctly laminated and possessing quite different types of neurons. For instance, in my opinion, the midget type of long-axon cell with few dendrites, giving off only a few branches and spreading only a short distance, is the most typical. These midget neurons are not found in the corpus striatum and, conversely, no helical or arachnoid short-axon cells are found in the lateral geniculate body.

Common features for both structures in primates are the marked differences in size of individual neurons and their differentiation into many types and varieties.

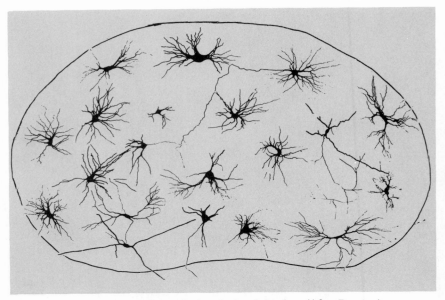

Fig. 131. Medial geniculate body of the dog. (After Popova.)

The work of Zhukova and of Popova (1960, 1961) makes it possible to compare several structures in the dog. The medial geniculate body (Fig. 131), for instance, differs considerably from the lateral geniculate body both in the structure of its neurons and in its architectonics. In the first place, a layer consisting only of large neurons cannot be distinguished in the medial geniculate body, whereas in the lateral geniculate body such a layer, containing large, long-axon, fusiform cells is present. Next, neurons of various sizes and shapes are scattered throughout the lateral geniculate body of the dog. Finally, among the large and medium-sized cells there are very small, long-axon cells mainly located in the parvocellular layer. These are completely absent in the medial geniculate body. On the whole, cells of the medial geniculate body are larger than those of the lateral geniculate body. I need not dwell on the most obvious difference between these two areas—the marked lamination of the lateral geniculate body and its complete absence in the medial geniculate body, because this is well known.

A further comparison of neurons of the subcortical structures already described with neurons of specific nuclei of the dog's thalamus reveals specific brushlike cells in the anterior nucleus of the thalamus (Leontovich, 1959b). These brush cells (Fig. 132) have dendrites emerging from the body as several thick trunks, suddenly breaking up some distance away from the cell body into a dense brush of uniformly thin, short, twisted branches. As

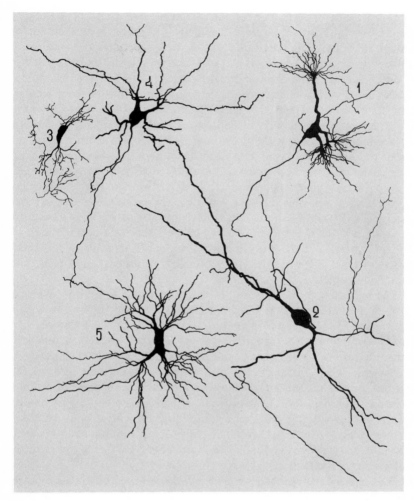

Fig. 132. Types of neurons of specific nuclei of the thalamus (Leontovich).
1, brushlike cell; 2, cell with few branches; 3, short-axon cell; 4, radial cell; 5,
shrublike cell.

can be very clearly seen from the illustrations I have given, no such cells are
present in the lateral geniculate body, medial geniculate body, or striopallidum.

The paleocortex (nuclei of the septum, the olfactory tubercle, region of
the diagonal band), representing a gradual transition from subcortical nuclei
to cortex (Leontovich, 1968a,b), differs considerably in the dog from the

lateral geniculate body in its neuronal structure. The region of the diagonal band and the nucleus of the stria terminalis, for instance, are composed of reticular neurons, while the other septal nuclei are composed of neurons similar to those of the striatum. In the olfactory tubercle, on the other hand, the deep layer is composed of reticular neurons, while the second layer includes areas with a nuclear type of structure and with neurons similar to those of the striatum, mixed with areas composed of primitive pyramidal cells. The neuronal structure of the islets of Calleja consisting of masses of very small cells, almost without cytoplasm, with short dendrites (evidently cells of the short-axon type) and single large neurons with long dendrites, giving dense branches at their ends, is even more distinctive. Such an organization, to some extent reminiscent of the outer layers of the olfactory bulb, suggests that these islets are the site of termination of a sensory nerve (Leontovich, 1968a). Neurons of all these primitive structures of the dog's telencephalon thus differ from neurons of the lateral geniculate body. Neurons of the magnocellular neurosecretory nuclei of the dog's hypothalamus, because of their few dendrites, resembling neuroblasts (Leontovich, 1969), are no less distinctive.

The structure of the sensory nuclei and reticular formation in the dog is also of great interest from this point of view. Neurons with a few straight, long, rarely branching dendrites, are characteristic, for instance, of all structures of the reticular formation starting from the spinal cord and ending in the diencephalon (Zhukova and Leontovich, 1964; Zhukova, 1959; Leontovich, 1959b; Leontovich and Zhukova, 1963). These cells with few branches, however, are found in small numbers in all specific nuclei of the thalamus (Robiner, 1957; Leontovich, 1959b), in the corpus striatum (Leontovich, 1952, 1954, 1959a), in the lateral geniculate body of the dog and man (Shkol'nik-Yarros, 1958b, 1959a, 1961b, 1962), and in the medial geniculate body (Popova, 1960). At lower levels of the brain stem these relationships are different.

It is only in the rostral and rostrolateral portions of the sensory complexes that the neurons differ sharply from reticular neurons, and most neurons of these complexes are to some extent similar to those of reticular type (Zhukova, 1959, 1964, 1965, 1966). In the nucleus of the descending root of the trigeminal nerve, single cells with few branches can be seen among the typical small cells of this nucleus with their dense ramifications. However, neither brush, midget, helical, nor arachnoid neurons are found in these structures.

An important subcortical structure—the inferior olive—was thoroughly studied by M. and A. Scheibel (1955a). In Golgi material they distinguished several varieties of neurons, the most typical being cells with numerous loops of dendrites winding spirally around their body. These cells are completely different from cells in all other subcortical structures. They also observed neurons with few branches, connected mainly with phylogenetically old parts of the olive and similar to reticular cells.

Comparison of the central visual system with two other systems thus suggests that specialized cells are present not only at receptor levels, but also in other structures of the brain.

Specialization at the periphery of sensory systems is very clearly expressed in all mammals, but the specialization of central neurons varies considerably and has received most study in monkeys and, more especially, in man. Specialization can be taken to mean a combination of all characteristics appearing in the course of adaptation to secure the best performance of a given function. Very little is yet known about specialization in brain centers. The most important factors here are the number and type of the connections, while structural properties of the neuron (its macro- and microstructure) and its chemical properties also play an important role.

In cytochemical analysis of retinal ganglion cells (Brodskii, 1960), the nucleus and cytoplasm reflect chemical changes in response to physiological stimulation. The intensity of protein synthesis affects the size of the nucleus and the nucleoplasmic ratio. Henschen's opinion that the nuclei of color-sensitive and photosensitive cells of the monkey's cortex are of different sizes can be explained, from the cytochemical point of view, by differences in the localization and intensity of protein synthesis in these two types of cells.

The work of Portugalov (1958) and his collaborators (Gershtein, 1958; Abdullakhodzhaeva, 1960; Savich and Yakovlev, 1957; Busnyuk, 1963), and also that of Roskin and Struve (1958) and others has demonstrated differences in the chemical properties of different parts of the brain and of individual neurons. Portugalov, Tsvetkova, and Yakovlev (1959) found differences not only in the protein content, but also in the activity of protein metabolism in different parts of the neuron. According to Portugalov, the metabolic level is determined by the type of function of the neuron as well as by phylogenetic principles.

Glezer (1960) studied neurons from the visual and motor cortex of rats with electron microscopy. Common features of these two areas were the presence of clearly defined membrane structures such as tubules and cisternae, hydration of the karyoplasm, and honeycombing of the nucleolus. The limiting membranes of the tubule in the motor cortex lie close together and are almost strictly parallel, resulting in stratification of the ergastoplasm, while in the visual cortex the ergastoplasm has a looped structure. He identified two types of structure in relation to the function performed by neurons of the central nervous system. Popova (1959c) had previously demonstrated the uneven distribution of ribonucleic acid in neurons of the motor and visual cortex in rats.

During the last few years the accumulation of data on the structure of synapses has continued intensively. A consideration of these new facts has shown that the specificity of a sensory system lies not only in the nature of its architectonics, connections, and chemical properties, but also in the distinctive structure of its synapses. For instance, connections of afferent fibers with neurons in layer IV of the visual cortex (Fig. 101) differ significantly from endings of afferent fibers in the lateral geniculate body (Figs. 56, 57, 58) and retina (Figs. 111 and 127). Differences visible under the optical microscope are naturally seen much more clearly in electron microscopic studies. If the ultrastructure of synapses in the visual cortex (Gray, 1961) is compared with the ultrastructure of synapses in the lateral geniculate body (Szentágothai, 1963b) and retina (Borovyagin, 1963; Sjöstrand, 1958; Kidd, 1962; and others) their very marked differences immediately become apparent.

Beritashvili (1963b) considers that reception of sensations of particular modalities by sensory neurons is determined not by the structure of the stellate cells, but by the phylogenetically evolved properties of the cytoplasm. However, somewhat earlier, Beritashvili (1963a) recognized the importance of external structural features of neurons.

It can be concluded from the facts described in this chapter that even the smallest structural features are important for the perception of sensations of different modalities. At the receptor level, for instance, besides the striking similarity in structure, chemical properties, and energy metabolism, differences related to the specific nature of their function are also found.

As was shown above, substantial differences are also found between different levels of the central portion of different systems. These are seen most clearly, perhaps, in the structure and length of the dendrites, determining the nonhomogeneity of perception and of synaptic connections.

SPECIFICITY OF STRUCTURE IN RELATION TO THE PROBLEM OF COLOR VISION

The classical three-component theory of color vision (Lomonosov, 1756; Young, 1802; Helmholtz, 1896) has been confirmed by the investigations of Marks (1965) and Marks, Dobelle, and MacNichol (1964). There are three types of cones in the retina of the goldfish, macaque, and man, each of which contains only one visual pigment.

It is thus an indisputable fact that color stimuli are transmitted by cones. The subsequent transmission of color information takes place through various types of retinal ganglion cells (Michael, 1968). The problem of which elements receive color sensations in the visual centers is less clear.

A number of theories have been put forward to explain the structure of visual centers in relation to the problem of finding a morphological basis for color vision. Henschen (1930), who published an extensive monograph on this subject, put forward an interesting theory. He studied visual centers in a number of monkeys, both nocturnal and diurnal. He found that only large cells, with a nucleus 6–8 μ in diameter, are found in layer IV of Area 17 of nocturnal monkeys. Since these monkeys do not possess color vision, Henschen concluded that these large cells are photosensitive. Diurnal monkeys, besides these large cells, also have small cells with a nucleus 4–5 μ in diameter. Henschen ascribes the function of color perception to the small cells present in the cortex of monkeys possessing color vision. The same state of affairs is found in the lateral geniculate body. In nocturnal members of the primates (*Perodicticus potto*, for example), large cells predominate in this nucleus, while small cells do so in diurnal species.

Le Gros Clark associated particular layers with the reception of a particular type of color stimulation: layers 1 and 2 are intermediate centers for pathways carrying the sensation of blue, layers 3 and 4 receive pathways carrying the sensation of red, and layers 5 and 6 receive the sensation of green. In this way, he hypothesized a link between the six-layered structure of the lateral geniculate body in many primates with the classical three-component theory of color vision.

However, this interesting theory has many weaknesses. For instance, Walls (1953) and Hartridge (1952) could justifiably ask where the rods were represented if all the six layers represent the cones of the retina. Chow (1955) could not confirm Le Gros Clark's results. In one of Le Gros Clark's experiments, neurons of the first two magnocellular layers of the lateral geniculate body developed atrophy after the monkeys had been kept in a room from which blue light was excluded. Under the same conditions Chow found no atrophy in these layers.

Kravkov (1951) and his pupils demonstrated the importance of subcortical structures for the perception of color stimuli. Shvarts (1950) considers that the physiological mechanisms affecting sensitivity to green and red light are to be found at the subcortical level. In pharmacological experiments, the action of nikethamide and veronal on the subcortex and of caffeine and chloral hydrate on the cortex was studied. Nikethamide caused a marked increase in sensitivity to green light and a decrease in the sensitivity to red. Veronal, on the other hand, increased sensitivity to red, but just about halved the sensitivity to green and blue. Substances acting on the cortex caused no dissociation of sensitivity: they either increased or decreased sensitivity to all wavelengths.

Chang (1952a) suggests that impulses carrying chromatic sensations are transmitted selectively by three visual pathways consisting of three sets of fibers of different size. On the basis of the work of O'Leary (1941) he identifies neurons of three sizes in the lateral geniculate body, and this coincides with the number of primary colors.

Feigenberg (1953) made an interesting comparison of the functions of the subcortical and cortical levels of the visual system with their structure. He concluded from many experiments on healthy human subjects that the visual cortex (area striata) plays the leading role in the formation of neuro-dynamic processes connected with the analysis of color and shape, while the subcortical level of the visual system (the lateral geniculate body) is concerned with the analysis of the intensity of light.

Walls (1953) criticizes Le Gros Clark and others studying the morphological basis of color vision, and considers that the number three has had a magical effect on them, for they have connected it directly with the three primary color stimuli and thus inevitably oversimplified the issue. Nobody has ever proved the existence of three retinogeniculate tracts. The cartographic theory of Walls corresponds to the complexity of human vision, but does little to explain the basic problem.

The discovery by Foerster (1928) and Penfield and Jasper (1954) that sparks and shapes of different colors can be obtained by electrical stimulation of the occipital cortex in man, and the many cases in which color vision is disturbed after injuries and tumors of the human occipital cortex (Henschen, 1890; Kononova, 1926; Preobrazhenskaya, 1954; Polyak, 1957; Luria, 1966, and his collaborators), are facts of considerable importance.

Finally, rare cases have been described in which hemiachromatopsia has been observed after injury to the occipital region (Kravkov, 1951; Polyak, 1957).

Extremely contradictory opinions and views are thus held on this problem of the morphological basis of color vision in the cortical and subcortical portions of the visual system.

To decide what part is played by neurons of the cortex and lateral geniculate body in the reception and analysis of color stimuli, I reexamined my material on neuron structure (pp. 12–100), and made a further study of the cytoarchitectonics of the visual centers in the mole, mouse, and cat, comparing these structural features with the state of color vision (see also Shkol'nik-Yarros, 1962).

1. The cytoarchitectonics of the central visual system in mammals differs with the degree of development of color vision. In animals with undeveloped or feebly developed color vision, the parvocellular layers in the lateral geniculate body are absent or poorly developed, and division of layer IV of the cortex in Area 17 into three sublayers, associated with the

formation of a wide parvocellular sublayer IVc, is absent. The greatest contrast in the size of different types of neurons was also observed cytoarchitectonically both in the cortex and the lateral geniculate body of primates possessing color vision.

These differences in the visual system must also be compared with the state of all other aspects of visual function (visual acuity, discrimination of details, shape, depth, and brightness, recognition of the meaning of events, and so on). The cytoarchitectonic features distinguishing the visual and other sensory systems are exhibited against a background of structural features of the central nervous system common to all these species.

2. A study of neurons of the different parts of the visual system revealed additional data shedding light on the problem of color vision. For instance, a very important cytoarchitectonic difference in neuron structure was found in the lateral geniculate body. The lateral geniculate body in primates is characterized not only by a well-marked lamination but also by the presence of midget neurons, with a small number of short dendrites, giving off few branches. No similar neurons are found in the subcortical structures of other systems. These cells are particularly numerous in the upper four layers of the lateral geniculate body in primates with well-developed colored vision. Only a few of these cells are present in dogs, which have poor color vision, and they are completely absent in the hedgehog which does not possess color vision. The main feature of the midget neurons is not the size of the cell body, but the very short range of their dendrites, the very small area of their distribution and, consequently, the low level of development of their axo-dendritic connections.

3. Neurons of layers IV of Area 17, the principal part of the visual cortex where fibers from the lateral geniculate body end, also differ considerably in the species of mammals described above and in man.

No concentrations of small, round neurons with dendrites winding spirally around their body and with axon collaterals resembling a weeping willow, characteristic of sublayer IVc of the cortex in monkeys, could be found in Area 17 of the hedgehog, rabbit, or dog. Likewise no large or small varieties of star cells with a long, descending axon were seen in the hedgehog, rabbit, and dog, but instead they are all uniformly equal in size. Typical double-tufted neurons and neurons with complex selectivity of their axons are also absent.

In the visual cortex of monkey and man, differentiation of neurons in layer IV is very sharply defined. Besides large cells with a long, descending axon, and with dendrites spreading far and wide (resembling a bird in flight), many small varieties of such neurons are present (Fig. 46). In sublayer IVc a concentration of small, round neurons with few dendrites, either ramifying close to the cell body or curving around the body, can be distinguished; the axon of these cells usually branches close to the cell body or among the ramifications of the dendrites, sometimes with the appearance of falling branches of a weeping willow. A much lower proportion of neurons from sublayer IVc send their axons upward. The very small number of widely branching axons is a typical feature which I observed for the dog's cortex.

The small, round neurons with few dendrites, concentrated in very large numbers in sublayer IVc of Area 17 of monkeys and man, bear some resemblance to my midget cells of the lateral geniculate body. The similarity lies in the density of their distribution, their size and shape, and their poorly developed dendrites. However, the differences between them are still considerable, for the midget cells of the lateral geniculate body have long axons transmitting visual impulses into the cortex, while the neurons of sublayer IVc have short axons and principally form synapses with other small neurons surrounding them.

4. No pyramidal neurons with an ascending arcuate axon could be found in cortical layers IV, V, and VI of the hedgehog. In the rabbit, where arcuate ascending collaterals from the descending axon are present, only isolated pyramidal neurons without a descending branch of their axon can be seen, and then only very rarely. In the dog's cortex fairly large and also smaller pyramidal cells with an arcuate descending axon and with no descending branch are observed. In the monkey there is a large concentration of typical small, round, pyramidal cells with an arcuate, ascending axon in sublayer IVc, but they are also present in layers V, VI, and VII. Their dendrites usually reach only as far as sublayer IVb, i.e., they lie in the region receiving the largest number of fibers from the lateral geniculate body. Terminal branches of the axon also lie in sublayer IVb. A similar arrangement is found in the human cortex. This pattern is a very clear distinguishing feature of cortical structure in primates. The presence of a few such neurons with an ascending arcuate axon in other layers and other areas does not alter the basic fact of their very high concentration in the lower layers of the visual cortex, especially in primates.

5. In sublayer IVc of Area 17 in monkeys and man, a particularly large number of visual fibers from the lateral geniculate body terminate, a smaller number terminating in layers III, IVa, IVb, and V. Among the specific afferent fibers which are identified in sublayer IVc, there were some of a special type, with the appearance of an umbrella, with numerous contacts with surrounding small neurons. There are no afferent fibers in the cortex of insectivores, rodents, and carnivores similar to the umbrellalike afferents found in the green monkey.

6. To obtain a more complete picture of neuron specialization, I compared my findings with studies of neurons by others at the Brain Institute. As described above, midget cells of the lateral geniculate body, which

are found in small numbers in dogs and in large concentrations in primates, are absent from the medial geniculate body of the dog. They are also absent from the striopallidum of the dog, monkey, and man, from the other nuclei of the thalamus, and also from other structures in the reticular formation of the brain stem.

7.   Finally, neurons of the visual cortex were compared with neurons of other cortical areas studied at the Brain Institute. Specialized neurons were also found in the cortex: the giant Betz cells of the motor cortex, the large, corkscrew-shaped spindles of the limbic cortex, the special, flattened stars of the visual cortex with winding, descending axons. In the visual cortex the specialized cells are the large star cells of sublayer IVb with a descending axon and also the concentrations of two types of neurons described above in sublayer IVc and the lower layers.

It can thus be concluded from a comparison of the structure of the central visual system in mammals possessing color vision and in those without it that considerable qualitative differences exist.

Similar qualitative differences have also been found in the structure of Area 17 of the squirrel (*Sciurus vulgaris*) (Shkol'nik-Yarros, 1968). Several authorities consider that the squirrel possesses color vision (Colvin and Burford, 1909; Meyer-Oehme, 1957; Orlov, 1965; Orlov and Maksimova, 1968). Orlov separates the color vision system of squirrels into a distinct group. According to his investigations, color discrimination is shown extremely clearly by these rodents under experimental conditions. The cytoarchitectonics of Area 17 in squirrels and the structure of its neurons (Fig. 132a) thus correspond completely to physiological functions. Gurevich, Bykhovskaya, and Uranovskii (1929) originally found that the cytoarchitectonics of Area 17 in the squirrel is similar to that of the corresponding area in higher mammals. The neuronal structure of layer IV, with its division into three sublayers, and the large cells of Cajal all point to the fact that the structure of area striata in the squirrel is of the primate type (Fig. 132a).

Comparison of the distinguishing features of the visual centers and their specific aspects with those of the retina on the lines described above, taking into account the presence or absence of color vision, revealed an extremely interesting detail, namely that midget cells are present in the retina of primates. Polyak (1941, 1957) found in the primate retina that, in addition to the well-known bipolar cells connected by synapses with the rods and sometimes with the cones of the retina, there are other bipolar cells, which he termed "midget" connected individually with each cone. This midget bipolar cell is connected, in turn, with a midget ganglion cell. The whole of this system (cone–midget bipolar–midget ganglion cell) is described by Polyak as the cone system. In comparing my own material with Polyak's I naturally was faced with the problem: must the midget

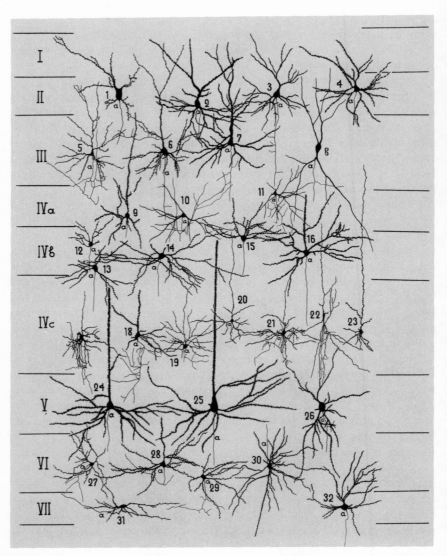

Fig. 132a. Composite drawing of neurons in Area 17 of the squirrel. a, axon. Cells: 1,
2, atypical pyramidal neurons; 3, 4, small pyramidal cells of layer II; 5, pyramidlike cell
with ascending arcuate axon in layer III; 6, 7, pyramidal cells of layer III; 8, fusiform
cell of layer III; 9, small pyramidal neuron of sublayer IVa; 10, 11, short-axon cells of
sublayer IVa; 12, small star cell of Cajal; 13, 14, star cells of Cajal in sublayer IVb of
semilunar type; 15, 16, star cells of Cajal of radial type in sublayer IVb; 17, 18, 19, 21,
short-axon neurons in sublayer IVc; 20, 23, small pyramidal cells in sublayer IVc; 24,

structures observed both in the retina and in central visual structures be regarded as a single cone–midget system? This system is well developed in primates possessing diurnal vision. It may be rudimentary in animals with undeveloped color vision, and completely absent in those following a nocturnal mode of life and with a retina consisting purely of rods.

To confirm this hypothesis, based on my comparative anatomical data, I consulted the literature amassed as a result of many years of work by numerous investigators. The first matter for consideration was the projection of parts of the retina on the lateral geniculate body in primates. It became clear that the macula lutea is represented in all layers of the lateral geniculate body (Polyak, 1957; Kupfer, 1962), but more extensively in the upper layers. Brouwer (1927) obtained results definitely showing that the macula lutea is represented mainly in the parvocellular layers. Consequently, elements in the center of the retina are mainly connected with neurons in the upper layers of the lateral geniculate body in primates.

What type of connection is this? I have already mentioned the interesting synaptic investigations of Glees and Le Gros Clark (1941), who felt that the visual afferent fiber divides in the lateral geniculate body into five branches, each of which terminates in one large synapse on the body of one of the cells.

Although Glees and Le Gros Clark were wrong when they stated that axo-dendritic contacts are absent and in the number of branches of the visual afferent fiber which they gave (see Figs. 40, 57), their underlying idea is in full agreement with my own hypothesis of the existence of a system with more individualized contacts. Glees and Le Gros Clark emphasize that it is more difficult to draw conclusions regarding the large neurons of the two magnocellular layers I and II, and that their observations of single synapses are concerned mainly with the small neurons of the upper four layers. Consequently, the synaptic and morphological data support the hypothesis that a special system is present in the visual analyzer of primates.

The exceptional ease and the rapidity with which transneuronal degeneration occurs in the lateral geniculate body of primates must be mentioned. This is a feature which can only be explained by the considerable individualization of synaptic endings on the neurons of this nucleus. This rapidly occurring transneuronal degeneration in the lateral geniculate body was first demonstrated by Minkowski (1913, 1920a,b), and not only in monkeys but in cats as well.

25, large pyramidal cells of sublayer IVc; 24, 25, large pyramidal cells of sublayer V; 26, short-axon neuron in layer V; 27, 29, short-axon cells of layer VI; 28, pyramid-shaped cell with ascending arcuate axon in layer VI; 30, cell with ascending axon in layer VI; 31, horizontal fusiform cell in layer VII; 32, pyramidal cell in layer VII. Golgi preparation; 100×. (Shkol'nik-Yarros, 1968.)

Observations on cortical structure in primates leading different modes of life, i.e., on nocturnal and diurnal monkeys, are of special interest. Solnitzky and Harman (1946), who compared the structure of the area striata in a large series of monkeys, found that it is divided into central and peripheral sectors.

In nocturnal primates (*Perodicticus potto*, for example), with no area centralis in their retina, the structure of Area 17 is uniform as it is in other mammals. Nocturnal primates, with an area centralis in their retina (*Galago demidovii*), have both central and peripheral sectors, but the latter is more highly differentiated. In diurnal monkeys, with a fovea centralis in their retina, differentiation of the cortical layers is finer and more discrete in the central sector of Area 17. The widest sublayer of the cortex in nocturnal monkeys is IVb (a) and in diurnal monkeys IVc (b).* Sublayer IVc (b) is narrower and less highly differentiated in nocturnal monkeys.

In all diurnal monkeys, sublayer IVc (IVb) has five subdivisions. Only in man is an additional subdivision present: IVc is divided further into three parts. A close correlation exists between the differentiation of the lateral geniculate body and of Area 17. In nocturnal monkeys the lateral geniculate body has the largest number of magnocellular layers (five in *Perodicticus potto* and *Galago*, four in lemurs); the nucleus is located dorsally in the diencephalon. In diurnal primates the structure of the lateral geniculate body is quite different: there are only two magnocellular layers and four parvocellular layers, while the nucleus is located ventrally in the diencephalon.

Ozhigova (1958, 1960), who studied the cytoarchitectonics of Area 17 in various monkeys, confirmed the division of Area 17 into two zones. Subarea 17a, located in the depth of the calcarine fissure and corresponding to peripheral vision, possesses a narrower cortex, its upper layers are wider than the lower layers, the large star cells are clearly distributed in the middle part of sublayer IVb, and sublayer IVc is homogeneous. Subarea 17b lies in the region of the operculum occipitale, on the walls of the superior occipital fissure. It has a more highly differentiated sublayer IVc and corresponds to macular vision.

The clinical cases described by Rønne (1910, 1913) also are important. In the first, ganglion cells were most severely affected in the retina. In the second case, one of diabetic amblyopia, Rønne observed that the large cells in the retina and the magnocellular layers 1 and 2 in the lateral geniculate body were intact, while considerable atrophy was present in the macular part

---

* The division of the cortex into layers used by these workers is similar to that used by von Bonin, and differs from Brodmann's method adopted at the Brain Institute. The terminology used by Solnitzky and Harman is given in parentheses.

of the retina. This patient was unable to see green, and with his left eye he could not see red.

Kravkov (1951), as already mentioned, describes his observations on two patients with head wounds with complete loss of color vision but with preservation of normal twilight vision. Earlier cases of lesions of the occipital lobes with loss of color vision were described by Henschen (1890–1896). Disturbances of color perception were shown by Preobrazhenskaya (1954) to be symptoms of damage to the occipital lobe in patients with head wounds. During recovery of vision by these wounded patients, perception of achromatic stimuli appeared before that of chromatic. Cases of hemiachromatopsia are described by Polyak (1957). Color agnosia has been described in cases of more extensive lesions.

After concussion, an artist immediately lost his sight, which returned in the following order: at first he began to distinguish between light and darkness, after which his whole environment appeared gray, to which different colors were gradually added. The patient recalls that recovery of perception of achromatic and chromatic stimuli took place separately.

Hence, different approaches to the problem of the morphological basis of color vision lead to similar conclusions. Specialization, while particularly conspicuous in the peripheral part of sensory systems, is also found in their central part.

It must be admitted that this account unavoidably is to some extent schematic, with the consequent oversimplification of very complex phenomena. Both the visual function itself and the structures corresponding to this function are extremely complex and varied and they differ considerably in animals and in man. However, the proven presence of midget cells (in the sense of the extent of their axo-dendritic connections, not of their size) in the central portion of the visual system and the fact that color vision may be lost in patients with brain lesions lead to the conclusion that a special cone–midget system exists in the visual analyzer of primates. The macular part of this system is the most extensive, and it is evidently concerned not only with the perception of color stimuli, but also with visual acuity, with the fineness and precision of visual discrimination, i.e., with the properties characteristic of macular vision. The peripheral part of this system (the rare midget cells in layers 1–2 of the lateral geniculate body, corresponding to the midget bipolars and ganglion cells at the periphery of the retina) is much less extensive.

According to Hassler (1966), who studied the visual system in primates and insectivores, layers 1 and 2 of the lateral geniculate body correlate in size and number of nerve cells with nocturnal activity, i.e., with scotopic vision. The conclusions from this comparative anatomical study agree with the results from studying neurons (Shkol'nik-Yarros, 1962, 1963).

NEW DATA ON THE STRUCTURE AND FUNCTION OF THE LATERAL GENICULATE BODY IN PRIMATES RELATIVE TO THE PROBLEM OF COLOR VISION

My hypothesis of the existence of a system for the special purpose of reception of color stimuli, first enunciated in 1958, has subsequently been confirmed by electrophysiological and histochemical investigations.

De Valois et al. (1958), De Valois (1960), and De Valois and Jones (1961) studied single neurons of the lateral geniculate body of primates with microelectrodes. Their results are extremely interesting.

Neurons of the lower layers 1 and 2 do not respond to color stimuli whereas neurons of layers 3, 4, 5, and 6 respond differentially to stimuli with different spectral characteristics. Within the parvocellular layers (3–6), if potentials are recorded from single neurons, strictly determined responses can be obtained. In layers 3 and 4 single neurons gave either on or off responses to a photic stimulus of definite wavelength. For example, a nerve cell gave an on response to blue light and an off response to yellow light, i.e., it responded to the complementary color. In layers 5 and 6 the cells gave simpler responses to color stimuli, giving both on and off responses to stimuli of the same color. Different neurons responded to stimulation with light of only a particular wavelength.

On the basis of these investigations De Valois is inclined to consider the system of layers 3 and 4 to be a mechanism working in accordance with Hering's four-component theory, while the system of layers 5 and 6 is a mechanism corresponding to the three-component theory of color vision.

According to De Valois, therefore, color vision in primates is represented by two simultaneously working systems.

Daniel et al. (1962) also obtained conclusive evidence of differences in spectral sensitivity for single small cells in the dorsal layers of the lateral geniculate body in monkeys, in contrast to the cells of the first two layers.

The orderly pattern of fundamental differences between layers 1–2 and 3–6 has been complicated by the interesting work of Hubel and Wiesel (1966). However, the type 1 cells which they found frequently in layers 3–6, characterized by differences in spectral sensitivity of the center and periphery of the receptive field, are completely absent in layers 1–2. Other interesting results which they obtained demonstrate the very large periphery of the receptive field in the lower layers. A relationship can be postulated between the size of the receptive fields and the range of dendritic branches of neurons in the corresponding layers (Fig. 39).

In a study carried out in conjunction with workers at the histochemistry laboratory of the Brain Institute (Ball', Portugalov, and Shkol'nik-Yarros,

1964), the histochemical characteristics of each layer of the lateral geniculate body were determined.

Localization of protein was examined by the methods of Danielli (tetrazonium reaction); Barnett and Seligman, in modifications adopted at the histochemistry laboratory, Brain Institute (reaction for SH- and COOH-groups); Weiss and co-workers (for amino groups); Brachet and Kresnik, for nucleic acids; Nachlas and co-workers for succinate dehydrogenase; and Gomori for acid phosphatase. The relative content of proteins and nucleic acids and the level of enzyme activity in each layer of the lateral geniculate body or in single neurons of these layers were estimated by direct photometry of sections. The results were expressed as percentages of the values for layer 1.

This investigation was carried out on 27 sexually mature and apparently healthy rhesus monkeys (*Macaca mulatta*) of both sexes. The proteins whose distribution and content were studied in each layer of the lateral geniculate body can be divided into two groups. The first includes proteins detectable by methods for SH- and NH_2-groups, the second includes proteins detectable by Danielli's tetrazonium reaction and by the reaction for COOH-groups. A common feature of both groups is their high content in all structures of layers 1 and 2. The lowest content of proteins detectable by methods for SH- and NH_2-groups is found in layers 3, 4, and 5, and in each layer the protein content is higher in the bodies of the nerve cells, other structures containing smaller concentrations of proteins. In layer 6 the differences between the bodies of neurons and structures surrounding them in their protein content are less marked than in other layers of the geniculate body. The relative content of all proteins assayed is identical in layer 6.

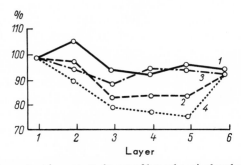

Graph 1. Protein content in separate layers of lateral geniculate body of rhesus monkey (as a percentage of layer 1). 1, tetrazonium reaction; 2, reaction for NH_2-groups; 3, reaction for COOH-groups; 4, reaction for SH-groups. (Ball', Portugalov, and Shkol'nik-Yarros, 1964.)

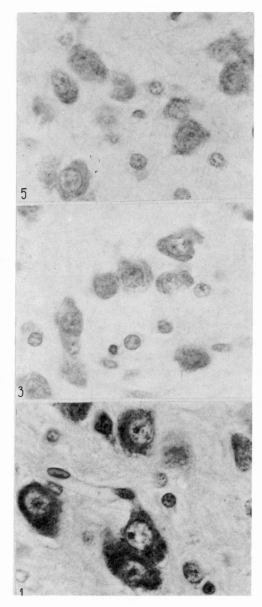

Fig. 133. Lateral geniculate body of a rhesus monkey. RNA content is highest in the cytoplasm of cells of layer 1 and lowest in the cytoplasm of neurons in layer 3; neurons of layer 5 in this respect occupy an intermediate position. (Ball', Portugalov, and Shkol'nik-Yarros, 1964.)

The individual layers differ from each other only very slightly in their content of proteins detectable by the method of Barnett and Seligman for COOH. The cytophotometric measurements show that the content of these proteins is only a little lower in layer 3. With Danielli's tetrazonium reaction, a very high concentration of protein is found in layer 1, and a still higher concentration in layer 2, while in the remaining layers their content is lower and more or less equal (Graph 1).

The bodies of single neurons in the same layer show substantial differences from each other in the content of proteins in their cytoplasm by all the tests used, although the differences between layers 1–2 and layers 3–6 are sufficiently clear (Graph 1).

The content of nucleic acids also varies in the neurons of the different layers. The largest RNA content per cell was found in layer 1. It was very slightly smaller in the neurons of layer 2. The lowest RNA content was found in the neurons of layers 3 and 4. Layers 5 and 6 occupy an intermediate position in this respect between layers 1–2 and 3–4 (Fig. 133 and Graph 2). The DNA concentration in the nuclei of the nerve cells corresponds to the size of the nuclei: the smaller the volume of the nucleus of the nerve cell, the higher its DNA concentration.

The level of acid phosphatase activity in the nerve cells is closely connected with their size, being higher in the larger neurons and lower in the small.

The distribution of the activity of an enzyme of the Krebs cycle—succinic dehydrogenase—in the lateral geniculate body is highest in the bodies of the neurons in layers 1 and 2. It is also fairly high in the processes of these cells, which can be traced, by the diformazan granules deposited in them in the sections, for considerable distances from their point of emergence from the neuron body. The general level of activity of the structures located in layers 1 and 2 between the bodies of the neurons is high. Succinic dehydrogenase activity is significantly lower in layers 3, 4, 5, and 6 (Fig. 134

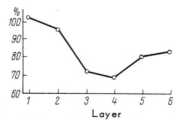

Graph 2. RNA content in cytoplasm of cells of lateral geniculate body of the rhesus monkey estimated by Brachet's method. (Ball', Portugalov, and Shkol'nik-Yarros, 1964.)

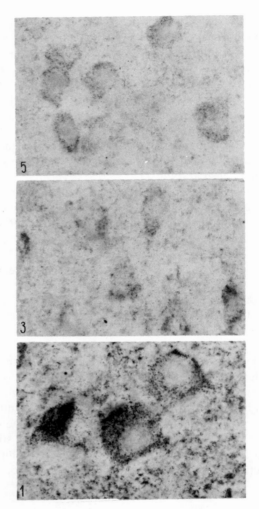

Fig. 134. Distribution of succinic dehydrogenase activity in layers 1, 3, and 5 of the lateral geniculate body of the rhesus monkey. Highest enzymatic activity located in bodies of neurons in layer 1; density of deposition of diformazan granules in them is also highest. High activity also present in processes of nerve cells and individual glial cells. Enzymatic activity in layers 3 and 5 much lower than in layer 1. Succinic dehydrogenase activity in 5 is mainly concentrated in bodies of nerve cells. Method of Nachlas *et al.* (Ball', Portugalov, and Shkol'nik-Yarros, 1964.)

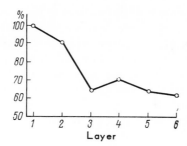

Graph 3. Level of succinic dehydrogenase activity in lateral geniculate body of rhesus monkey determined by Nachlas's method. (Ball', Portugalov, and Shkol'nik-Yarros, 1964.)

and Graph 3). In these layers the activity of this enzyme, while its general level in the bodies of the neurons is low by comparison with the magnocellular layers, is considerably higher than its activity in other structures.*

Consequently, neurons of the two magnocellular layers differ from those of the four parvocellular layers not only in size, shape, organization of their Nissl substance, and number and length of dendrites, but also in the content and composition of their proteins. Compared with the other layers, the highest content of proteins and a higher activity of succinic dehydrogenase and acid phosphatase are found in layers 1 and 2.

Neurons of individual layers of the lateral geniculate body can be subdivided into three groups depending on their RNA content. The highest RNA content is found in cells of layers 1 and 2, the lowest in cells of layers 3 and 4; neurons of layers 5 and 6 in this respect occupy an intermediate position.

The basic morphological and histological differences thus revealed in primates between layers 1 and 2, on the one hand, and the other layers of the lateral geniculate body on the other hand, can be compared with the electrophysiological data described above, revealing fundamental differences in

---

* Fundamental differences between the structure and connections of layers 1–2 and 3–6 of the lateral geniculate body of diurnal primates were revealed most clearly in an original investigation carried out by Figurina (1965). After removal of both eyes and other receptors the upper layers atrophied (transneuronal degeneration), while in the lower magnocellular layers, particularly in the caudal portions of the nucleus, the large cells remained intact.

No better confirmation could be obtained of the more extensive connections of the large neurons in the lower layers of the lateral geniculate body by comparison with the limited connection of neurons in the upper layers than is afforded by these experiments.

the responses of single neurons of this nucleus to color stimuli. This suggests that there are definite connections between the functional, histochemical, and structural features distinguishing neurons of different layers of the lateral geniculate body. In other words, the coding of different visual stimuli and the transmission of visual information to the cortex are carried out by highly differentiated systems of neurons, some of which are specially adapted for the transmission of color.

The neurons of the lower layers 1 and 2 have the following characteristics: large size, large volume of distribution of axo-dendritic contacts, high concentration of proteins and acid phosphatase, and high RNA content. The neurons of layers 3, 4, 5, and 6, whose responses to color stimuli show a complex pattern of differentiation, are characterized by small size, a smaller range of axo-dendritic contacts, and by different relative contents and absolute concentrations of individual proteins in their cytoplasm compared with the neurons of the magnocellular layers, and also by very low activity of oxidative enzymes and a low RNA content. It can be concluded from these findings that the cytoplasm of neurons (as well as some aspects of their structure) responding to color stimuli differs from that of neurons not so responding.

A close correlation exists between the structure, function, and chemical properties of particular neuron complexes (Byzov, 1961, 1966; Utina, 1960; Brodskii and Nechaeva, 1959; Brodskii, 1960; Portugalov *et al.*, 1963; Svanidze, 1963; Busnyuk, 1963; Chekunov, 1964). In my opinion this important hypothesis is confirmed by our observations on the structure and chemical properties of the functionally differentiated layers of the lateral geniculate body.

BIBLIOGRAPHY

Abdullakhodzhaeva, M. (1960). Abstracts of proceedings of a conference of scientific workers from the Proletarskaya District of Moscow [in Russian], Moscow, pp. 21–23.

Adrianov, O. S. (1951). "Morphological differentation of the nucleus of the motor analyzer in dogs and its participation in the act of vision." Dissertation, Moscow.

Adrianov, O. S. (1953). *Zh. Vyssh. Nervn. Deyat.* **3**:428.

Adrianov, O. S., and T. A. Mering (1959). *Atlas of the Dog's Brain* [in Russian], Moscow.

Akimoto, H., and O. Creutzfeldt (1958). *Arch. f. Psych.* **196**:494.

Alouf, I. S. (1929). *J. Psych. u. Neurol.* **38**:5.

Andersen, P., J. C. Eccles, and Y. Løyning (1964). *J. Neurophysiol.* **27**:608.

Andersen, P., J. C. Eccles, and P. E. Voorhoeve (1964). *J. Neurophysiol.* **17**:1138.

Anokhin, P. K. (1965). "Mechanisms of functional system arranged for autoregulation." *Reflexes of the Brain.* Moscow. (In: *Brain Reflexes. Progress in Brain Research, Vol. 22.* E. A. Asratyan, ed., Amsterdam, Elsevier, 1968, pp. 230–251.)

Anokhin, P. K. (1968). *Biology and Neurophysiology of the Conditional Reflex.* Meditsina, Moscow. **1**:23

Armstrong, P., and J. Z. Young (1957). *J. Physiol.* **137**:10.

Arvanitaki, A. (1942). *J. Neurophysiol.* **5**(2):89.

Babayan, S. A. (1955). "Efferent pathways of the parietal cortex of the dog." Author's abstract of dissertation, Moscow.

Bailey, P., and G. von. Bonin (1951). *The Isocortex of Man.* Urbana, Ill.

Ball', T. V., V. V. Portugalov, and E. G. Shkol'nik-Yarros (1964). *Zh. Vyssh. Nervn. Deyat.* **4**:707. (*Fed. Proc. Transl. Suppl.* **24**: T781–T785, 1965.)

Balmasova, Z. N. (1950). "Histological investigation of interneuronal connections in the optic nerve system of some mammals and man." Author's abstract of dissertation, Leningrad.

Barris, R. E., W. R. Ingram, and S. W. Ranson (1935). *J. Comp. Neurol.* **62**:117.

Bekhterev, V. M. (1890). *Arkh. Psikhiat. Nevrol. Sud. Psikhopatol.* **15**:1.

Bekhterev, V. M. (1896a). In: *Selected Works* [in Russian], Moscow (1954), pp. 76–80.

Bekhterev, V. M. (1896b). *Obozr. Psikh. Nevrol. i Éksper. Psikhol.* **1**:12.

Bekhterev, V. M. (1896c). *Obozr. Psikh. Nevrol. i Éksper. Psikhol.* **1**:23.

Bekhterev, V. M. (1896–1898). *Conducting Pathways of the Spinal Cord and Brain* [in Russian], Vols. I, II, St. Pertersburg. (Translation available in German.)

Bekhterev, V. M. (1903–1907). *Fundamentals of the Study of Brain Function* [in Russian], Nos. 1–7, St. Petersburg. (Translation available in German.)

Bekhterev, V. M. (Bechterew, W.) (1911). *Die Funktionen der Nervencentra.* Vol. III, Verlag von Gustav Fischer, Jena.

Belenkov, N. Yu., and T. E. Kalinina (1963). In: *Electrophysiology of the Nervous System*. Proceedings of the 4th All-Union Electrophysiological Conference [in Russian], Rostov-on-Don.

Beresford, W. A. (1962). *J. f. Hirnforschung* **5**(3):210.

Beritashvili, I. S. (1956). *Gagrskie Besedy (Tbilisi)* **2**:201.

Beritashvili, I. S. (1963a). *Gagrskie Besedy (Tbilisi)* **4**:111.

Beritashvili, I. S. (1963b). Abstracts of proceedings of an international conference to commemorate the centenary of I. M. Sechenov's book *Reflexes of the Brain* [in Russian], Moscow. (In: *Brain Reflexes. Progress in Brain Research, Vol.* 22. (E. A. Asratyan [ed.], Amsterdam, Elsevier 1968, 600 pp.)

Beritashvili, I. S. (1968). *Vertebrate Memory, Its Characteristics and Genesis* [in Russian], Metsniereba, Tbilisi.

Beritov, I. S. (1960). *Arkh. Anat.* **8**:3.

Beritov, I. S. (1961). *Nervous Mechanisms of Higher Vertebrate Behavior* [in Russian], Moscow. (Translated by W. T. Liberson, Boston; Little Brown, 1965. 384 pp.)

Berkley, M., E. Wolf, and M. Glickstein (1967). *Exper. Neurol.* **19**(2):188.

Betz (Bets), V. A. (1873–1874). *Vrach. Vestn.* **25**:426.

Biryuchkov, Yu. V. (1963). "Topographical-anatomical investigation of conducting pathways in the peripheral portion of the visual analyzer." Author's abstract of dissertation, Moscow.

Bishop G. H., and R. Davis (1953). *Science* **118**:241.

Bishop, G. H., and M. H. Clare (1955). *J. Comp. Neurol.* **103**:269.

Bishop, P. O., D. Jeremy, and J. G. McLeod (1953). *J. Neurophysiol.* **16**(4):437.

Blinkov, S. M. (1941). *Nevropatol. i Psikhiat.* **10**(2):48.

Blinkov, S. M. (1955). *Structural Features of the Human Brain. The Temporal Lobe of Man and Monkeys* [in Russian], Moscow.

Bodian, D. (1940). *J. Comp. Neurol.* **37**(2):323.

Bodian, D. (1952). *Cold Spring Harbor Symp. Quant. Biol.* **17**:14.

Bogolepov, N. N. (1964). *Zh. Nevropatol.* **3**:326.

Bogoslovskii, A. I., and E. N. Semenovskaya (1959). *Byull Éksperim. Biol. i Med.* **27**(3):3.

Bongard, M. M., E. A. Liberman, and M. S. Smirnov (1957). Abstracts of proceedings of a conference on the physiology of reception [in Russian], Moscow, pp. 3–6.

Bongard, M. M., and M. S. Smirnov (1959). *Priroda* **5**:13.

Bonin, G. von. (1942). *J. Comp. Neurol.*, **77**:405.

Borovyagin, V. L. (1963). "Electronmicroscopy of nervous and glial elements of the peripheral nerve and retina of vertebrates." Author's abstract of dissertation, Moscow.

Borovyagin, V. L. (1966). *Biofizika* **11**(5):810.

Boycott, B. B., E. G. Gray, and R. W. Guillery (1960). *J. Physiol.* **152**:3P.

Brazovskaya, F. A. (1951). "Corticopontine tracts." Author's abstract of dissertation, Moscow.

Brazovskaya, F. A. (1953). *Vopr. Neirokhir.* **2**:22.

Brindley, G. S., and D. I. Hamasaki (1961). *J. Physiol.* **159**(2):88.

Brindley, G. S., and D. I. Hamasaki (1966). *J. Physiol.* **184**(2):444.

Brodmann, K. (1909). *Vergleichende Localisationslehre der Grosshirnrinde in ihren Prinzipien dargestellt auf Grund des Zellenbaues*, Leipzig.

Brodskii, V. Ya. (1956). *Dokl. Akad. Nauk SSSR* **111**(6):1340.

Brodskii, V. Ya. (1960). *Dokl. Akad. Nauk SSSR* **130**(1):189.

Brodskii, V. Ya., and N. V. Nechaeva (1959). *Tsitologiya* **1**(2):172.

Brouwer, B. (1923). *Schweiz. Arch. Neurol. Psych.*, **13**:118.

Brouwer, B. (1927). *Anatomical, Phylogenetic and Clinical Studies on the Central Nervous System*. Baltimore, Maryland.

Brouwer, B. (1936). In: *Handbuch der Neurologie*, Vol. 6 (O. Bumke and O. Foerster, eds.) pp. 449–532.

Brouwer, B., and W. P. Zeeman (1926). *Brain* **49**:1.

Bruesch, S. R., and L. B. Arey (1942). *J. Comp. Neurol.* **77**(3):631.

Busnyuk, M. M. (1963). *Zh. Vyssh. Nervn. Deyat.* **4**:731.

Byzov, A. L. (1961). *Fiziol. Zh. SSSR* (1):71.

Byzov, A. L. (1966). *Electrophysiological Investigations of the Retina.* Nauka, Moscow.

Cajal, S. Ramon Y. (1889). *Anat. Anz.* **4**:111.

Cajal, S. Ramon Y. (1891). *La Cellule* **7**:125.

Cajal, S. Ramon Y. (1892). *La Cellule* **9**:119.

Cajal, S. Ramon Y. (1896). *Rev. Trimest. Microgr.* **2**:123.

Cajal, S. Ramon Y. (1900–1906). *Studien über die Hirnrinde des Menschen*, No. 1–5, Leipzig.

Cajal, S. Ramon Y. (1903). *Trabajos del Labor. de Invest. Biol. de la Univ. de Madrid* **2**:129.

Cajal, S. Ramon Y. (1909). *Histologie du Système Nerveux de l'Homme et des Vertébrés*, Vol. 1, Paris.

Cajal, S. Ramon Y. (1911). *Histologie du Système Nerveux de l'Homme et des Vertébrés*, Vol. 2, Paris.

Cajal, S. Ramon Y. (1935). *Handbuch der Neurologie*, Vol. 1. (O. Bumke and O. Foerster, ed.), pp. 887–994.

Campbell, A. W. (1905). *Histological Studies on the Localization of Cerebral Function*, Cambridge.

Chang Hsiang-Tung (1952a). *J. Neurophysiol.*, **15**(1):5.

Chang Hsiang-Tung (1952b). *Cold Spring Harbor Symp. Quant. Biol.* **17**:189.

Chekunov, A. S. (1964). "Histochemical investigation of proteins and nucleic acids in cellular structures of the rabbit and guinea pig visual analyzer in ontogenesis." Author's abstract of dissertation, Moscow.

Cholokashvili, E. S. (1958a). Abstracts of Proceedings of the 6th All-Union Congress of Anatomists, Histologists, and Embryologists [in Russian], Khar'kov, pp. 433–434.

Cholokashivili, E. S. (1958b). *Trud. Inst. Fiziol. im. I. S. Beritashvili (Tbilisi)* **11**:207.

Chow, K. L. (1950). *J. Comp. Neurol.* **93**(3):313.

Chow, K. L. (1955). *J. Comp. Neurol.* **102**:597.

Chow, K. L., and P. J. Hutt (1953). *Brain* **76**(4):625.

Chow, K. L., J. S. Blum, and R. A. Blum (1950). *J. Comp. Neurol.* **92**:227.

Chusid, J. G., O. Sugar, and J. D. French (1948). *J. Neuropath. Exper. Neurol.* **7**(3):439.

Clark, W. E. Le Gros (1932). *Brit. J. Ophthalmol.*, **16**:264.

Clark, W. E. Le Gros (1940). *Nature* **146**:558.

Clark, W. E. Le Gros (1941). *J. Anat.* **75**(2):225.

Clark, W. E. Le Gros (1942). *Physiol. Rev.* **22**:205.

Clark, W. E. Le Gros, and G. G. Penman (1934). *Proc. Roy. Soc. Ser. B.* **114**:291.

Clark, W. E. Le Gros, and S. Sunderland (1939). *J. Anat.* **73**(3):563.

Colonnier, M. (1966). In: *Brain and Conscious Experience*, (J. C. Eccles, ed.), Springer, New York, pp. 1–23.

Colonnier, M. (1968). *Brain Res.* **9**:268.

Colonnier, M., and R. W. Guillery (1964). *Z. Zellforsch. Mikr. Anat.* **62**:333.

Colvin, S., and Burford, C. C. (1909). *Psych. Monogr.* **11**:1.

Conel, J. LeRoy (1939–1959). *Postnatal Development of the Human Cerebral Cortex*, Vols. 1–6, Cambridge.

Cords, R. (1926). *Graefe's Arch. f. Ophthalm.* **117**(1):58.

Cragg, B. G. (1962). *Exper. Neurol.* **5**(5):406.

Creutzfeldt, O., and H. Akimoto (1958). *Arch. f. Psychiat.* **196**(5):520.

Creutzfeldt, O., G. Baumgartner, and R. Jung (1956). *Electroenceph. Clin. Neurophysiol.* **8**:163.

Crinis, M. de (1933). *J. Psych. Neurol.* **45**(6):439.

Crosby, E. C., and J. W. Henderson (1948). *J. Comp. Neurol.* **88**:53.

Daniel, P. M., D. I. B. Kerr, K. M. Seneviratne, and D. Whitteridge (1962). *J. Physiol.* **159**(2):87P.

Daniel, P. M., and D. Whitteridge (1962). *J. Physiol.* **159**(2):203.

Davidenkov, S. N., and S. N. Dotsenko (1956). *Zh. Vyssh. Nervn. Deyat.* **4**:525.

Davydova, T. V., and L. N. D'yachkova (1962). *Dokl. Akad. Nauk SSSR* **147**(5):1191.

Demirchoglyan, G. G. (1961). *Biofizika* **4**:499.

Detwiler, S. R. (1955). *Proc. Amer. Philos. Soc.* **99**(4):224.

Dodt, E. (1956). *J. Neurophysiol.* **19**(4):301.

Dogel', A. S. (1892). *Izv. Tomsk. Univ.* **4**:214.

Dogel', A. S. (1895). *Arch. Mikr. Anat.* **44**:622.

Dolgo-Saburov, B. A. (1956). *The Neuron Theory—The Basis of Modern Ideas on Structure and Function of the Nervous System* [in Russian], Moscow.

Dolgo-Saburov, B. A., V. V. Astachova, V. M. Godinov, A. S. Gusev, N. N. Zlatitskaya, I. F. Konkin, I. D. Lev, and Z. U. Pervushin (1958). Abstracts of Proceedings of the 6th All-Union Congress of Anatomists, Histologists, and Embryologists [in Russian], Khar'kov.

Doty, R. W. (1958). *J. Neurophysiol.* **21**:437.

Doty, R. W. (1961). In: *The Visual System, Neurophysiology and Psychophysics*. Berlin, pp. 228–247.

Dowling, J. E. (1968). *Proc. Roy. Soc. B* **170**:205.

Dowling, J. E., and B. B. Boycott (1966). *Proc. Roy. Soc. B* **166**:80.

Dowling, J. E., and W. M. Cowan (1966). *Z. Zellforsch. Mikr. Anat.* **71**(1):14.

Dusser de Barenne, J. G., and W. S. McCulloch (1938). *J. Neurophysiol.* **1**(1):69.

Dzugaeva, S. B. (1949). "Macroscopic investigation of certain association, commissural, and optico-thalamo-cortical pathways in the human brain." Doctoral dissertation, Moscow.

Dzugaeva, S. B. (1958). *Zh. Vyssh. Nervn. Deyat.* **6**:942.

Eccles, J. C. (1959). *The Physiology of Nerve Cells* [Russian translation], Moscow (Baltimore, Johns Hopkins Press, 1957, 270 pp.).

Eccles, J. C. (1961). *Ergebn. Physiol.* **51**:229.

Eccles, J. C. (1964). *The Physiology of Synapses*, New York.

Economo, C. von, and G. N. Koskinas (1925). *Die Cytoarchitektonik der Hirnrinde des Erwachsenen Menschen*. Berlin.

Élinson, A. (1896). *On Vasomotor Nerves of the Retina* [in Russian], Kazan'.

Engelmann, T. W. (1885). *Pflüg. Arch. Ges. Physiol.* **35**:498.

Éntin, T. I. (1950). *Nauchn. Byull. Leningrad. Gos. Univ.* **26**:27.

Éntin, T. I. (1952). Abstracts of proceedings of a scientific conference of Leningrad State University [in Russian], Leningrad, pp. 59–64.

Éntin, T. I. (1954a). *Arkh. Anat.* (4):25.

Éntin, T. I. (1954b). *Nauchn. Byull. Leningrad. Gos. Univ.* p. 28.

Éntin, T. I. (1956). In: *Problems in Morphology of the Nervous System* [in Russian], Leningrad, pp. 59–64.

Éntin, T. I. (1959). *Trudy Leningrad. Obshch. Estestvo.* **70**(1):66.

Éntin, T. I. (1960). *Z. Mikr.-Anat. Forsch.* **66**(3):341.

Éntin, T. I. (1966). *Arkh. Anat., Gistol. Émbriol.* **50**(4):87.

Erlanger, J., and H. S. Gasser (1937). *Electrical Signs of Nervous Activity*. Philadelphia.

Estable, C. (1961). In: *Brain Mechanisms and Learning*. Symposium, Springfield, Ill., pp. 309–334.

Feigenberg, I. M. (1953). In: *Problems in Physiological Optics* [in Russian], No. 8, Moscow, pp. 230–237.

Fel'dman, N. G. (1951). *Ontogenesis and Histopathology of the Retina. Experimental Changes in its Neural Elements* [in Russian], Moscow.

Fessard, A. (1958). In: *International Conference on Electroencephalography and Higher Nervous Activity*, Moscow. In: *Electroenceph. Clin. Neurophysid., Suppl.* 13 (H. H. Jasper and G. D. Smirnov, eds.), publ. 1960.

Figurina, I. I. (1965). *Dokl. Akad. Nauk SSSR* **161**(1):248.

Filimonov, I. N. (1928). *J. Psychol. Neurol.* **36**:22.

Filimonov, I. N. (1932). *J. Psychol. Neurol.* **44**:1.

Filimonov, I. N. (1933). *J. Psychol. Neurol.* **45**:69.

Filimonov, I. N. (1949). *Comparative Anatomy of the Mammalian Cerebral Cortex* [in Russian], Moscow.

Filimonov, I. N. (1951). *Klin. Med.* (6):5.

Filimonov, I. N. (1957). In: *Textbook of Neurology in Several Volumes* [in Russian], Vol. 1, Part 2, Moscow, pp. 20–29.

Foerster, O. (1928). *J. Psychol. Neurol.* **39**:4.

Foerster, O. (1936). In: *Handbuch der Neurologie*, Vol. 6 (O. Bumke and O. Foerster, eds.), pp. 1–357.

Fomin, V. A. (1967). In: *The Organization of Interneuronal Connections* [in Russian], Moscow, p. 113.

Forel, M. (1887). *Arch. f. Psych.* **18**:162.

Fox, C. A., and J. W. Barnard (1957). *J. Anat.* **91**(3):299.

French, J. D., R. Hernández-Peón, and R. B. Livingston (1955). *J. Neurophysiol.* **18**:74.

Frolov, Yu. P. (1918). *Trudy Petrograd. Obshch. Estestvo.* **49**(1):3.

Galambos, R. (1956). *J. Neurophysiol.* **19**:424.

Garey, L. J., and T. P. S. Powell (1968). *J. Anat.* **102**(2):189.

Geier, T. A. (1904). "Data on the shape and development of protoplasmic processes of nerve cells of the spinal cord." Dissertation, Moscow.

Gershtein, L. M. (1958). *Histochemical Methods in Normal and Pathological Morphology* [in Russia] Moscow, pp. 81–95.

Gershuni, G. V. (1960). Abstracts of Proceedings of the 3rd Conference on Electrophysiology of the Nervous System [in Russian], Moscow, pp. 107–108.

Gerver, A. V. (1899). "The brain centers for movements of the eyes." Dissertation, St. Petersburg.

Gerver, A. V. (1937). *Nevropat. i Psikhiat.* **6**(2):21.

Gibson, W. C. (1937). *Arch. Neurol. Psych.* **38**(6):1145.

Glees, P. (1941). *J. Anat.* **75**(4):434.

Glees, P. (1942). *J. Anat.* **76**(3):313.

Glees, P. (1946). *J. Neuropath. Exper. Neurol.* **5**:54.

Glees, P. (1958). *Verhandl. der Anat. Gesellsch. auf der 55 Versammlung im Frankfurt am Main*, pp. 60–69.

Glees, P., and W. E. Le Gros Clark (1941). *J. Anat.* **75**(3):295.

Glees, P., T. A. Marsland, C. Pearson, and A. C. Smith (1958). *J. Physiol.* **143**:3P.

Glezer, I. I. (1958). "Quantitative characteristics of some stages of development of the frontal cortex in human postnatal ontogenesis." Author's abstract of dissertation, Moscow.

Glezer, I. I. (1966). Abstracts of Proceedings of the 3rd All-Union Conference on Electron Microscopy [in Russian], Leningrad.

Glezer, V. D. (1966). *The Mechanisms of Identification of Visual Images.* Nauka, Moscow.

Globus, A., and A. B. Scheibel (1967). *Exper. Neurol.* **19**(3):331.

Granit, R. (1956). *Receptors and Sensory Perception,* New Haven.

Grashchenkov, N. I. (1948). *Interneuronal Connections—Synapses and Their Role in Physiology and Pathology* [in Russian], Minsk.

Gray, E. G. (1959). *J. Anat.* **93**:420.

Gray, E. G. (1961). In: *Electron Microscopy in Anatomy,* pp. 54–73.

Gray, E. G. (1962). *Nature* **193**:82.

Gray, E. G. (1963). *J. Anat. (Lond.)* **97**(1):101.

Grether, W. E. (1939). *Comp. Psych. Monogr.* **15**(4):38.

Grundfest, H. (1958). *Electroenceph. Clin. Neurophysiol.* Suppl. **10**:22.

Guillery, R. W. (1967a). *Am. J. Anat.* **120**(3):583.

Guillery, R. W. (1967b). *J. Comp. Neurol.* **130**(3):197.

Gurevich, M. O., G. Kh. Bykhovskaya, and Ya. Uranovskii (1929). In: *Higher Nervous Activity* [in Russian], No. 1, pp. 3–38.

Hamlyn, L. H. (1962). *J. Anat. (London)* **96**(1):112.

Hamlyn, L. H. (1963). *J. Anat. (London)* **97**(2):189.

Hartridge, H. (1952). *Recent Advances in the Physiology of Vision.* [Russian translation], Moscow.

Haschke, W. (1963). *J. Hirnforsch.* **6**(3):165.

Hassler, R. (1966). In: *Evolution of the Forebrain,* Stuttgart, Georg Thieme Verlag, pp. 419–434.

Hayhow, W. R. (1958). *J. Comp. Neurol.* **110**(1):1.

Hayhow, W. R. (1959). *Acta Anat.* **37**(4):281.

Hayhow, W. R. (1966). *J. Comp. Neurol.* **126**(4):653.

Hayhow, W. R., A. Sefton, and C. Webb (1962). *J. Comp. Neurol.* **118**(3):295.

Helmholtz, H. (1896). *Handbuch der Physiologischen Optik.*

Henschen, S. E. (1890). *Klinische und Anatomische Beiträge zur Pathologie des Gehirns,* Vol. 1, Uppsala.

Henschen, S. E. (1892). *Klinische und Anatomische Beiträge zur Pathologie des Gehirns,* Vol. 2.

Henschen, S. E. (1894–1896). *Klinische und Anatomische Beiträge zur Pathologie des Gehirns,* Vol. 3.

Henschen, S. E. (1923). *Z. Ges. Neurol. Psychiat.* **87**:505.

Henschen, S. E. (1925). *Trabajos del Labor. de Invest. Biol. de la Univ. de Madrid.* **23**:217.

Henschen, S. E. (1926). *Arch. Ophthalm.* **117**(3):403.

Henschen, S. E. (1930). *Klinische und Anatomische Beiträge zur Pathologie des Gehirns,* Vol. 8. Lichtsinn und Farbensinnzellen in Gehirn, Stockholm.

Hoff, E. C. (1932). *Proc. Roy. Soc. B* **111**:175.

Holubar, J., B. Hanke, and V. Malik (1967). *Exper. Neurol.* **19**(3):257.

Honrubia, F. M., and J. H. Elliot (1968). *Arch. Ophthalm.* **80**(1):98.

Hubel, D. H., and T. N. Wiesel (1963). *J. Physiol.* **165**:559.

Hubel, D. H., and T. N. Wiesel (1965). *J. Neurophysiol.* **28**(2):229.

Hubel, D. H., and T. N. Wiesel (1966). *J. Neurophysiol.* **29**(6):1115.

Iontov, A. S., and V. Yu. Ermolaeva (1961). Abstracts of proceedings of a conference on the physiology of analyzers [in Russian], Leningrad, pp. 35–36.

Ivanitskii, A. M. (1958). *Byull. Éksper. Biol. i Med.* (10):87.

Ivanov, I. I. (1901). *Voprosy Nervno-Psikh. Med.* **6**(1):56.

Jampel, R. S. (1960). *J. Comp. Neurol.* **115**(3):371.

Jasper, H., C. A. Marsan, and J. Stoll (1952). *Arch. Neurol. Psych.* **67**(2):155.

Jung, R. (1958). In: *Reticular Formation of the Brain*, (H. Jasper, ed.), Boston, pp. 423–434.

Jung, R. (1961). In: *Neurophysiologie und Psychophysik des Visuellensystems* (*Symposium, Freiburg, 1960*), Berlin, pp. 410–434.

Kaplan, L. L. (1952). *Arkh. Anat.* (2):18.

Kaplan, L. L. (1958). Abstracts of Proceedings of the 6th All-Union Congress of Anatomists, Histologists, and Embryologists [in Russian], Khar'kov, pp. 393–394.

Kappers, C. U. A., G. C. Huber, and E. C. Crosby (1936). *The Comparative Anatomy of the Nervous System of Vertebrates including Man*, Vol. 2, New York, pp. 865–1845.

Khananashvili, M. M. (1960a). *Fiziol. Zh. SSSR* (2):156.

Khananashvili, M. M. (1960b). *Annual Report of the Institute of Experimental Medicine, AMN SSSR, for 1959* [in Russian], Leningrad, pp. 28–32.

Khananashvili, M. M. (1962). *Experimental Investigation of the Central Mechanisms of Visual Function,* [in Russian], Leningrad.

Kiernan, J. A. (1967). *J. Comp. Neurol.* **131**(3):405.

Kidd, M. (1962). *J. Anat.* **96**(2):179.

Klosovskii, B. N. (1939). "Mechanisms of vestibular nystagmus and its participation in cortical movements of the eyes." Doctoral dissertation.

Klosovskii, B. N. (1958). *Vopr. Neirokhir.* **4**:3.

Koelliker, A. (1896). *Handbuch der Gewebelehre des Menschen*, Vol. 2, Leipzig.

Kolmer, W. (1936). In: *Handbuch der Mikroskopischen Anatomie des Menschen*, Vol. 2, Part 2, (Auge), Berlin, pp. 295–466.

Kononova, E. P. (1926). *Anatomy and Physiology of the Occipital Lobes on the Basis of Clinical, Pathologico-anatomical, and Experimental Data* [in Russian], Moscow.

Kononova, E. P. (1935). *Transactions of the Brain Institute* [in Russian], Vol. 1, Moscow, pp. 49–118.

Kononova, E. P. (1938). *Transactions of the Brain Institute*, Vol. 3–4, Moscow, pp. 213–274.

Kononova, E. P. (1940). *Transactions of the Brain Institute*, Vol. 5, Moscow, pp. 73–121.

Kononova, E. P. (1962). *The Frontal Region of the Brain* [in Russian], Leningrad, Medgiz.

Kositsyn, N. S. (1962). *Dokl. Akad. Nauk SSSR* **147**(2):77.

Kostyuk, P. G. (1963). Proceedings of the 4th All-Union Electrophysiological Conference [in Russian], Rostov-on-Don, p. 203.

Kravkov, S. V. (1951). *Color Vision* [in Russian], Moscow.

Krieg, W. J. S. (1947). *J. Comp. Neurol.* **86**(3):267.

Krol', V. M. (1968). "Organization of multichannel specific afferent projections in the cat visual cortex." Author's abstract of dissertation, Moscow.

Krushinskii, L. V. (1967). *Zh. Vyssh. Nervn. Deyat.* **17**(5):880.

Kukuev, L. A. (1953). *Zh. Vyssh. Nervn. Deyat.* **5**:765.

Kukuev, L. A. (1955). *Zh. Nevropat. i Psikhiat.* **12**:890.

Kupfer, C. (1962). *Am. J. Ophthalmol.* **54**(4):597.

Kusama, T., K. Otani, and E. Kawana (1966). *Progr. Brain Res.* **21A**:292.

Lashley, K. S. (1933). *Physiol. Rev.* **13**:1.

Lashley, K. S. (1934a). *J. Comp. Neurol.* **59**:341.

Lashley, K. S. (1934b). *J. Comp. Neurol.* **60**(1):57.

Lashley, K. S. (1941). *J. Comp. Neurol.* **75**(1):67.

Larionov, V. E. (1907). *Proceedings of the Second Congress of Russian Psychiatrists* [in Russian], Kiev, pp. 271–298.

Laties, A. M., and J. M. Sprague (1966). *J. Comp. Neurol.* **127**(1):35.

Lavdovskii, M. D. (1879–1880). *Proceedings of the 4th Congress of Russian Naturalists and Physicians* [in Russian], St. Petersburg.

Lavdosvskii, M. D. (1889). *Zapiski Akad. Nauk (SPb).* **61**:38.

Lavdovskii, M. D. (1902). *Russk. Vrach.* **12**:449.

Lavdovskii, M. D., and F. V. Ovsyannikov (1887–1888). *Fundamentals of the Study of Microscopic Anatomy of Man and Animals* [in Russian], Vols. 1–2, St. Petersburg.

Lavrent'ev, B. I., and E. K. Plechkova (1955). In: *Textbook of Neurology in Several Volumes* [in Russian], Vol. 1, Part 1, Moscow, pp. 89–218.

Lavrov, K. A. (1949). *Proceedings of a Histological Conference* [in Russian], Moscow, p. 140.

Leboucq, G. (1909). *Arch. f. Anat. Microsk.* **10**:555.

Lennox, M. A. (1956). *J. Neurophysiol.* **19**(3):271.

Leonova, O. V. (1896). *Arch. Psych. u. Nervenkrankh.* **28**:53.

Leontovich, T. A. (1952). "The neuronal structure of the striopallidum of certain mammals." Author's abstract of dissertation, Moscow.

Leontovich, T. A. (1954). *Zh. Nevropat. i. Psikhiat.* **2**:168.

Leontovich, T. A. (1958). *Arkh. Anat.* (2):17.

Leontovich, T. A. (1959a). In: *Development of the Central Nervous System* [in Russian], Moscow, pp. 185–204.

Leontovich, T. A. (1959b). In: *Structure and Function of the Reticular Formation and Its Place in the System of Analyzers* [in Russian], Moscow, pp. 91–126.

Leontovich, T. A. (1968a). In: *Structure and Function of the Archipaleocortex*, Vol. 5 in the series "Discussions at Gagra." Nauka, Moscow, pp. 56–87.

Leontovich, T. A. (1968b). *Uspekhii Sovr. Biol.* **65**:34.

Leontovich, T. A. (1969). *J. f. Hirnforsch.* In press.

Leontovich, T. A., and G. P. Zhukova (1963). *J. Comp. Neurol.* **121**(3):347.

Leushina, L. I. (1961). Abstracts of Proceedings of a Conference on the Physiology of Analyzers [in Russian], Leningrad, p. 39.

Leushina, L. I. (1963). In: *Electrophysiology of the Nervous System.* Proceedings of the 4th All-Union Electrophysiological Conference [in Russian], Rostov-on-Don, pp. 229–230.

Levin, G. Z. (1953). "Comparative embryology of the visual and auditory centers of the diencephalon and mesencephalon in reptiles and mammals." Doctoral dissertation, Leningrad.

Livanov, M. N., and V. M. Anan'ev (1955). *Fiziol. Zh. SSSR* (4):461.

Livanov, M. N., and V. M. Anan'ev (1960). *Electroencephaloscopy* [in Russian], Moscow.

Locke, S. (1960). *J. Comp. Neurol.* **115**(2):155.

Lomonosov, M. V. (1756). *Collected Works* [in Russian], Vol. 4, St. Petersburg (1898), pp. 392–424.

Loos, H. van der. (1959). *International Meeting of Neurobiology, Amsterdam*, p. 41.

Loos, H. van der. (1964). *Progr. Brain Res.* **6**:43.

Lorente de Nó, R. (1922). *Trabajos del Lab. de Invest. Biol. de la Univ. de Madrid.* **20**:1.

Lorente de Nó, R. (1933). *J. Psychol. Neurol.* **45**(6):381.

Lorente de Nó, R. (1934). *J. Psychol. Neurol.* **46**(2–3):113.

Lorente de Nó, R. (1938). In: J. F. Fulton, *Physiology of the Nervous System*, Chap. 14, Oxford.

Luria, A. R. (1966). *Higher Cortical Function in Man.* Translated by B. Haigh, New York, Consultants Bureau, 513 pp.

Luria, A. R., C. Pribram, and E. D. Khomskaya (1966). In: *The Frontal Lobes and Regulation of Psychological Processes* [in Russian], Moscow University Press, Moscow, pp. 554–575.

Lyubimov, N. N. (1963). In: *Electrophysiology of the Nervous System.* Proceedings of the 4th All-Union Electrophysiological Conference [in Russian], Rostov-on-Don p. 242.

Lyubimov, N. N. (1964). *Zh. Vyssh. Nervn. Deyat.* **14**(2):287.

Maiorov, V. N. (1960). *Trudy. Leningrad. Obshch. Estestvo.* **21**(1):69.

Markova, A. Ya. (1961). *Vopr. Antropol.* **6**:44.

Marks, W. B. (1965). In: *Colour Vision. Physiology and Experimental Psychology*, Churchill, London, pp. 208–216.

Marks, W. B., W. H. Dobelle, and E. F. MacNichol, Jr. (1964). *Science* **143**:1181.

Matthews, M. R. (1964). *J. Anat. (London)* **98**(2):255–263.

Menner, E. (1929). *Z. Vergl. Physiol.* **8**(5):761.

Mering, T. A. (1951). "Conditioned reflexes in dogs after removal of the nuclear zone of the auditory analyzer." Dissertation, Moscow.

Mering, T. A. (1954). *Zh. Vyssh. Nervn. Deyat.* **3**:448.

Mering, T. A. (1962). In: *Structure and Function of the Nervous System* [in Russian], Moscow, pp. 178–185.

Meshcherskii, R. M. (1963). Abstracts of Proceedings of an International Conference to Commemorate the Centenery of Publication of I. M. Sechenov's Book, *Reflexes of the Brain*, Moscow, pp. 39–41. (In: *Brain Reflexes Progress in Brain Research*, Vol. 22. E. A. Asratyan [Editor] Amsterdam Elsevier, 1968, pp. 312–339.)

Mettler, F. A. (1935). *J. Comp. Neurol.* **61**(2):221.

Meyer-Oehme, D. (1957). *Zeitschrift f. Tierpsychol.* **14**:473.

Meynert, T. (1867). *Vierteljahrschr. f. Psychiat.*, Leipzig, pp. 77–93.

Meynert, T. (1869). *Vierteljahrschr. f. Psychiat.*, Leipzig, pp. 88–113.

Michael, C. R. (1968). *J. Neurophysiol.* **31**(2):268.

Minkowski, M. A. (1911). *Dtsch. Z. f. Nervenheilk.* **41**:109.

Minkowski, M. A. (1913). *Arbeiten aus dem Hirnanatomischen Inst. in Zürich.* **7**:255.

Minkowski, M. A. (1920a). *Schweiz. Arch. f. Neurol. Psych.* **6**:291.

Minkowski, M. A. (1920b). *Schweiz. Arch. f. Neurol. Psych.* **7**:268.

Mokhova, T. M., E. N. Popova, and S. A. Sarkisov (1960). In: *Structure and Function of the Nervous System.* Proceedings of a scientific conference [in Russian], Moscow, pp. 44–56.

Monakow, C. von (1885). *Arch. f. Psychiat.* **16**:151.

Monakow, C. von (1889). *Arch. f. Psychiat.* **20**:714.

Mountcastle, V. B. (1957). *J. Neurophysiol.* **20**(4):408.

Narikashvili, S. P., and D. V. Kadzhaya (1963). Abstracts of Proceedings of an International Conference to Celebrate the Centerary of Publication of I. M. Sechenov's book *Reflexes of the Brain.* Moscow, pp. 41–43. (In: *Brain Reflexes Progress in Brain Vol. 22.* E. A. Asratyan [ed.] Amsterdam, Elsevier, 1968, pp. 340–352.)

Nathan, P. W., and M. C. Smith (1955). *Brain* **78**(2):248.

Nauta, W. J. H., and V. M. Bucher (1954). *J. Comp. Neurol.* **100**(2): 257.

Novokhatskii, A. S. (1956). "Anatomical connections of the visual pathways with the hypothalamus." Author's abstract of dissertation, Khar'kov.

Novokhatskii, A. S. (1957). *Ophthalmol. J.* **2**:100.

Novokhatskii, A. S. (1964). *Vopr. Neirooftal'm.* **11–12**:59.

Obukhova, G. P. (1958). "Synaptic endings in the lateral geniculate body." Author's abstract of dissertation, Leningrad.

Obukhova, G. P. (1959). *Trudy Leningrad. Obshch. Estestvo.* **70**(1):63.

Obukhova, G. P. (1960). *Annual Report of the Institute of Experimental Medicine, Academy of Medical Sciences of the USSR, for* 1919 [in Russian], Leningrad, pp. 65–69.

Ogden, T. E. (1968). In: *Structure and Function of Inhibitory Neuronal Mechanisms*, Oxford, p. 89.

O'Leary, J. L. (1940). *J. Comp. Neurol.* **73**(3)405.

O'Leary, J. L. (1941). *J. Comp. Neurol.* **75**(1):131.

O'Leary, J. L., and G. H. Bishop (1938). *J. Comp. Neurol.* **68**:423.

Orbeli, L. A. (1908). "Conditioned reflexes from the eye in dogs." Doctoral dissertation, St. Petersburg.

Orbeli, L. A. (1913). *Vopr. Nauchn. Med.* **1**(5–6):513.

Orlov, O. Yu. (1965). *Byull. Mosk. Obshch. Ispytat. Prirody. Otdel. Biol.* **70**(6):163.

Orlov, O. Yu., and E. M. Maksimova (1968). "Problems in the evolution of mechanisms of color vision in vertebrates." Abstracts of Proceedings of the 5th Scientific Conference on Evolutionary Physiology in Memory of L. A. Orbeli [in Russian], Leningrad, p. 193.

Ostrovskii, M. A. (1962). "Descending influences on the retina in amphibians." Author's abstract of dissertation, Moscow.

Ozhigova, A. P. (1958). *Sov. Antropol.* **2**(4):37.

Ozhigova, A. P. (1960). "Architectonics of the occipital cortex in primates." Author's abstract of dissertation, Moscow.

Palay, S. L. (1958). *Exper. Cell Res. Suppl.* **5**:275.

Pavlov, I. P. (1927). *Lectures on the Operation of the Cerebral Hemispheres* [in Russian], Second Edition, Moscow; p. 372.

Pavlov, I. P. (1951). *Twenty Years Experience in Objective Study of Higher Nervous Activity (Behavior) of Animals. Conditioned Reflexes.* 7th ed., Moscow. *Pavlov's Wednesdays.* (1949). Vols. I, II, and III, Moscow, Academy of Sciences Press, USSR.

Pchelina, L. A. (1951). *Scientific Memoir*, Vol. 2, Moscow, pp. 203–209.

Penfield, W., and H. Jasper (1954). *Epilepsy and the Functional Anatomy of the Human Brain*, Boston.

Peters, A., and S. L. Palay (1966). *J. Anat. (London)* **100**(3):451.

Pigareva, Z. D. (1958). Abstracts of Proceedings of a Conference on the Physiology and Pathology of the Nervous System of Animals and Man [in Russian], Moscow, pp. 41–42.

Pigareva, Z. D., and N. N. Shilyagina (1960). *Proceedings of the 4th Scientific Conference on Age Morphology, Physiology, and Biochemistry* [in Russian], Moscow, pp. 99–105.

Pilipenko, V. I. (1961). *Zh. Vyssh. Nervn. Deyat.* **5**:884.

Pines, L. Ya., and I. E. Prigonikov (1936). In: *Problems in Morphology of the Cerebral Cortex* [in Russian], pp. 57–97.

Pines, L. Ya., and I. E. Prigonikov (1939). *Transactions of the V. M. Bekhterev Institute for Study of the Brain* [in Russian], Vol. 11, pp. 66–71.

Plechkova, E. K. (1961). *Reaction of the Nervous System of the Organism to Chronic Injury of a Peripheral Nerve* [in Russian], Moscow.

Poemnyi, F. A. (1940). "Relationship between the visual cortex and lateral geniculate body of mammals during phylogenesis." Dissertation, Moscow.

Polyak, S. (1927). *J. Comp. Neurol.* **44**(2):197.

Polyak, S. (1932). *The Main Afferent Fiber Systems of the Cerebral Cortex in Primates*, Berkeley, Calif.

Polyak, S. (1933). *J. Comp. Neurol.* **57**:541.

Polyak, S. (1941). *The Retina*, Chicago.

Polyak, S. (1957). *The Vertebrate Visual System*, Chicago.

Polyakov, G. I. (1937). *The Early and Middle Ontogenesis of the Human Cerebral Cortex* [in Russian], Moscow.

Polyakov, G. I. (1949). In: *Cytoarchitectonics of the Human Cerebral Cortex* [in Russian], Moscow, pp. 33–91.

Polyakov, G. I. (1951). *Proceedings of the 5th All-Union Congress of Anatomists, Histologists, and Embryologists* [in Russian], Leningrad, pp. 535–539.

Polyakov, G. I. (1953). *Arkh. Anat.* (5):48.

Polyakov, G. I. (1954). *Zh. Vyssh. Nervn. Deyat.* **1**:123.

Polyakov, G. I. (1955). *Arkh. Anat.* (2):15.

Polyakov, G. I. (1956). *Zh. Vyssh. Nervn. Deyat.* **3**:469.

Polyakov, G. I. (1959). *Vestn. Akad. Med. Nauk SSSR* **9**:27.

Polyakov, G. I. (1961a). *Zh. Nevropat. Psikhiat.* (1):3.

Polyakov, G. I. (1961b). *Zh. Nevropat. i. Psikhiat.* (2):271.

Polyakov, G. I. (1963). Abstracts of Proceedings of an International Conference to Commemorate the Centenary of Publication of I. M. Sechenov's book *Reflexes of the Brain*, Moscow, pp. 15–16. (In: *Brain Reflexes. Progress in Brain Research Vol. 22*, E. A. Asratyan [Editor] Amsterdam, Elsevier, 1968, pp. 98–106.)

Polyakov, G. I. (1965). *Principles of Neuronal Organization of the Brain* [in Russian], Moscow University Press, Moscow.

Polyakov, G. I., and S. A. Sarkisov (1949). In: *Cytoarchitectonics of the Human Cerebral Cortex* [in Russian], Chap. IV, Moscow.

Pomerat, C. M. (1952). *Texas Rep. Biol. Med.* **10**(4):885.

Popova, E. N. (1959a). *Dokl. Akad. Nauk SSSR* **125**(5):1130.

Popova, E. N. (1959b). *Arkh. Anat.* (6):11.

Popova, E. N. (1959c). *Proceedings of the 1st Scientific Conference of Junior Research Workers at Moscow Morphological Laboratories* [in Russian], Moscow.

Popova, E. N. (1968). *The Action of Certain Neurotropic Drugs on Brain Structures* [in Russian], Meditsina Press, Leningrad.

Popova, N. S. (1960a). *Zh. Vyssh. Nervn. Deyat.* (1):80.

Popova, N. S. (1960b). *Zh. Vyssh. Nervn. Deyat.* (5):764.

Popova, N. S. (1961). *Zh. Vyssh. Nervn. Deyat.* (4):690.

Portugalov, V. V. (1958). *Zh. Nevropat. i. Psikhiat.* (6):641.

Portugalov, V. V., M. M. Busnyuk, and L. M. Gershtein (1963). *Discussions at Gagra* [in Russian], Vol. 4, Tbilisi, pp. 87–110.

Portugalov, V. V., I. V. Tsvetkova, and V. A. Yakovlev (1959). *Tsitologiya* (4):422.

Preobrazhenskaya, N. S. (1939). "Postnatal ontogenesis of the occipital region in man." Dissertation, Moscow.

Preobrazhenskaya, N. S. (1948). *Transactions of the Brain Institute* [in Russian], Vol. 6, Moscow, pp. 44–76.

Preobrazhenskaya, N. S. (1952). *Zh. Nevropat. i. Psikhiat.* **4**:21.

Preobrazhenskaya, N. S. (1954). "Disturbance and recovery of visual functions after gunshot wounds of the occipital lobes of the brain." Author's abstract of dissertation, Moscow.

Preobrazhenskaya, N. S. (1955). Proceedings of the Second Scientific Conference on Age Morphology and Physiology [in Russian], Izd. APN, Moscow, pp. 47–55.

Preobrazhenskaya, N. S. (1962). In: *Structure and Function of the Nervous System* [in Russian], Moscow, pp. 295–305.

Preobrazhenskaya, N. S. (1966). *J. f. Hirnforschung* **8**(3):269.

Preobrazhenskaya, N. S., and I. N. Filimonov (1949). In: *Cytoarchitectonics of the Human Cerebral Cortex* [in Russian], Moscow, pp. 240–262.

Prigonikov, I. E. (1949). In: *Ontogenesis of the Human Brain* [in Russian], Leningrad, pp. 99–118.

Probst, M. (1902). *Arch. f. Psychiat.* **35**:22.

Purpura, D. P. (1958). In: *Reticular Formation of the Brain*, (H. Jasper, ed.), Boston, pp. 435–458.

Purpura, D. P., and H. Grundfest (1956). *J. Neurophysiol.* **19**:573.

Rabinovich, M. Ya. (1961). *Zh. Vyssh. Nervn. Deyat.* (3):463.

Rabinovich, M. Ya. (1964). "Electrical responses of individual layers of the cerebral cortex during conditioned reflex formation." Author's abstract of disseration, Moscow.

Ramon-Moliner, E. (1962). *J. Comp. Neurol.* **119**(2):211.

Ramon-Moliner, E., and W. J. H. Nauta (1956). *J. Comp. Neurol.* **126**(3):311.

Retzius, G. (1894). *Biologische Untersuchungen* **6**:29.

Rioch, D. (1929–1930). *J. Comp. Neurol.* **49**:1.

Robiner, I. S. (1957). *Arch. Anat.* (3):20.

Roginskii, G. Z. (1947–1948). *Scientific Memoirs of Leningrad University, No. 109, Series of Philosophical Sciences* [in Russian], Vol. 2, Leningrad, pp. 207–215.

Roitbak, A. I. (1956). *Discussions at Gagra* [in Russian], Vol. 2, Tbilisi, pp. 165–187.

Roitbak, A. I. (1963). Abstracts of Proceedings of an International Conference to Commemorate the Centenary of Publication of I. M. Sechenov's Book *Reflexes of the Brain*. Moscow, pp. 19–20. (In: *Brain Reflexes. Progress in Brain Research* Vol. 22, E. A. Asratyan [Editor] Amsterdam, Elsevier, 1968, pp. 123–137.)

Rönne, H. (1910). *Arch. f. Ophthalm.* **77**:1.

Rönne, H. (1913). *Arch. f. Ophthalm.* **85**:489.

Rose, J. E., and L. I. Malis (1955). *J. Comp. Neurol.* **125**(1):121.

Roskin, G. I., and M. E. Struve (1958). Abstracts of Proceedings of the 6th All-Union Congress of Anatomists, Histologists, and Embryologists [in Russian], Khar'kov.

Rossi, G. F., and A. Brodal (1956). *J. Anat. (London)* **90**(1):42.

Rubino, A., and A. Scoppa (1955). *Acta Neurol.* **10**(5):603.

Sarkisov, S. A. (1939). *Nevropat. i. Psikhiat.* **8**(2/3):11.

Sarkisov, S. A. (1948). *Some Aspects of the Structure of Neuronal Connections in the Cerebral Cortex* [in Russian], Moscow.

Sarkisov, S. A. (1956). Paper read at the 20th International Congress of Physiologists in Brussels [in Russian], Moscow.

Sarkisov, S. A. (1960). Proceedings of the International Meeting of Neurologists, 1959, Amsterdam, p. 81.

Sarkisov, S. A. (1964). *Outlines of the Structure and Function of the Brain* [in Russian], Moscow.

Sarkisov, S. A., and T. M. Mokhova (1958). *Zh. Nevropat. i. Psikhiat.* (8):907.

Savich, K. V., and V. A. Yakovlev (1957). *Vopr. Med. Khimii* **3**(2):121.

Scheibel, M. E., and A. B. Scheibel (1955a). *J. Comp. Neurol.* **102**(1):77.

Scheibel, M. E., and A. B. Scheibel (1955b). *J. Neurophysiol.* **18**:309.

Scheibel, M. E., and A. B. Scheibel (1958a). *Electroenceph. Clin. Neurophysiol. Suppl.* **10**:43.

Scheibel, M. E., and A. B. Scheibel (1958b). In: *Symposium: Reticular Formation of the Brain*, Boston, pp. 131–155.

Scheibel, M. E., and A. B. Scheibel (1968). *Communications in Behavioral Biology*, Part A, Vol. 1, pp. 231–265.

Scheibel, M., A. Scheibel, A. Mollica, and G. Moruzzi (1955). *J. Neurophys.* **18**:309.

Sechenov, I. M. (1901). In: *Selected Philosophical and Psychological Works* [in Russian], Moscow (1947), pp. 392–397.

Sepp, E. K. (1949). *History of Development of the Nervous System of Vertebrates from the Acrania to Man* [in Russian], Moscow.

Shapiro, B. I. (1957). *Data on Evolutionary Physiology* [in Russian], Vol. 2, Moscow, pp. 127–136.

Shenger-Krestovnikova, N. R. (1921). *Izvest. Petrograd. Nauchn. Inst. im. I. F. Lesgafta*, Vol. 3.

Shevchenko, Yu. G. (1938). *Nevrol. i. Psikh.* **7**(5):53.

Shibkova, S. A. (1956). In: *Problems in Morphology of the Nervous System* [in Russian], Leningrad.

Shibkova, S. A., and L. V. Koroleva (1964). *Arkh. Anat.* (2):36.

Shkol'nik-Yarros, E. G. (1950a). *Nevropat. i. Psikhiat.* **19**(1):51.

Shkol'nik-Yarros, E. G. (1950b). *Byull. Eksperim. Biol. i Med.* **30**(11):379.

Shkol'nik-Yarros, E. G. (1954). *Zh. Vyssh. Nervn. Deyat.* (2):289.

Shkol'nik-Yarros, E. G. (1955a). *Probl. Fiziol. Optiki* **11**:162.

Shkol'nik-Yarros, E. G. (1955b). Abstracts of Proceedings of a Conference on Interneuronal Connections [in Russian], Leningrad, pp. 23–24.

Shkol'nik-Yarros, E. G. (1955c). Abstracts of Proceedings of the 4th Conference on Physiological Optics [in Russian], Leningrad, pp. 125–126.

Shkol'nik-Yarros, E. G. (1956). *Problems in Morphology of the Nervous System* [in Russian], Leningrad, pp. 51–58.

Shkol'nik-Yarros, E. G. (1958a). *Zh. Vyssh. Nervn. Deyat.* (1):123.

Shkol'nik-Yarros, E. G. (1958b). *Probl. Fiziol. Optiki* (12):429.

Shkol'nik-Yarros, E. G. (1958c). Abstracts of Proceedings of the 6th All-Union Congress of Anatomists, Histologists and Embryologists [in Russian], Khar'kov, pp. 437–438.

Shkol'nik-Yarros, E. G. (1959a). In: *Structure and Function of the Reticular Formation and Its Place in the System of Analyzers* [in Russian], Moscow, pp. 317–319.

Shkol'nik-Yarros, E. G. (1959b). In: *Development of the Central Nervous System* [in Russian], Moscow, pp. 169–184.

Shkol'nik-Yarros, E. G. (1960). *Arkh. Anat.* (2):24.

Shkol'nik-Yarros, E. G. (1961a). *Zh. Vyssh. Nervn. Deyat.* (4):680.

Shkol'nik-Yarros, E. G. (1961b). "Neurons of the visual analyzer. Cortex and lateral geniculate body. Neurons and interneuronal connections in some mammals." Dissertation, Moscow.

Shkol'-nik-Yarros, E. G. (1961c). Abstracts of Proceedings of a Conference on the Physiology of Analyzers [in Russian], Leningrad, pp. 70–71.

Shkol'nik-Yarros, E. G. (1962). *Arkh. Anat.* (42):12. (*Fed. Proc. Transl. Suppl.* **22**: T389–T400, 1963.)

Shkol'nik-Yarros, E. G. (1963). *Discussions at Gagra* [in Russian], Vol. 4, Tbilisi, pp. 35–58.
Shkol'nik-Yarros, E. G. (1965). *Zh. Vyssh. Nervn. Deyat.* **15**(6):1063.
Shkol'nik-Yarros, E. G. (1968). *Arkh. Anat., Gistol., i Embriol.* **52**(11):35.
Sholl, D. A. (1953). *J. Anatomy* **87**(4):387–406.
Sholl, D. A. (1955). *J. Anatomy* **89**(1):33–46.
Sholl, D. A. (1956). *The Organization of the Cerebral Cortex.* London.
Shumilina, A. I. (1949). In: *Problems of Higher Neuron Activity.* Moscow, pp. 628–652, 653–673.
Shvarts, L. A. (1950). In: *Problems in the Physiology and Pathology of Vision* [in Russian], Moscow, pp. 61–65.
Sikharulidze, N. I. (1962). "The receptive functions of central area 17 and peripheral areas 18 and 19 of the visual cortex." Author's abstract of dissertation, Tbilisi.
Silva, P. S. (1956). *J. Comp. Neurol.* **106**(2):463.
Sjöstrand, F. S. (1958). *Ergebn. Biol.* **21**:128.
Skrebitskii, V. G. (1960). *Fiziol. Zh. SSSR* (12):1429.
Skrebitskii, V. G., and E. G. Shkol'nik-Yarros (1964). *Zh. Vyssh. Nervn. Deyat.* **14**:277. (*Fed. Proc. Transl. Suppl.* **24**: T437–T442, 1965.)
Skrebitskii, V. G., and E. G. Shkol'nik-Yarros (1967). In: *The Visual and Auditory Analyzers.* Proceedings of a Symposium [in Russian], Moscow, pp. 178–181.
Skrebitskii, V. G., and L. L. Voronin (1965). *Dokl. Akad. Nauk SSSR* **160**(4):972.
Smith, E. M. (1912). *Brit. J. Psych.* Vol. 2.
Smythies, J. R., and O. R. Inman (1960). *J. Anat.* (*London*) **94**(2):241.
Snesarev, P. E. (1950). *Theoretical Basis of the Pathological Anatomy of Mental Diseases* [in Russian], Moscow.
Snyakin, P. G. (1948). *The Functional Mobility of the Retina* [in Russian], Moscow.
Snyakin, P. G., A. P. Anisimova, A. I. Esakov, N. S. Zaiko, L. M. Kurilova, and N. A. Suchovskaya. (1961). Abstracts of proceedings of a conference on the physiology of analyzers [in Russian], Leningrad, pp. 63–65.
Sokolov, E. N. (1958). *Perception and Conditioned Reflex* [in Russian], Moscow.
Solnitzky, O., and P. J. Harman (1946). *J. Comp. Neurol.* **85**:313.
Sperry, R. W., N. Miner, and R. E. Myers (1955). *J. Comp. and Physiol. Psych.* **48**(1):50.
Sprague, J. M. (1966). In: *The Thalamus*, Columbia University Press, New York, pp. 391–417.
Stankevich, I. A. (1938). *Transactions of the Brain Institute* [in Russian], Vol. 3/4, Moscow, pp. 107–154.
Stankevich, I. A. (1949). In: *Cytoarchitectonics of the Human Cerebral Cortex* [in Russian], Moscow, pp. 263–272.
Stefanovskaya, M. (1897). *Soc. Biol., Séanse du 13 Novembre.*
Stefanovskaya, M. (1898). *Bull. Soc. Sci.* Bruxelles.
Stefanovskaya, M. (1900). *J. Neurol.* (*Bruxelles*), March 20, 6.
Stefanovskaya, M. (1901). *Trav. de l'Inst. Solvay* Vol. 1.
Stefanovskaya, M. (1906). *J. Neurol.* (*Bruxelles*), p. 313.
Sukhanov, S. A. (1896). *Vopr. Filosof. i Psikhol.* Vol. 34.
Sukhanov, S. A. (1898). *La Cellule* **14**(2):387.
Sukhanov, S. A. (1899). "Data on the beaded appearance of protoplasmic processes of nerve cells in the cerebral cortex." Dissertation, Moscow.
Sukhanov, S. A. (1903). *Le Nevraxe* **4**:224.
Sukhanov, S. A., T. A. Geier, and M. O. Gurevich (1904). *Le Nevraxe* **6**:119.

Svanidze, I. K. (1960). Abstracts of Proceedings of the First Conference on Problems in Cytochemistry and Histochemistry [in Russian], Moscow, pp. 95–96.

Svanidze, I. K. (1963). *Arkh. Anat.* (2):18.

Svanidze, I. K. (1964). *Dokl. Akad. Nauk SSSR* **158**(3):743.

Svetukhina, V. M. (1959). In: *Development of the Central Nervous System* [in Russian], Moscow, pp. 115–138.

Szentágothai, J. (1943). *Arch. f. Psychiat.* **116**(4):721.

Szentágothai, J. (1958). *Acta Morph. Acad. Sci. Hung.* **8**(3):297.

Szentágothai, J. (1960). Abstracts of Proceedings of a Conference on Structure and Function of the Nervous System [in Russian], Moscow, p. 67.

Szentágothai, J. (1963a). Abstracts of Proceedings of an International Conference to Commemorate the Centenary of Publication of I. M. Sechenov's Book *Reflexes of the Brain* [in Russian], Moscow, pp. 22–23. (In: *Brain Reflexes. Progress in Brain Research* Vol. 2, E. A. Asratyan [Editor] Amsterdam, Elsevier, 1968, pp. 148–160.)

Szentágothai, J. (1963b). *Acta Anat.* **55**:166.

Szentágothai, J. (1965). In: *Modern Trends in Neuromorphology*, Budapest, pp. 251–265.

Szentágothai, J. (1967). In: *Recent Development of Neurobiology in Hungary*, Vol. 1, Budapest, pp. 9–46.

Szentágothai, J. (1968). In: *Structure and Function of Inhibitory Neuronal Mechanisms*, Oxford, p. 15.

Szentágothai, J., B. Flerkó, B. Mess, and B. Halász (1962). *Hypothalamic Control of the Anterior Pituitary*, Budapest.

Szentágothai, J., J. Hamori, and T. Tömböl (1966). *Exper. Brain Res.* **2**(4):283.

Taboada, R. P. (1927–1928). *Trab. Lab. Invest. Biol. Univ. Madrid* **25**:319.

Tello, F. (1904). *Trab. Lab. Invest. Biol. Univ. Madrid* **3**:36.

Thuma, B. D. (1928). *J. Comp. Neurol.* **46**:173.

Tikh, N. A. (1947). "The communal life of monkeys and means of their communication in the light of the problem of anthropogenesis." Doctoral dissertation [in Russian].

Tikh, N. A. (1949). *Advances in Medicine. Higher Nervous Activity* [in Russian], Vol. 14, pp. 48–53.

Tolgskaya, M. S. (1954). *Byull. Éksperim. Biol. i Med.* (12):53.

Tolgskaya, M. S. (1957). *Byull. Éksperim. Biol. i Med.* (1):104.

Troitskaya, S. A. (1954). *Arkh. Anat.* (1):15.

Tron, E. Zh. (1955). *Diseases of the Optic Pathway* [in Russian], Leningrad.

Tsinda, N. I. (1959). In: *Development of the Central Nervous System* [in Russian], Moscow.

Tsinda, N. I. (1960). "Development of the limbic region of the human brain after birth." Author's abstract of dissertation, Moscow.

Uchizono, K. (1965). *Nature* **207**:642.

Utina, I. A. (1960). *Biofizika* **5**(5):626.

Valkenburg, C. J. van (1913). *Brain* **36**:119.

De Valois, R. L. (1960). In: *Mechanisms of Color Discrimination* (Proceedings of the International Symposium, 1958), pp. 111–114.

De Valois, R. L., R. J. Smith, S. T. Kitai, and A. J. Karoly (1958). *Science* **127**:238.

De Valois, R. L., and A. E. Jones (1961). In: *The Visual System. Neurophysiology and Psychophysics.* (*Symposium*, 1960), Berlin, pp. 178–191.

Valverde, F. (1967). *Exper. Brain Res.* **3**:337.

Vastola, E. F. (1961). *J. Neurophysiol.* **24**(5):469.

Vatsuro, E. G. (1948). *Trudy Fiziol. Lab. im. I. P. Pavlova* **14**:192.

Veize, L. G., and G. M. Frank (1960). *Biofizika* (1):34.

Viktorov, I. V. (1965). In: *Structure and Function of the Nervous System* [in Russian], Moscow, pp. 38–41.

Viktorov, I. V. (1968). *Arkh. Anat.* **54**(2):45.

Vinnikov, Ya. A. (1947). *The Vertebrate Retina* [in Russian], Moscow.

Vinnikov, Ya. A. (1962). In: *Structure and Functions of the Nervous System.* (S. A. Sarkisov, ed.) [in Russian], Moscow, p. 42.

Vinnikov, Ya. A. (1963). Abstracts of Proceedings of an International Conference to Commemorate the Centenery of publication of I. M. Sechenov's book *Reflexes of the Brain* [in Russian], Moscow, pp. 48–50. (In: *Brain Reflexes, Progress in Brain Research* Vol. 22, E. A. Asratyan [Editor] Amsterdam, Elsevier, 1968, pp. 518–526.)

Vogt, C., and O. Vogt (1919). *J. Psych. Neurol.* **25**(1):279.

Voitonis, N. Yu. (1949). *Prehistory of the Intellect* [in Russian], Moscow.

Voronin, V. V., and M. R. Kuparadze (1958). Abstracts of Proceedings of the 6th All-Union Congress of Anatomists, Histologists, and Embryologists [in Russian], Khar'kov, pp. 376–377.

Walberg, F., and A. Brodal (1953). *Brain* **76**(3):491.

Walls, G. L. (1942). *The Vertebrate Eye and its Adaptive Radiation*, Michigan.

Walls, G. L. (1953). *The Lateral Geniculate Nucleus and Visual Histophysiology*, Univ. Calif. Press.

Weber, A. (1945). *Schweiz. Med. Wschr.* **75**:631.

Winkler, C., and A. Potter (1911). *An Anatomical Guide to Experimental Researches on the Rabbit's Brain*, Amsterdam.

Wilson, M. E., and B. G. Cragg (1967). *J. Anat.* (*London*) **101**:677.

Wolter, J., and L. Liss (1956). *Arch. f. Ophthalm.* **58**:1.

Young, J. Z. (1958). *Electroenceph. Clin. Neurophysiol. Suppl.* **10**:9.

Young, T. (1802). "Lecture on the theory of light and colours." *Phil. Trans. Roy. Soc.* Vol. 21.

Yuvchenko, A. I. (1954). "Synapses in the occipital cortex of the dog." Author's abstract of dissertation, Minsk.

Zambrhitskii, I. A. (1954). "Cytoarchitectonics and neuronal structure of the superior limbic region in mammals." Author's abstract of dissertation, Moscow.

Zambrzhitskii, I. A. (1959). In- *Development of the Central Nervous System* [in Russian], Moscow.

Zavarzin, A. A. (1950). *Selected works, Vol. 3. Essays on the Evolutionary Histology of the Nervous System* [in Russian], Moscow.

Zhukova, G. P. (1950). "Neuronal structure of the motor cortex of some mammals." Dissertation, Moscow.

Zhukova, G. P. (1953). *Arkh. Anat.* **30**(1):32.

Zhukova, G. P. (1959). In: *Structure and Function of the Reticular Formation and Its Place in the System of Analyzers* [in Russian], Moscow, p. 71.

Zhukova, G. P. (1960). *Arkh. Anat.* (12):72.

Zhukova, G. P. (1961). *Arkh. Anat.* (7):58.

Zhukova, G. P. (1964). *Zh. Vyssh. Nervn. Deyat.* **14**(4):714.

Zhukova, G. P. (1965). *Arkh. Anat.* **49**(7):65.

Zhukova, G. P. (1966). *Zh. Nevropat. i. Psikhiat.* **46**(8):1195.

Zhukova, G. P., and T. A. Leontovich (1964). *Zh. Vyssh. Nervn. Deyat.* (1):122.

Zurabashvili, A. D. (1947). *Synapses. Introduction to Synapse Artchitectonics* [in Russian], Tbilisi.

Zurabashvili, A. D. (1951). *Synapses and Reversible Changes in Nerve Cells* [in Russian], Moscow.

Zvorykin, V. P. (1954). "Cytoarchitectonics of the medial geniculate body in a comparative-anatomical series of mammals and its origin." Author's abstract of dissertation, Moscow.

Zvorykin, V. P. (1960). *Arkh. Anat.* (4):22.

Zvorykin, V. P., and E. G. Shkol'nik-Yarros (1953). *Arkh. Anat.* (5):43.

INDEX